D1537657

MARKETING
HEALTH
SERVICES

MARKETING
HEALTH
SERVICES

Richard K. Thomas

Health Administration Press, Chicago
AUPHA Press, Arlington, VA

AUPHA
HAP

Your board, staff, or clients may also benefit from this book's insight. For more information on quantity discounts, contact the Health Administration Press Marketing Manager at (312) 424-9470.

09   08   07   06   5   4   3   2

Library of Congress Cataloging-in-Publication Data

Thomas, Richard K., 1944–
   Marketing health services / Richard K. Thomas.
     p. cm.
   Includes bibliographical references and index.
   ISBN 1-56793-234-7 (alk. paper)
   1. Medical care—Marketing.   I. Title.
   RA410.56.T48 2004
   362.1'068'8—dc22

                                       2004059852

The paper used in this publication meets the minimum requirements of American National Standard for Information Sciences—Permanence of Paper for Printed Library Materials, ANSI Z39.48-1984. ⊗™

Acquisitions editor: Audrey Kaufman; Project manager: Jane C. Williams; Cover designer: Trisha Lartz

Health Administration Press
A division of the Foundation
   of the American College of
   Healthcare Executives
One North Franklin Street
Suite 1700
Chicago, IL 60606
(312) 424-2800

Association of University Programs
   in Health Administration
2000 N. 14th Street
Suite 780
Arlington, VA 22201
(703) 894-0940

CONTENTS IN BRIEF

Part IV Managing and Supporting the Marketing Effort

Part V The Future of Healthcare Marketing

DETAILED CONTENTS

Part III Healthcare Marketing Techniques

Part IV Managing and Supporting the Marketing Effort

INTRODUCTION

Most observers consider 1977 the "official" launch data of marketing as a component of healthcare. The first conference on healthcare marketing was sponsored by the American Hospital Association, and the first book on the topic was published in 1977. While formal marketing activities became common early on among retail-oriented healthcare organizations like health insurance, pharmaceuticals, and medical supplies, health services providers had long resisted the incorporation of formal marketing activities into their operations. Of course, hospitals and other healthcare organizations had been doing "marketing" under the guise of public relations, physician relationship development, community services, and other activities, but few health professionals equated these with marketing. To many, marketing meant advertising, and, until the 1970s, advertising on the part of health services providers was considered inappropriate.

The formal recognition in the 1980s of marketing as an appropriate activity for health services providers represented an important milestone for healthcare. The acceptance of marketing by health professionals opened the door for a variety of new activities on the part of healthcare organizations. This development led to the establishment of marketing budgets and the creation of numerous new positions within the organizations, culminating with the establishment of the position of vice president for marketing in many organizations. This development opened healthcare up to an influx of concepts and methods from other industries and helped to introduce modern business practices into the healthcare arena.

While most would agree that, after years of grudging acceptance, marketing has become reasonably well established as a legitimate healthcare function, the process has not been without its fits and starts. Healthcare has demonstrated surges of interest in marketing, followed by periods of retrenchment when marketing, and marketers, were considered unnecessary and/or inappropriate. Periods of prosperity for marketing have alternated with periods of neglect over the past 25 years. There have been periods of exuberant, almost reckless, marketing frenzy and periods of retrenchment. There has been ongoing tension between those who eagerly accepted marketing as a function of the healthcare organization and those who doggedly resisted its intrusion into their realm. With each revival of marketing in healthcare, new wrinkles have been added that made the "new" marketing, if not better, at least different from previous approaches.

Once the dam broke and marketing made its initial incursion into healthcare, a stampede ensued as healthcare organizations, led by major hospitals, established aggressive marketing campaigns. Urged forward by marketers recruited from other industries, hospitals and other healthcare organizations embarked on a whirlwind of marketing activity. The effectiveness of these initial marketing campaigns did not match their proponents' enthusiasm, and it was soon realized that marketing healthcare was not the same as marketing hamburgers. The approaches required for the healthcare arena were not easily adapted from other industries, and much of what was effective elsewhere was not necessarily effective in the healthcare industry. The evolution of marketing in healthcare is discussed in a later section within the context of developments in the healthcare field.

Today, healthcare is still struggling to find the appropriate role for marketing, and marketers continue to strive to find their niche within healthcare. The industry still suffers from a lack of standardization when it comes to marketing, and this has not been helped by the fact that few graduate programs offer coursework in healthcare marketing. Today, healthcare marketing appears poised to play a greater role in the new healthcare environment. But, as the chapters illustrate, this is likely to be a different kind of marketing than that envisioned in the mid-1970s when the first marketing efforts were introduced into healthcare.

Before the 1980s, marketing campaigns targeting healthcare consumers were relatively rare. In fact, the marketing activity that existed was primarily on the part of industry segments that were not involved in patient care (e.g., pharmaceuticals and insurance) and whose targets were not patients but other players in the healthcare arena (e.g., physicians and employers). Healthcare organizations did not need to market their services. The industry was product driven and most "producers" of services operated in semimonopolistic environments. There was an almost unlimited flow of customers (patients), and revenues were essentially guaranteed by third-party payers.

This situation began to change in the early 1980s. Along with a number of other significant changes in healthcare, competition was introduced for the first time. Healthcare organizations began to realize that to survive in this new world, they would have to adopt business practices long established in other industries. This involved, among other things, a shift from a product orientation to a service orientation. For the first time, then, the market became a factor for the industry. These developments resulted in the introduction of marketing as a legitimate function in healthcare.

By the mid-1980s, marketing departments had been established in most of the large healthcare organizations. Once introduced to each other, marketing and healthcare passed through a tentative getting-to-know-you period. By the mid-1980s, however, it was a romance in full bloom with the two being seen everywhere together. Healthcare organizations were spending feverishly on their newfound consort, and marketers rushed to take advantage of the sudden burst of interest. Those without formal departments started developing marketing functions through other mechanisms. However, the introduction of marketing into healthcare resembled a shaky romance.

Hospitals were among the first to embrace marketing as a part of their operations. Other healthcare organizations followed their lead. As new forces emerged in the industry, often led by entrepreneurs rather than clinicians, the use of marketing techniques proliferated. Innovative healthcare programs, such as urgent care centers and freestanding diagnostic centers, began using marketing as a means of attracting patients from the established sources of care.

Unfortunately, in the early years healthcare executives did not see marketing for what it really was, and many expensive mistakes were made by the organizations pioneering healthcare marketing. Healthcare organizations failed to do their market research homework, rushed headlong into expensive media advertising, became obsessed with image rather than substance, and failed to evaluate their hastily contrived marketing initiatives. Perhaps the gravest error of all was to equate advertising with marketing.

As a result of these mistakes, by the late 1980s healthcare organizations were slashing their marketing budgets, disbanding marketing staff, and generally scaling back this relationship. Healthcare did not want to break it off altogether, but it did not want to continue spending on initiatives with uncertain benefits.

Both parties—healthcare and marketing—could probably be blamed for the shaky initial relationship. The marketers that healthcare imported from other industries failed in their effort to convert existing marketing techniques to healthcare uses. The first rule of marketing, of course, is to know your market, and marketers did not. They were offering quick fixes and short-run answers in an industry that required long-term initiatives.

By the early 1990s, healthcare executives realized that marketing did not consist of spending truckloads of money on mass-media advertising. Progressive healthcare organizations began to assess their marketing objectives in a more reasonable light. They began to try to understand the market, their customers, and their customers' motivations.

Marketers, too, had learned some important lessons. Few marketing techniques could be transferred unmodified from other industries. The messages and the methods had to be tailored to healthcare. Sensitive issues that are not factors in other industries had to be addressed in healthcare. Furthermore, marketers were faced with the unique situation in which certain consumers were "desirable" and others were not.

Today, healthcare marketers have a much better understanding of the market and their customers. Fairly sophisticated market research techniques have been put into place. An appreciation for what works and does not work in terms of marketing initiatives has evolved. New techniques have been developed specifically for the healthcare market, and a core of professional healthcare marketers have emerged.

The rest of this book will be devoted to the development of an understanding of marketing as a field and its application to healthcare. The chapters introduce the reader to the concepts, methods, and data used in healthcare marketing, providing the information required for developing an appreciation of the role of marketing in healthcare along with the tools necessary to plan and implement marketing initiatives.

The book provides sound grounding in basic marketing concepts, along with background on the factors that drive marketing approaches and consumer behavior in healthcare. It presents nuts-and-bolts information on the marketing process and its management. It also critiques the marketing techniques currently in use in healthcare and introduces emerging techniques being adapted for healthcare.

The Audience

This book is designed primarily for use by students of healthcare administration and by those studying marketing (typically in MBA programs). Under various guises (e.g., healthcare administration, hospital management, public administration), most programs offered for those with an interest in healthcare administration include a component on healthcare marketing. This text should provide the core of information necessary for those courses.

Many business administration programs offer healthcare marketing as a component of their marketing concentrations; this book should serve that audience as well. It should also serve as a reference work for academicians involved in healthcare administration or marketing but who are not directly involved in the healthcare marketing arena.

This book is also a useful reference work for practitioners in the field. Healthcare administrators who require an understanding of the marketing process, health planners, and those directly involved in marketing activities are expected to benefit from its contents. Marketing firms and advertising agencies with an interest in healthcare should find the book useful as an introduction to the unique aspects of healthcare marketing.

Organization of the Book

Designed to serve as a comprehensive guide for students in marketing and healthcare administration, the text surveys the field of healthcare marketing, beginning with basic marketing concepts (as applied to healthcare) and exploring all components of healthcare marketing.

Part I provides an overview of marketing and its applications to healthcare. Chapter 1 addresses the history of marketing overall and its recent experience within healthcare. Chapter 2 follows up on this discussion with a description of the unique aspects of healthcare that create challenges for marketers. The changing context of healthcare is described in Chapter 3 to provide the marketer with an appreciation of the volatile nature of the contemporary healthcare arena. Chapter 4 introduces and defines the basic marketing concepts that are used throughout the text, exposing the student to the language of marketing as a prerequisite to further study. Chapter 5 describes the current status of marketing in healthcare and identifies the contexts in which marketing is presently taking place.

Part II introduces the reader to the nature of healthcare markets, the consumers who populate them, and the factors that influence the demand for health services. Chapter 6 provides an overview of the "market" for health services and examines the ways in which healthcare differs from other industries in this regard. Chapter 7 focuses on the nature of healthcare consumers and the variety of constituents healthcare organizations serve. It notes the unique characteristics of the end users of health services and the manner in which healthcare decision making differs from this process in other industries. Chapter 8 addresses the notion of "product," describing healthcare products and services and distinguishing them from the products and services that marketers generally promote. Chapter 9 introduces the notions of healthcare "need," "want," and "utilization" and discusses the factors that influence the demand for health services and the ultimate level of utilization.

Part III focuses on the practical aspects of healthcare marketing, describing marketing strategies and marketing techniques—both traditional and cutting edge—as they relate to healthcare. Chapter 10 discusses the notion of marketing strategies, describing the strategy-development process and indicating means of implementing strategies. Chapter 11 distinguishes between public relations, advertising, and other traditional marketing activities. Chapter 12 presents contemporary marketing techniques, often adopted from other industries, and their potential contribution to healthcare marketing.

Part IV presents a practical guide to managing and supporting the marketing process in healthcare. Just as the concept of marketing is relatively new in healthcare, so is the notion of "managing" the process. Chapter 13 provides an overview of the marketing process, tying together various components discussed earlier in the text. It provides an overview of the issues involved in managing and evaluating marketing initiatives. Part IV also describes the various functions that are necessary to support the marketing effort, from the initial market research to technology-based approaches to managing the customer base. Chapter 14 presents an overview of the marketing research process, describing the uses of research by marketers and reviewing basic research techniques with application of healthcare. Chapter 15 introduces the reader to marketing planning. Notwithstanding its late introduction in the book, marketing planning should be an early and constant consideration in the marketing process. Chapter 16 examines the categories of data that are used for marketing research and planning, indicating the manner in which these data are generated and the sources from which they can be obtained.

Part V includes a single chapter—Chapter 17—on the future of healthcare marketing. The current status of the field is summarized and prospects for the future are considered. The factors that are likely to influence the future course of marketing are considered, and speculation on the future characteristics of healthcare marketing, and marketers, is offered.

I

HEALTHCARE MARKETING: HISTORY AND CONCEPTS

Part I describes the overall context necessary for an understanding of the field of marketing and its applications to healthcare. One cannot understand where the field is going unless one knows where it has been, so the evolution of the field requires review. Ultimately, this section places healthcare marketing solidly within the frameworks of both the healthcare industry and the marketing profession and provides insights into what had been tried in the past.

Chapter 1 presents an overview of the history of marketing, ultimately focusing on its more recent history in the healthcare arena. It describes the factors that led to a shift from a production orientation to a service orientation in healthcare, with the concomitant growing awareness of market demands. The stages in the development of healthcare marketing are outlined, and the changes that occurred in the field are noted at each stage. The factors that have contributed to successive periods of healthcare marketing successes and setbacks during the past quarter of a century are reviewed.

Chapter 2 addresses marketing within a context that was initially resistant to any type of business principles in general and "formal" marketing in particular. The chapter describes the ways in which healthcare is different from other industries and in which healthcare marketing is different from other types of marketing. The factors that have contributed to the acceptance of marketing in healthcare are identified, along with the contribution that marketing can make to the industry.

Chapter 3 reviews the developments that have occurred in healthcare in recent years and describes their implications for marketing. The importance of the transformation experience by healthcare in the 1980s for the emergence of marketing as a function within healthcare organizations is noted. The halting evolution of marketing as a legitimate healthcare endeavor is outlined.

Chapter 4 introduces the concepts basic to the marketing endeavor. Key terms and concepts are defined, and the special treatment of these notions in healthcare is reviewed. The application of the four Ps of marketing to healthcare is discussed. The challenge of adopting marketing concepts and techniques from other industries to healthcare is explored.

Chapter 5 examines the current status of marketing in healthcare, identifying the types of organizations that are most actively involved in promotional activities. The regard with which marketing is held in healthcare today is noted, and current trends in the application of marketing techniques in healthcare are reviewed.

THE HISTORY OF MARKETING IN HEALTHCARE

Despite its short history, healthcare marketing has experienced many twists and turns. Since the notion of marketing was introduced to healthcare providers during the 1970s, the field has gone through various periods of growth, decline, retrenchment, and renewed growth. This chapter reviews the history of marketing in the U.S. economy in general and traces its evolution in healthcare over the last quarter of the twentieth century.

The History of Marketing

Marketing as we use the term today is a modern concept. It was first used around 1910 to refer to what would be called *sales* today. It is a uniquely American concept, and the English word "marketing" has been adopted by other languages that lack a word for this concept.

Although the 1950s is considered to mark the beginning of the "marketing era" in the United States, the establishment of the marketing function within the U.S. economy took several decades, and marketers had to overcome a number of factors that retarded its development. Many of these factors reflected characteristics of the U.S. economy carried over from the World War II period. In the 1950s, America was still in the Industrial Age, and the U.S. economy was production oriented until well after the war. Because essentially all aspects of the U.S. economy were geared to production, the prevailing mind-set emphasized the interests of the producer over those of the consumer (as epitomized by Henry Ford's maxim, "You can paint it any color, so long as it's black"). This production orientation assumed that the producer knew a priori what the consumer needed. Products were produced to the specification of the manufacturer, and then customers were sought. A "here is our product, take it or leave it" approach characterized most industries during this period. The mind-set was that a good product would sell itself; thus, there would be no need for marketing even if the field had existed.

During the postwar period, considerable product (i.e., brand) differentiation continued to exist. In the days before the standardization of production, there was enough variation among products offered by different producers that the differences generally spoke for themselves (without benefit of marketing). Furthermore, until the prosperity of the 1950s, the concept of *consumer* was poorly developed. The existence of a weak consumer segment lacking consumer credit and an acquisitive mind-set was not conducive to the development of the marketing enterprise.

Stage One: Product Differentiation and the Consumer Mentality

The postwar period witnessed the emergence of a wide variety of new products, particularly in the consumer-goods industries. Newly empowered consumers demanded a growing array of goods and services, even if existing goods and services had adequately served previous generations. This development contributed to the emergence of marketing for at least two reasons. First, consumers had to be introduced to and educated about these new goods and services. Second, new market entrants introduced a level of competition unknown in the prewar period. This meant that mechanisms had to be developed to both make the public aware of a new product and to distinguish that product from those of competitors' in the eyes of potential customers.

Consumers had to be made aware of purchase opportunities and then convinced to buy a certain brand. The standardization of existing products that occurred during this period further contributed to the need to convince newly empowered consumers to purchase a particular good or service. Marketers gained a foothold in U.S. industry when they were enlisted to highlight and, if necessary, "create" differences between similar products.

These developments resulted in a shift away from a seller's market to a buyer's market. Once the consumer market began to be tapped, it was realized that the demand for many types of goods was highly elastic. The prewar mentality had emphasized the meeting of consumer *needs* and assumed that a finite amount of goods and services could be purchased by a population. With the increase in discretionary income and the introduction of consumer credit after World War II, consumers began to satisfy *wants*. Fledgling marketers found out that they could not only influence consumers' decision-making processes but could even *create* demand for certain goods and services.

The emergence of marketing was aided by changes in the cultural aspects of U.S. society. The postwar period was marked by a growing emphasis on consumption and acquisition. The frugality of the Depression era gave way to a degree of materialism that was shocking to older generations. The availability of consumer credit and a mind-set that emphasized "keeping up with the Joneses" generated a demand for a growing range of goods and services. America had given rise to the first generation of citizens with a consumer mentality.

By the 1970s, there was a growing emphasis on self-actualization in American culture, often carried to the point of narcissism in the minds of many observers. Not only were individuals coming to be identified in terms of their material possessions, but the cultural environment encouraged people to "do their own thing." This called for additional goods and services and served to boost a fledgling market for consumer health services (e.g., psychotherapy, cosmetic surgery). A growing consumer market with expanding needs, coupled with a proliferation of products, created a fertile field for the emergence of marketing.

Underlying these developments was the growing emphasis being placed on change itself. Traditional societies (including the United States until World War II) emphasized stability; the status quo; and, as the name implies, tradition. A premium was placed on the old ways of doing things, and impending change engendered skepticism, if not outright resistance. Clearly, previous generations were oriented to the present (or even the past) in terms of their cultural moorings. The prospect of change had always threatened deep-seated convictions that had survived for generations.

By the 1970s, not only had change become accepted as inevitable as society underwent major transformations, but change began to take on a positive connotation. Newly empowered consumers demanded a growing array of goods and services. The future-oriented outlook emerging within U.S. society further underscored the importance of change in forging a path to a better future. Individuals began switching jobs, residences, and even spouses at a rate that shocked their forefathers. It became a maxim that the American dream involved the advancement of each generation over the previous one.

Stage Two: The Emerging Role of the Sales Representative

The second stage of marketing evolution focused on sales. Many U.S. producers had enjoyed regional monopolies (or at least oligopolies) since the dawn of the Industrial Age. Under these conditions, sales representatives took orders from what was essentially a captive audience. Marketing would have been considered an unnecessary expense under this scenario. However, as competition increased in most industries following World War II, these regional monopolies disintegrated, especially with the increased mobility available to sales forces.

The emphasis on sales characterizing the U.S. economy during the last third of the twentieth century continued to reflect to a great extent the production aspects of society. However, sales representatives eventually served as a bridge between the production economy and the service economy as they developed and maintained relationships. Sales representatives progressed from their roles as "order takers" to become "consultants" to their clients. This created a conduit for information to flow from customers back to producers, thereby facilitating the emergence of a market orientation for U.S. business.

Stage Three: A Customer-Driven Approach

The third stage in the evolution of the field actually focused on marketing per se. By the end of the twentieth century, the industrial economy had given way to a service economy and the remaining production industries became increasingly standardized. This shift from a product orientation to a service orientation represented a sea change vis-à-vis marketing. Service industries tend to be market driven, and U.S. corporations began abandoning their father-knows-best mind-set in favor of a market orientation. For the first time, progressive managers in a wide range of industries sought to determine what consumers wanted and then strove to fulfill those needs. This opened the door for market research and the emergence of professional marketers to exploit consumer desires. These new market-driven firms adopted an *outside-in* way of thinking that considers service delivery from the point of view of the customer.

The emergence of a service economy had important implications for both marketing and healthcare. Services are distinguished from products because they are generally produced as they are consumed and cannot be stored or taken away. For example, an x-ray machine is a product that is used to provide a service (medical diagnostics); the service is provided as the patient "consumes" it (by being subjected to the procedure). Unlike a tangible product, the standard of service may differ each time it is produced (e.g., one radiologist may be more expert at interpreting x-rays than another).

The marketing of services is different from the marketing of products; this creates a challenge for marketers in any field. The development of capabilities for marketing services occurred slowly as the United States became a service-oriented economy. There are considerable differences between marketing goods and marketing services, and a new mind-set and new promotional approaches had to be developed. (See Chapter 2 for additional discussion of the challenge of marketing services.)

Marketing in Healthcare

Healthcare adopted marketing approaches well after most other industries, and the marketing era was not considered to begin in healthcare until the 1980s. This does not mean that certain healthcare organizations in the retail and supplier sectors had not been involved in marketing activities. Pharmaceutical companies, consumer-product vendors, and health plans have a long history of marketing activities; indeed, some of these organizations devote an inordinate proportion of their budgets to marketing. These types of organizations are addressed throughout this book, although the emphasis is on marketing on the part of healthcare providers.

While marketing was noticeably absent from the functions of most healthcare providers until the 1980s, precursors to marketing had long been established. Every hospital and many other healthcare organizations had well-established public relations (PR) functions. PR involved disseminating information concerning the organization and announcing new developments (e.g., additions to staff, purchase of equipment). The main interface for PR staff was with the media. They disseminated press releases, responded to requests for information, and served as the interface with the press should some negative event occur.

Large provider organizations also typically had communication functions, although they were often carried out under the auspices of the PR department. Communications staff would develop materials for dissemination to the public and the employees of the organization. Internal (and, later, patient-oriented) newsletters and patient-education materials were frequently developed by communications staff.

Some of the larger organizations (and certainly the major retail firms and professional associations) established government-relations offices. These staff members were responsible for tracking regulatory and legislative activities that might affect the organization. They served as the interface with government officials and provided lobbying efforts as appropriate. The government-relations office frequently became involved in certificate-of-need activities. This function has historically been critical for many healthcare organizations because of the constant pressure on not-for-profit healthcare organizations to justify their tax-exempt status.

In addition to these formal precursors of marketing, healthcare organizations of all types were involved in informal marketing activities to a certain extent. This occurred when hospitals sponsored health education seminars, held an open house for a new facility, or supported a community event. Hospitals marketed by making their facilities available to the community for public meetings and by otherwise attempting to be good corporate citizens. Physicians marketed themselves through networking with their colleagues at the country club or medical-society–sponsored events. They sent letters of appreciation to referring physicians and provided services to high school athletic teams.

Ultimately, low-budget PR departments were transformed into multimillion-dollar marketing programs. This did not happen overnight, and a number of developments had to occur before healthcare came to appreciate the relevance of marketing. Some of these developments are addressed below, and others are discussed in Chapter 2. See Box 1.1.

Box 1.1: Pioneers in Healthcare Marketing

Although the 1970s marked the formal emergence of marketing in the health services industry, few healthcare organizations—as organizations—had yet bought into marketing. True, the for-profits like Columbia and HCA (Healthcare Corporation of America) had more of a marketing orientation and may even have given an incentive to their administrators to perform marketing activities. Despite the fact that Evanston (Indiana) Hospital claimed a vice president of marketing in 1976, many professionals would cite the publication of Philip Kotler's *Marketing for Non-Profits* a few years later as the advent of marketing in health services.

Interestingly, the emergence of marketing in healthcare was not driven at the corporate level. Ultimately, it came down to a handful of assertive and creative individuals who took the initiative and, often against great odds, established marketing programs. Organizations like the Mayo Clinic and the Cleveland Clinic developed permanent marketing programs, but the inroads marketing made were a result of the tenacity of a handful of true believers.

To the extent that marketing was incorporated into healthcare in the 1970s and 1980s, it was a result of the hard work of people, like Bernie Lachner in Evanston Hospital; Kent Seltman at the Mayo Clinic; and William Gombeski at the Cleveland Clinic, rather than any commitment on the part of their organizations. Seltman entered the healthcare field in 1984, when marketing was in its infancy, and went on to develop innovative marketing programs at Loma Linda University Medical Center and the Mayo Clinic. Gombeski guided the early development of marketing initiatives at the Cleveland Clinic and established the organization as a textbook example of successful marketing.

The Stages of Healthcare Marketing

The stages through which marketing has evolved can be viewed as they relate to healthcare (Berkowitz 1996). Box 1.2 indicates the progression and its implications for the hospital industry as an example. The stages through which marketing has evolved within the healthcare setting are outlined below.

The 1950s

Although the 1950s was viewed as the marketing era outside healthcare, marketing was essentially not on the radar screen in healthcare during this period. True, the emerging pharmaceutical industry was beginning to market to physicians and the fledgling insurance industry was beginning to market health plans. In the healthcare trenches, however, healthcare providers

Other pioneers included Ann Fyfe and Judith S. Neiman, who carried the marketing banner often in the face of strong resistance. Fyfe served as a top marketing and strategy administrator for several healthcare systems. She served as a member of the American Marketing Association's board and assisted the association with the formation of a healthcare section, the Academy of Health Services Marketing. Neiman served as the executive director of the Society for Healthcare Strategy and Market Development of the American Hospital Association. Among other marketing practitioners were pioneers like Dan Beckham and Scott MacStravic. Beckham played an early role in the establishment of organizations for healthcare marketing professionals.

MacStravic (1977) can trace his pioneering marketing activities to the mid-1970s and is credited with the first book on healthcare marketing. MacStravic served as a marketing executive for hospitals and health systems all over the United States and pioneered some of the early healthcare marketing initiatives.

In the academic arena Eric Berkowitz, a long-time professor of marketing at the University of Massachusetts, built on the early work of Kotler to help establish healthcare marketing as a legitimate component of academic marketing. Berkowitz has published numerous books on healthcare marketing, including *Essentials of Health Care Marketing*. Other academics who contributed to the establishment of healthcare marketing were Steve Brown and Roberta Clark.

This brief discussion cannot include all those who contributed to the development of healthcare marketing as a separate field, but it does pay tribute to a few of the pioneers who, often in the face of great odds, advanced the cause of healthcare marketing in its early days.

were light-years away from formal marketing activities. Hospitals and physicians for the most part considered marketing (i.e., advertising) to be inappropriate and even unethical. This did not preclude marketing on the part of hospitals through free educational programs and PR activities, nor did it prevent physicians from cozying up to potential referring physicians and networking at the country club with their colleagues. These activities were not considered to be marketing in the parlance of the day.

As the hospital industry came of age and large numbers of new facilities were established, the industry continued to reflect the production orientation that was waning throughout the rest of the U.S. economy. The demand for physician and hospital services was considered inelastic, and no attention was paid to the patient, much less the consumer. The empha-

Box 1.2: The Evolution of Marketing	Business Orientation	Manufacturer	Hospital
	Production	Produce quality product	Deliver quality care
	Sales	Generate volume	Fill hospital beds
	Marketing	Satisfy needs/wants	Satisfy needs/wants

sis was on providing quality care, and most providers held monopolies or oligopolies in their markets.

The 1960s

As the health services sector expanded during the 1960s, the role of PR was enhanced. While the developments that would force hospitals and other healthcare organizations to embrace marketing were at least a decade away, the field of PR was flourishing. This relatively basic marketing function was the healthcare organization's primary means of keeping in touch with its various publics.

The publics of this period were primarily the physicians who admitted or referred patients to a healthcare organization's facilities and the donors who made charitable contributions to the organization. Consumers were not considered an important constituency because they did not directly choose hospitals but were referred by their physicians. The use of media to advance strategic marketing objectives had not evolved, and media relations in this era often consisted of answering reporters' questions about patient conditions.

Print was the medium of choice for communications throughout the 1960s, in spite of the increasingly influential role the electronic media were playing for marketers in other industries. This was the era of polished annual reports, informational brochures, and publications targeted to the community. Health communications became a well-developed function, and hospitals continued to expand their PR function.

Some segments of the healthcare industry entered the sales stage during this decade. Sales forces were established to solicit physicians on the part of pharmaceutical companies and individuals on the part of insurance plans. Sales forces in the employ of healthcare providers, however, were still a development for the future.

The 1970s

During the 1970s, hospitals felt a growing urgency to take their case to the community. This was coupled with the growing conviction that, in the future, healthcare organizations were going to have to be able to attract patients. Legal restrictions on marketing were loosened, and many organizations extended their PR functions to include a broader marketing mandate. Such activity appeared to be particularly strong in parts of the country where health maintenance organizations (HMOs) were emerging.

The 1970s witnessed the growing importance of the for-profit hospital sector. With few limits on reimbursement, both not-for-profit and for-profit hospitals expanded services. Continued high demand for health services and the stable payment system created by Medicare made healthcare attractive to investor-owned companies. Numerous national for-profit hospital and nursing home chains emerged during this period.

Much of the early interest in healthcare marketing was generated from outside the industry, principally by academic marketers who saw an opportunity to expand marketing's scope into industries where it was rare. Philip Kotler was an early proponent of healthcare marketing from this perspective. Some early attempts at advertising health services were made, and interest in market research was beginning to emerge. Official recognition of marketing came with a conference on the topic sponsored by the American Hospital Association in 1977, and the movement was given impetus by rulings that allowed healthcare providers to advertise.

For hospitals, the sales era began in the mid-1970s with the changes that occurred in reimbursement. Under cost-based reimbursement (a la Medicare), competition with other hospitals was not a major concern. Hospitals had ample patients, lengths of stay were not a concern, and occupancy rates were high. Hospitals treated patients and passed along the actual costs, along with an appropriate profit margin, to third-party payers for reimbursement. The first and top priority was to acquire as many patients as possible. Traditionally, this goal was accomplished by attracting as many physicians as possible to admit patients to the hospital. The hospital wanted to maximize the number of patients that were admitted into the facility when directed by their doctors. Hospitals tried to entice doctors to admit to a particular facility, developed physician-relations programs to bond with the providers, and offered other enticements to encourage physician loyalty (Berkowitz 1996).

When hospitals recognized that patients might play a role in the hospital-selection decision, a second strategy for selling to the public emerged. In the mid-1970s many hospitals adopted mass-advertising strategies to promote their programs, including the use of billboard displays and television and radio commercials touting a particular service. The advertising goal was to encourage patients to use the hospital facilities when the doctor presented a choice or to self-refer if necessary (Berkowitz 1996). These developments reflected healthcare's evolution to the sales stage.

Marketing as we know it today still had not taken root in hospitals by the decade's end. Competition for patients was increasing, and hospitals and other providers turned to the familiar PR function for their promotional efforts. Communications efforts were beginning to be targeted toward patients, and patient satisfaction research grew in importance. Even so, marketing as a mechanism for managing the flow of services between an organization and its customers was still not a recognized function in most healthcare organizations.

The 1980s

If healthcare marketing was born in the 1970s, it came of age in the 1980s. The healthcare industry had evolved from a seller's market to a buyer's market, a change that was to have a profound effect on the marketing of health services. Employers and consumers had become purchasers of healthcare, and the physician's role in referring patients for hospital services was beginning to diminish. The 1980s witnessed the continued growth of the hospital industry, as centrally managed health systems (both for profit and not for profit) expanded. The dramatic growth of megachains of hospitals and other facilities was initiated during this period, and this development was to have a profound effect on marketing.

Marketers had to begin looking at audiences in an entirely different way, and the importance of consumers was heightened by the introduction of the prospective payment system. Hospitals began to think of medical care in terms of product or service lines, a development that was to have major consequences for the marketing of health services. Hospitals realized that marketing directly to consumers for services such as obstetrics, cosmetic surgery, and outpatient care could generate revenue and enhance market share.

Many providers became convinced that they could bring about shifts in market share through marketing initiatives; like many movements in healthcare, once a few hospitals started marketing many others followed suit. However, many healthcare organizations felt that they were in a class by themselves and thus did not need to advertise. Often, when they did advertise, it was mainly in response to marketing initiatives by other providers. Even when providers conceded that they did have competitors, marketing was not necessarily their first response.

Although marketing was beginning to be accepted, healthcare suffered from a lack of professional marketing personnel. Many marketers during this period were not familiar with healthcare and had limited expertise in transferring techniques from other industries to healthcare. There was no way for healthcare administrators to link marketing efforts to return on investment, and many saw marketing (especially advertising) as an expensive PR gimmick. Marketing was simply not considered an integral component of operations; at that time (and even today) marketers were considered outsiders by other health professionals.

The rise of service-line marketing launched the great hospital advertising wars of the 1980s. Barely a blip on the healthcare marketing radar screen a decade earlier, advertising's growth during this decade was dramatic. In 1983, the year the prospective payment system was launched, hospitals spent $50 million on advertising; in 1986 that figure had risen to $500 million, a tenfold increase in three years. Once a medium of dubious respectability, advertising was now hailed as a marketing panacea for hospitals (Berkowitz 1996).

The proliferation of hospital advertising was fueled by an increasingly competitive marketplace and a belief among marketing professionals that advertising was the key to competitive success. Whatever the problem, advertising was viewed as the solution. In fact, many marketing directors defined their marketing programs in terms of the size of their advertising budget.

However, much of the advertising of the mid- to late 1980s was ineffectual at best and disastrous at worst. Many of the campaigns involved poorly conceived strategies and led to an enormous waste of dollars. Ad copy tended to be institutionally focused, and healthcare marketing initiatives lacked the impact of the advertising produced in other industries. This was due to a great extent to the conservative, risk-averse culture of hospitals.

Although marketing involves a great deal more than advertising, certainly this was the activity that epitomized marketing for many in healthcare during this period. Marketers themselves contributed to the perpetuation of this notion, and even today many healthcare executives equate marketing with advertising. Ultimately, this surge in advertising was both a blessing and a curse. The perception of marketing as advertising certainly helped get the ball rolling. Advertising campaigns were something relatively concrete in which the organization could invest. Establishing advertising budgets and developing advertising initiatives were the quickest ways to get marketing incorporated into healthcare and gain some visibility for this function. On the other hand, the lack of success of much healthcare advertising and the often negative fallout it generated were definitely setbacks for healthcare marketing.

The perception of marketing as advertising ultimately had a serious negative effect on healthcare marketing. After the initial rush generated by seeing their billboard and television commercials, hospital administrators began to question the expense and, more important, the effectiveness of the marketing initiatives they were funding. Many health professionals and consumers considered hospital advertising as distasteful at best.

Despite the misplaced emphasis on advertising, the explosion in healthcare advertising probably did more to establish marketing as a legitimate force in the industry and attract the attention of both professionals and consumers than any other development. At the same time, the reckless advertising that characterized the 1970s and 1980s ultimately contributed to the discrediting of marketing in the late 1980s. Even during the 1980s, there was a great deal of residual resistance to marketing among health professionals, especially physicians, as well as a public reaction to marketing expenditures in the face of rising costs for consumers.

Already skeptical about the merits of marketing, especially advertising, healthcare organizations faced serious financial retrenchment in the 1980s. In addition, managed care was becoming a factor, and many thought this would obviate the need for marketing. Hospitals were looking for cuts wherever they could find them, and marketing expenditures were easy targets. Budgets were cut, and marketing staff were laid off. While the marketing function was not entirely eliminated, it was often incorporated into business development or strategic planning. In many places marketing went underground, and dedicated marketing professionals kept the field alive. In some healthcare organizations marketing essentially disappeared as a corporate function and was never brought back. On the positive side, this retrenchment allowed healthcare marketers to reassess the field and concentrate on developing the baseline data that could be used when a marketing revival inevitably occurred.

Consumer research grew in importance as the emphasis on the consumers of health services increased. While most hospitals had conducted patient satisfaction research for some time, consumer research was virtually unknown until the 1970s. By the mid-1980s, two-thirds of hospitals were conducting physician and consumer research. The latter was crucial in developing advertising messages and monitoring the success of marketing programs (Berkowitz 1996).

The 1990s

As healthcare became market driven in the 1990s, the marketing function grew in importance within healthcare organizations. The institutional perspective that had long driven decision making gave way to market-driven decision making. Hospital policies and procedures that had been established for the convenience of the hospital staff, not for the benefit of the patient, were reexamined and looked at from the point of view of customers and other external audiences. The popularity of guest-relations programs during the 1990s solidified the transformation of *patients* into *customers*. The 1990s represented a turning point in developing a real marketing perspective in healthcare. Every hospital was now trying to win the "hearts and minds" battle for the healthcare consumer.

Changes in the marketplace created new paradigms for marketing professionals. The rise of integrated delivery systems dictated a new approach to institutional marketing. Whereas physicians were the dominant audience in pre–managed-care marketing, suddenly *purchasing groups* (e.g., employers, business coalitions) increased in importance.

Although the integrated delivery systems movement ran out of steam, advertising thrived in the mid-1990s, spurred by the massive wave of hospital mergers. Mergers and consolidations resulted in the creation of larger organizations that had more resources and more sophisticated management. Executives entered the field from outside healthcare, bringing a more businesslike atmosphere.

The marketing of the emerging megasystems demanded more than advertising. PR achieved new status as the positioning tool of choice. To gain credibility for newly merged health systems or reinforce positioning for established ones, healthcare organizations turned to various print and electronic media. The media-relations function became a strategic tool for showcasing clinical centers of excellence or institutional programs. The rise in healthcare media and the interactive technology of the Internet combined to create an *informed consumer* who was more empowered with information than at any other time in human history.

The consumer was rediscovered during this process, and the direct-to-consumer movement was an outgrowth of these developments. As consumers gained influence, marketing became increasingly integrated into the operations of healthcare organizations. The consumers of the 1990s were better educated and more assertive about their healthcare needs than consumers of the previous generation. The emergence of the Internet as a source of health information furthered the rise of consumerism. Newly empowered consumers were taking on an increasingly influential (if informal) role in reshaping the U.S. healthcare system. Consumers were beginning to challenge physicians and their health plans armed with unprecedented knowledge.

Accountability became a hallmark of the new consumerism and was evidenced by the *report cards* issued on health plans and healthcare providers. Increasingly, employer groups and consumers were beginning to demand measurable clinical-outcomes data on providers and health plans. Empowered consumers demanded information on the services and pricing of health plans, hospitals, and physicians as they sought to make informed decisions. The backlash against managed care and consumer's rights legislation further improved the standing of the consumer. Indeed, the reaction to managed care has provided marketers with the challenge of damage control and image building for managed care plans.

During the 1990s, health professionals developed a new perspective on the role of marketing, aided by a new generation of healthcare administrators who were more business oriented. A more qualified corps of marketing professionals, who brought ambitious but realistic expectations to the industry, emerged. Pharmaceutical companies began advertising directly to consumers, and this development made everyone in the industry more aware of marketing. In addition, virtually everyone in healthcare was becoming more consumer sensitive, and data that allowed for a better understanding of the healthcare customer were becoming available.

Marketing research grew in importance during this decade. The need for information on consumers, customers, competitors, and the market demanded expansion of the research function. Patient and consumer research was augmented, and newly developed technologies brought the research capabilities of other industries to healthcare.

Business practices in general came to be more accepted in healthcare during this period, and marketing was an inevitable beneficiary. Marketing was repackaged in a more professional guise, and the shift away from advertising was noticeable. Marketing ended the decade as a more mature discipline, emphasizing market research and sensitivity to the needs of the consumer. Healthcare had finally reached the third stage in the evolution of the marketing function.

The Future of Healthcare Marketing

The marketing that characterizes healthcare today is different from that of the early years in a number of ways. In the 1990s, the emphasis shifted from sick people to well people in response to the emergence of managed care and capitated payments. Patient satisfaction became a new focus, and efforts at generating consumer data increased. The baby boomers who were coming to dominate the healthcare landscape viewed marketing more as a source of valuable information than as hucksterism and were disinclined to utilize an organization that did not cater to their interests.

Image advertising was deemphasized in favor of targeted promotions for specific services, making for more content and less fluff. Techniques from other industries, like customer relationship marketing, started being explored. A new generation of healthcare administrators seem to be more comfortable with marketing, considering this function an inherent aspect of healthcare operations.

With the repackaging and maturation of marketing in the 1990s, the field became more sophisticated overall. The market was in many ways more competitive, and even the managed care environment held opportunities for promotional activities. In addition, the mergers that occurred not only created more potential marketing clout but often involved for-profit healthcare organizations that were inherently more marketing oriented.

A new cohort of healthcare administrators is certainly contributing to a greater acceptance of business practices, including marketing. The

1990s witnessed a massive turnover in hospital administrators through retirement, mergers, and downsizing. Many of these new administrators have come from other, often more profit-oriented industries where marketing is considered a normal corporate function. These administrators are instilling a marketing mind-set in keeping with the more strategic orientation they bring to the industry.

While some still focus primarily on advertising and sales, marketing executives today are expanding their toolbox with a renewed emphasis on research, measurement, planning, analysis, forecasting, targeting, segmentation, and strategy. Reliable and effective public, media, and community relations; customer service; and reputation and relationship management are making a comeback, demonstrating the effectiveness of carefully designed, low-cost methods in reaching audiences and swaying public opinion.

Evidence of the Acceptance of Marketing

Today, what evidence exists that marketing has been accepted as a legitimate function by the healthcare industry? Beyond the traditional marketing-oriented sectors (e.g., pharmaceuticals, consumer products, health plans), have healthcare organizations embraced marketing? A number of indicators bear witness to this acceptance.

The healthcare industry has witnessed a continuous, if unsteady, advance in the role and status of marketing over the past quarter century. During the period following World War II the concept of marketing was unknown in healthcare. The PR role was expanded over time, and communications and government-relations functions were added. By the late 1970s formal marketing activities were being initiated, and advertising on the part of healthcare providers was becoming common. Even during the 1980s, however, marketing was still seen by many as an external function, not something inherent to healthcare but a supportive service that was called on when needed.

By the end of the 1980s marketing was being incorporated into the structure of healthcare organizations. Marketing departments were being established and marketing expenses factored into organizational budgets. Marketers were being promoted to managers, directors, and ultimately vice presidents. Marketing was moving from the periphery of the organization to the boardroom. Marketers were transformed from technical resources called on as needed to full partners in the corporate decision-making process. The most progressive healthcare organizations developed a marketing mind-set that ensured that marketing was a consideration with every initiative and that marketers had input into the direction of the enterprise.

A survey of nearly 300 hospitals by the Society for Healthcare Strategy and Market Development (SHSMD) found that in 2002 hospital marketing departments averaged 5.7 staff members with budgets of $1.2 million (SHSMD 2002). Larger hospitals reported 10 or more staff members and budgets in excess of $3 million. The majority of marketing executives were at the director or manager level of the organization, although nearly one-third of marketing managers held the title of vice president or senior vice president (SHSMD 2002). Another SHSMD study of 706 marketing, communications, and strategy staff reported in 2003 an average salary for marketing executives of $122,000. This compares favorably to the compensation of healthcare executives in other departments (SHSMD 2003).

The importance of marketing for healthcare is also reflected in the emergence of publications devoted to the topic. These include *Marketing Health Services,* the healthcare publication of the American Marketing Association, and *Health Marketing Quarterly.* Articles on healthcare marketing regularly appear in other marketing journals as well. Numerous newsletters are devoted to healthcare marketing or some component of it such as health communications or PR.

Associations devoted to healthcare marketing such as SHSMD, sponsored by the American Hospital Association, have been established. The American Marketing Association has an active healthcare marketing constituency, and one of its eight special-interest groups is devoted to healthcare.

Textbooks on healthcare marketing began appearing in the 1980s, and healthcare marketing courses are taught as part of many marketing curricula in U.S. universities. Courses on the topic are now standard in healthcare administration programs. Specialized training programs on various aspects of healthcare marketing are offered by numerous universities and other training programs.

These developments reflect both the growing importance of marketing in the healthcare arena and its changing role. The ways in which marketing is being transformed as it matures within the healthcare industry will be discussed throughout this book. Case Study 1.1 demonstrates the hard lessons learned from an early attempt at healthcare marketing.

Summary

Since the notion of marketing was introduced to healthcare providers during the 1970s, the field has gone through various periods of growth, decline, retrenchment, and renewed growth. Although the 1950s is considered to mark the beginning of the "marketing era" in the United States, the establishment of the marketing function within U.S. healthcare took several decades.

During the post-World War II period, U.S. society underwent a number of changes that facilitated the growth of marketing. The healthcare industry eventually progressed through the stages of production, sales, and marketing, adopting many of the concepts and techniques of other industries along the way. Building on their experience in public relations and communications, healthcare organizations expanded their range of marketing techniques to encompass a variety of different approaches.

Early in this process, marketing was often equated with advertising, and, beginning in the 1980s, many healthcare organizations initiated major advertising campaigns. The limitations (and costs) of traditional advertising were eventually realized, and healthcare organizations began developing a more balanced approach to marketing. Over time, direct sales capabilities were added and technology-based marketing techniques were adopted. A new generation of health professionals offered a more mature approach to marketing as the twentieth century drew to a close.

Once marketing became accepted as an essential business function, healthcare organizations allowed marketers an expanded role. During this period of growth and development, marketing moved from the periphery of the corporation (and its status as a necessary evil) to a core function for determining the direction of the corporation. Marketers were given high-level administrative positions and the opportunity to sit in the corporate boardroom. By the beginning of the twenty-first century, marketing was poised to have a major impact on the future direction of healthcare.

Discussion Questions

- Why was marketing not considered important by healthcare professionals until the 1980s?
- What factors mitigated against the introduction of marketing into healthcare?
- What factors ultimately forced the incorporation of marketing into healthcare?
- Why is today's healthcare environment more hospitable to marketing and marketers than past environments?
- In what ways have marketers become better prepared to address the needs of healthcare?

References

Berkowitz, E. N. 1996. *Essentials of Health Care Marketing.* Gaithersburg, MD: Aspen.

MacStravic, R. E. S. 1977. *Marketing Healthcare.* Gaithersburg, MD: Aspen.

Society for Healthcare Strategy and Market Development. 2002. *Marketing by the Numbers.* Chicago: American Hospital Association.

———. 2003. *Salary, Compensation and Work Satisfaction Study.* Chicago: American Hospital Association.

Additional Resources

American Marketing Association. www.ama.org.

Health Marketing Quarterly, published by The Haworth Press.

Herzlinger, R. E. 1997. *Market-Driven Health Care.* Reading, MA: Addison-Wesley.

Marketing Health Services, published by the American Marketing Association.

Society for Healthcare Strategy and Market Development. http://www.hospital-connect.com/shsmd.

AN EARLY ATTEMPT AT HEALTHCARE MARKETING

n the late 1970s healthcare providers engaged in little discussion of marketing. Indeed, early pioneers in the field of healthcare marketing were just emerging. Ann Fyfe was an aggressive 28-year-old owner of a small advertising agency in Colorado. Her clients included a western clothing manufacturer, an irrigation system company, and an international food distributor. Fyfe subscribed to Philip Kotler's marketing formula based on the four Ps—product, price, place, and promotion (see Box 4.3 in Chapter 4), an approach that had worked well for her in the past.

In 1978, Fyfe was enticed by a visionary CEO at a major hospital in San Francisco to bring her marketing formula and suitcase of implementation strategies to a hospital setting. Fyfe jumped at the opportunity to bring what appeared to be a virtually bulletproof system for generating revenue into a field that seemed to be rich with possibility and amazingly untouched by the whole notion of marketing.

Fyfe and her colleagues rolled up their sleeves and got to work. They surveyed consumers using both qualitative and quantitative methods. They found out what consumers wanted and what approaches they would respond to. They designed innovative programs built around customer-friendly products. They established among others an executive physicals program called Vital, an urgent care center in the hospital called CliniCare, and one of the first sports-medicine programs in the United States.

In the area of promotions, no expense was spared. A sales force was established, and a major ad agency was engaged to develop clever collateral materials and radio spots. They used direct mail and radio for both public service announcements and paid advertising. They also implemented a full program of community services, from dinners for seniors to wellness programs at health clubs to educational seminars. The marketing initiative was so impressive that it could boast Charles Schwab as the chair of the board's marketing committee and was considered newsworthy enough to be featured on the *Today Show*.

All of the hospital's innovative programs had respectable returns on investment despite (or maybe because of) the fact that they spared no expense on promotions. Corporations were eager to offer a suite of health services to their executives, consumers loved the urgent care clinic, and sports medicine boomed along with the wellness craze of the 1970s.

Despite the apparent success of the hospital's aggressive marketing program, the process soon experienced an ironic twist. Within two years of pulling off this marketing miracle, one that nearly every other U.S. hospital was eager to copy, Fyfe and the hospital's CEO were summarily fired by the physician-dominated hospital board.

As a fledgling healthcare marketer, no one had said anything to Fyfe about physicians. She was busy listening to customers, and they loved what the hospital was doing. However, the medical staff was an entirely different type of hospital customer. To some physicians, the hospital represented direct competition in that physical exams and urgent care patients were being diverted away from their practices. Most staff doctors, however, experienced a more visceral reaction: this slick marketing approach felt sleazy, commercial, and inappropriate, and the culture of medicine was simply not ready for it.

Meanwhile, hospitals everywhere were lining up to learn how to replicate this organization's dubious success. In response to overwhelming demand, Fyfe assisted the American Marketing Association in the formation of a healthcare section. She also formed and became president of the Northern California Health Care Marketing Association. Fyfe received one of the first *Modern Healthcare* "up and comer" awards and was presented with a cash prize by the HealthCare Forum for her article on CliniCare. (Unfortunately, a hospital CEO in the audience at the award ceremony actually stood up and reminded Fyfe's enthusiastic fan club that her activities had managed to get her CEO fired.)

Fyfe is still active in healthcare marketing and believes that she has helped shape a profession and contributed to a more mature approach to marketing. Over time her contributions have made healthcare organizations smarter about their business decisions, more cautious about advertising, and more sensitive to the needs of their customers. The experience has made Fyfe smarter too. Today she works closely with her primary strategic partner in the marketing enterprise—the physician.

THE CHALLENGE OF HEALTHCARE MARKETING

The marketing of healthcare goods and services is not comparable to the marketing that takes place in any other industry. For that reason, healthcare marketing presents special challenges. The extent to which healthcare is different from other industries, and the implications of this for marketing, cannot be overemphasized. This situation requires a specialized approach to the marketing endeavor in healthcare, along with a need to develop healthcare-specific techniques to complement marketing techniques adopted from other industries.

The conditions that historically surrounded healthcare mitigated the need for and interest in marketing for the majority of organizations involved in patient care. The slow acceptance of marketing in healthcare described in Chapter 1 reflects a number of characteristics of the healthcare industry as well as the attributes of healthcare organizations, products and services, professionals, and consumers. The historical challenges that have faced healthcare marketing are described in the sections that follow, and the developments that are now encouraging healthcare organizations to overcome these challenges are reviewed.

Why Healthcare Is Different

Even a cursory knowledge of U.S. healthcare would lead an observer to note that healthcare is truly different from other institutions in American society. Healthcare as an industry is set apart from the other sectors of economy because of its unique characteristics. The characteristics of healthcare organizations stand in contrast to the characteristics of firms in other industries, with healthcare providers in particular behaving in a manner often inconsistent with that of organizations in other fields. Health professionals, especially clinicians, fall into a special category, and the fact that clinicians—not administrators or businesspeople—make most of the decisions with regard to patient care creates a dynamic unique to healthcare.

The nature of healthcare goods and services sets them apart from the goods and services offered in other industries. Furthermore, significant differences exist between healthcare consumers and the consumers of virtually any other good or service. These differences are particularly apparent with regard to the consumer decision-making process. Each of the factors that makes healthcare different is discussed below.

The Healthcare Industry

The development of a marketing culture in any industry is predicated on the existence of certain assumptions about that industry and the marketing enterprise. These assumptions include the existence of a rational market for the goods and services proffered by the organizations in that industry. It is presumed that the market involves organized groups of sellers, informed buyers, an orderly mechanism for carrying out transactions between sellers and buyers, and a straightforward process for transferring payment for products between buyers and sellers.

The existence of a true market in an economic sense in healthcare has been much debated. It could be argued that, to the extent that any type of market for health services exists, it is not rational in the sense of the markets for other goods and services. The operation of a market further assumes that consumers have adequate, if not perfect, knowledge concerning the available goods and services, that a rational system of pricing exists, and that the laws of supply and demand operate.

Furthermore, the existence of a market is predicated on assumptions about the motives and activities of buyers and sellers in the market. For example, the assumption that buyers are driven primarily, if not exclusively, by economic motives does not fit well with what we know about the behavior of healthcare organizations. Another assumption from economic theory—that buyers seek to maximize their benefits from the exchange—is also an uncomfortable fit. Thus, a number of factors operate to prevent the buyers of health services from operating in the same manner as the buyers of lawn services or accounting services.

The existence of a market also presumes that sellers compete for the consumer's resources and that this competition determines the price of the goods and services offered. In healthcare, however, it is not unusual for healthcare providers to maintain a monopoly over a particular service within a particular market. It is even more common for oligopolies of healthcare organizations to dominate a particular market. Thus, the buyer of health services is frequently limited in her choice of medical personnel or facilities.

As an industry, healthcare also differs from other sectors of society in terms of the diverse goals of its key organizations. The packaged goods industry, for example, has the unitary goal of producing, marketing, and distributing products directly to the consumer. The goals are straightforward whether the product is detergent, cereal, or office supplies. The intent is to sell as many units as possible while extracting the maximum profit from the transaction. This does not mean that retailers do not serve other purposes. They provide employment and benefits for their employees and profits for their shareholders, and they usually contribute to the community in the form of donations, sponsorship of events, and so on, but these activities are secondary to their single-minded goal of selling consumer products. The diffuse goals of most healthcare organizations distinguish them from other firms.

Many healthcare organizations suffer from a lack of *seller discretion*. In other industries, potential buyers who do not have the ability to pay or who for some other reason are considered to be undesirable customers can be refused service. Most healthcare organizations, on the other hand, are obligated to accept clients even though the clients are unable to pay for the services and are deemed "undesirable." Hospitals are bound by law in most cases to accept patients regardless of the patient's ability to pay. While providers may have some discretion in acceptance of patients with stable, routine conditions, emergency departments essentially cannot turn away any patient needing emergency care until the patient has at least been stabilized. While physician offices may require some payment on the front end for those patients without insurance, there are ethical considerations associated with turning a clearly symptomatic patient away.

This situation means that healthcare organizations often provide services that are not profitable. In some cases, this reflects the fact that certain services (e.g., emergency rooms at hospitals) may be legally mandated or otherwise controlled through regulation; in other situations, it reflects the fact that hospitals, and to a lesser degree physicians, must offer the comprehensive services required by the community to remain competitive. Thus, the economic considerations that apply to other industries may be moderated by factors unique to healthcare.

The healthcare industry also tends to be much less organized than other industries in the United States. Often referred to as a *nonsystem,* healthcare lacks the coordination and centralized (albeit often informal) systems of control found in other industries. Even industries characterized by cutthroat competition typically have a central clearinghouse of industry data and mechanisms for cooperating for the benefit of the industry overall. In contrast, the healthcare industry is characterized by fragmentation, discontinuity, and a lack of coordination. It is also characterized by a dismaying lack of information on the industry itself and on its key players. As a result, healthcare lacks the organization typically characteristic of an established market.

Unlike other industries, healthcare lacks a straightforward means of financing the purchase of goods and services, particularly for patient care services. Consumers in other industries typically pay directly for the goods and services they consume, either out of pocket or through some method of credit. In healthcare, while some small portion of the cost may be paid out of pocket by the consumer, the majority of the fees are likely to be paid by a third party. This may be a private insurance plan or a government-sponsored plan such as Medicare or Medicaid. The seller may have to deal with thousands of different insurance plans, and the services may be paid for using a combination of different payment mechanisms. Thus, it is not unusual for an elderly patient to pay for a hospital visit with Medicare reimbursement, supplementary private insurance reimbursement, and out-of-pocket payments. This type of situation cannot be found in any other industry and results in a much more complicated financial picture for healthcare than for other industries.

Finally, healthcare is different from other industries in that generally accepted laws of supply and demand seldom apply. An increase in the supply of health services, for example, does not necessarily result in a decrease in prices, nor does increased demand invariably drive up prices. Because the demand for health services is relatively elastic, the normal rules do not apply. For one thing, the availability (supply) of services dictates, to a certain extent, the demand for these services. In fact, the historical maxim was, "A bed built is a bed filled." Pent-up demand for health services often surfaces when more facilities become available. As a result, neither the increased supply of beds nor the increase in demand has a significant effect on prices.

The factors that govern supply, demand, and price in healthcare are complex and unique to this industry. The supply of health services is affected by the vagaries of health professional training programs, restrictions brought to bear by certificate-of-need processes and other regulations, and even fads that affect the healthcare industry. The level of demand, arguably the most problematic of the three governing factors, is typically not controlled by the end user. Except for elective procedures for which the consumer pays out of pocket, most of the decisions that affect the demand for health services are made by gatekeepers such as physicians and health plans. Thus, the level of demand is more often a function of such factors as insurance plan provisions, availability of resources, and physician practice patterns than the level of sickness within the population.

Healthcare Organizations

A number of characteristics set healthcare organizations apart from the sellers in other industries. Many healthcare organizations, particularly hospitals, still linger in the production stage of their evolution. Many such organizations argue that their goal is the provision of high-quality medicine. They feel that by providing state-of-the-art technology and the physicians, nurses, and allied health personnel to support it, they will be able to attract customers.

As with the early industrialists, many of these healthcare organizations have historically maintained oligopolistic or even monopolistic control over their markets. Because of their dominance in the market or arrangements with competitors, health services providers have often been able to ensure a steady flow of patients without having to solicit them. Today, however, few organizations can command that type of loyalty. Virtually all healthcare organizations face some competition, and innovations like telemedicine have broadened the scope of would-be competitors.

Healthcare organizations tend to be multipurpose organizations. While some purveyors of healthcare goods or services are single minded in their intent, large healthcare organizations like hospitals are likely to pursue a number of goals simultaneously. Indeed, the main goal of an academic medical center may not be the provision of patient care at all; it may be education, research, or community service, with direct patient care being a secondary concern. Even large specialty practices are likely to be involved in teaching and research, and, while they are not likely to neglect their core activity, they often have a more diffuse orientation than organizations in other industries.

Not-for-profit organizations have historically played a major role in healthcare; even today, not-for-profits continue to control a large share of the hospital-bed inventory. Although physician groups are usually incorporated as for-profit professional corporations, large numbers of community-based clinics, faith-based clinics, and government-supported programs operate on a nonprofit basis. This not-for-profit orientation creates an environment much different from that characterizing other industries. The fact that many health facilities and programs operate with government support also creates a different dynamic. For some organizations the unpredictability of government subsidy is an unsettling factor. For others the assurance of government support allows them to operate perhaps less efficiently than they would otherwise.

Another factor that sets healthcare organizations apart from their counterparts in other industries is the emphasis placed on referral relationships. Hospitals depend on admissions from their medical staffs, and their staff members in turn depend on referrals from other physicians. Indeed, except in emergency situations, patients can only gain hospital admission through a referral. Many specialists will not accept self-referred patients but rely on other physicians to send them patients. The same types of referral relationships exist with regard to other services (e.g., home healthcare, nursing homes).

This situation has become more complicated in that health plans may exert some level of influence over the referral process. Not only do health plans determine which providers can be seen under a particular coverage plan, they may require patients to be referred to specialists and may even seek to authorize any such referrals. In no other industry do parties who are not the end user exert such an influence on the process (see Box 2.1).

Box 2.1: The Importance of Referral Relationships

Healthcare is distinguished from other industries because of its reliance on referral relationships. *Referral relationships* as used here include any mechanism for the steering of consumers by a third party into the distribution channels of a healthcare organization or any use of an intermediary to promote goods and services to healthcare consumers. The importance of such relationships in healthcare is reflected by the fact that the end users of health services frequently do not make the consumption decision themselves. The purchase decision may be made by a physician, health plan, or some other party. This means that the marketer is more likely to target physicians, provider networks, health plans, and other gatekeepers that may influence the referral process rather than the end user.

There are situations in which the end user is targeted in healthcare. A wide range of consumer health products are marketed like any other retail product, and over-the-counter pharmaceuticals are marketed in the same manner as other goods. Individual health insurance policies are regularly sold directly to the consumer. With the advent of Internet-purchase options, an increasing range of health-related products are offered directly to consumers. Elective procedures are often promoted directly to prospective patients, with the organizations offering them using standard promotional techniques to attract customers.

Nevertheless, the bulk of health services utilization is a function of referral relationships and intermediaries. The most entrenched example of this is the requirement of a physician referral for hospital admission. Patients cannot present themselves directly to a hospital for purposes of admission; they must have an admitting physician. Even emergency cases require that a physician take responsibility for admitting the patient before he or she will be accepted into the hospital. If a physician does not have admitting privileges at a particular hospital, he or she cannot admit a patient there or treat patients hospitalized by other physicians. Other institutions, such as nursing homes and hospices, may depend on referrals from physicians as well.

Physicians themselves often depend on referrals from other physicians and, in some cases, health or social service agencies for customers. Medical and surgical spe-

Healthcare Products

The goods and services that constitute healthcare products are also somewhat unique to healthcare. While many healthcare consumer goods (e.g., Band Aids, fitness equipment, over-the-counter drugs) may be marketed just as any other product, most healthcare products do not fall into this category. Indeed, even the most common of consumer-oriented healthcare products—pharmaceuticals—must be prescribed by a middleman before they can be acquired and consumed.

cialists, for example, may be unwilling to accept a patient "off the street," who may or may not be a suitable candidate for their services. Instead, they rely on referrals from other physicians who are usually generalists. With most contemporary health insurance arrangements, a referral from a primary care physician to a specialist may be required before the insurer will cover the treatment episode. Depending on their specialty, physicians may also depend on referrals from nonphysician providers. Providers such as psychologists, optometrists, and chiropractors may make referrals to psychiatrists, ophthalmologists, and neurosurgeons, respectively, if the treatment requirements exceed their capabilities. Mental health centers and social service agencies may be major sources of patients for some specialists, as these agencies represent the front line of contact with many potential patients.

Prescription drugs are becoming an increasingly important aspect of patient care, and this area also involves indirect access to the end user. Except in the case of over-the-counter drugs, pharmaceutical companies cannot deal directly with patients. The patient must have a prescription written by a physician to obtain the drug from a pharmacist, and numerous safeguards prevent unauthorized access to prescription drugs. The pharmaceutical company relies on the physician to recommend its brand of drug, and, understandably, the main thrust of pharmaceutical marketing is toward physicians.

A final example of the referral process involves the steering of patients on the part of health insurance plans. Whether a plan is offered by a traditional indemnity insurer, health maintenance organization, preferred provider organization, or employer with a self-insured plan, there will virtually always be restrictions placed on providers that can be used. Typically, a health plan will have an arrangement with a network of providers, and the plan enrollee will be channeled to one of these providers rather than an out-of-network provider. Thus, the choice of physician, hospital, home health agency, and other providers is likely to be essentially outside the control of the end user. In these cases it is more important for the provider to develop relationships with the various health plans than to market directly to patients.

Healthcare providers are generally concerned with the promotion of a service, yet the nature of their services is difficult to describe. While a physician may break services down by procedure code (e.g., CPT codes), few services stand alone in reality. Services come in *bundles*—the group of services that surrounds a particular surgical procedure, for example. While clinicians (and their billing clerks) may see them as discrete services, the patient perceives them as a complex mix of services related to heart care, diabetes management, or cancer treatment.

As will be seen in the discussion of healthcare products in Chapter 8, the "products" generated by a healthcare organization are difficult to conceptualize. The things that providers are likely to think they provide (e.g., quality care, prolongation of life, elimination of pathology) are often hard to define or measure. The difficulty in specifying the services provided becomes obvious to the marketer who asks a hospital department head what services the department provides.

Healthcare products are also characterized by a lack of substitutability. A *substitute* is a good or service that can be used in place of another good or service. While one form of transportation may be substituted for another, for example, the opportunity to substitute one surgical procedure for another seldom exists. Unlike other industries, healthcare often provides only one solution for a particular need.

Health Professionals

The healthcare industry has been historically dominated by professionals rather than administrators. Clinical personnel (usually physicians, but other clinicians as well) define much of the demand for health services and are responsible directly or indirectly for the majority of healthcare expenditures. This is comparable to a situation in other industries in which technicians rather than administrators run the industry. However, this situation in healthcare is more significant in that the clinicians may not have the same goals and objectives as the administrators.

The medical ethics that drive the behavior of health professionals exist independent of the operation of the system. Clinicians are bound by oath to do what is medically appropriate, whether or not it is cost effective or contributes to the efficiency of the organization. Decisions made in the best interests of the patient may not reflect the best interests of the organization. Although health professionals have had to become somewhat more realistic with regard to indiscriminate use of resources, clinical interests continue to outweigh financial considerations in most cases. Conflict between the respective goals of clinicians and administrators is an inherent feature of the healthcare organization, and no comparable situation can be found in any other industry.

The conflict between the clinical and business sides of the health-care operation is augmented by an antibusiness orientation that character-izes many health professionals. Most health workers entered the field because they wanted to be in a profession, not a business, and many physicians and other clinicians hold a distorted perception of the business world. If health professionals cannot appreciate the business side of the operation, they are not likely to appreciate the importance of marketing. Even among non-clinicians, many business practices have been considered inappropriate for the not-for-profit healthcare world.

Healthcare Consumers

Consumers refers to those individuals with the potential to consume a par-ticular good or service; that is, anyone who has a want or need for (and presumably the ability to pay for) a product could be thought of as a poten-tial buyer. The good news for healthcare is that virtually everyone is a prospect for the consumption of health services. Many individuals in the United States do not own lawnmowers, computers, or even automobiles. Many also will never take a cruise vacation, hire an accountant, or attend a rock concert. This means that large segments of the population are not potential customers for these goods and services.

This is clearly not the case for healthcare. Virtually everyone is likely to utilize healthcare goods or services at some time, and literally everyone will be involved in the healthcare system even if they never do anything but experience childbirth in a hospital or receive the childhood immu-nizations required for admission to elementary school. Viewed in this light, the entire U.S. population represents a market for at least some type of healthcare good or service.

Despite this unique attribute of healthcare consumers, healthcare organizations have failed to perceive consumers in this manner. The tradi-tional notion that individuals are not true consumers of health services until they become sick has hampered the development of marketing in health-care. Until recently, the assumption was that none of the 285 million U.S. citizens is a prospect for health services *until* they are sick. Thus, health-care providers made no attempt to develop relationships with nonpatients. They were not considered paying customers until they presented them-selves for treatment. (This does not mean that there are not numerous par-ties catering to nonpatients. Major industries have developed around prevention, fitness, and lifestyle management. Indeed, much of the social marketing that takes place in U.S. society is geared toward nonpatients.)

This situation is in stark contrast to the approach taken by consumer-goods industries. The marketers of food products and household goods make the assumption that virtually everyone must have a need (or at least a want) that could be exploited. In fact, if consumers do not need baking soda to cook with, they can be encouraged to put it in the refrigerator to reduce odors. Marketers in other industries do not wait for a decision point to occur to address the potential needs of the consumer population. When the time comes to make a purchase, the intent is to have a consumer prepared to become not just someone's customer but *their* customer.

Healthy people, it could be argued, do not need health services. Would it not be a waste of marketing resources to solicit business from individuals who do not need your goods or services? How do you convince someone to undergo heart surgery if they do not have heart problems? These questions reflect some misconceptions about healthcare that need to be addressed. First, a misconception of what constitutes healthcare products exists: one immediately thinks of "heroic" surgical procedures, trauma care, and other life-saving efforts or conditions that typically occur unexpectedly and require an immediate response and the infusion of extensive resources on the part of the healthcare system. In many ways the types of clinical procedures the layperson is likely to associate with healthcare are among the least marketable of services. In a life-and-death situation factors other than the image presented by a marketer determine where patients are sent for treatment, which will typically be the closest facility (in the case of emergency care) or the best facility (in the case of trauma care). These are decisions made by clinicians or emergency medical personnel, not by the consumer.

The most important consideration here, though, is the fact that these are rare events. When they do occur, they tend to be traumatic and require inordinate resources. Fewer than 1 in 11 Americans are admitted to a hospital each year, and only a minority of these cases involve life-threatening conditions. Common causes for hospital admission include childbirth, management of chronic conditions, diagnostic tests, and other conditions unlikely to be matters of life and death.

In comparison, the majority of the population visits a physician at least once during the year, and most of those who do use physician services report more than one visit. Virtually everyone buys health-related products from a pharmacy. A large portion of the population is under pharmaceutical management, and virtually everyone purchases over-the-counter drugs at some point. This is not to mention those who purchase fitness equipment, self-help books, health food, and a variety of other supportive goods and services.

Ultimately, many healthcare purchases are not in response to a health *need* (and certainly not an urgent need), but in response to a *want*. One has only to look at the hot areas in the provision of health services today: business is booming for cosmetic surgery, laser eye surgery, skin care, and medically supervised weight-loss programs. None of the conditions these procedures address are life threatening or even medically necessary. The fact that virtually none of these services are covered by standard insurance plans reflects the elective nature of these procedures. Astute marketers recognize a want when they see one; it is not necessary to wait until a need is discovered.

Healthcare consumers are perhaps most distinguished from consumers of other goods and services by their insulation from the price of the products they consume. Because of the unusual financing arrangement characterizing healthcare and the lack of access to pricing information, healthcare consumers seldom know the price of the services they are consuming until after they have consumed them. In the typical case the physician or clinician providing the service is also not likely to know the price of the service being provided. Because the end user is seldom required to pay directly for the service provided—this is typically left up to third-party payers—he or she may not even notice how much his or her care costs.

While the positive effect of this situation is that clinicians are likely to provide or recommend the services they believe to be medically necessary independent of price, at least two problematic consequences arise from this situation. First, consumers are not likely to limit resource utilization to prevent running up the cost of care. If they do not know the amount of the fees being charged, and do not have to pay them anyway, no incentive to use services wisely exists. Similarly, providers have no incentive to provide services efficiently if this is the case. Indeed, under traditional fee-for-service arrangements the incentives available to physicians contributed to greater use of resources.

Second, few healthcare providers are able to use price as a means of competition or as a basis for marketing. With the exception of those organizations that provide elective services or serve a retail market, there is no way to compete based on price. Few healthcare organizations make their fee schedules public; even when they do, widely varying mechanisms for determining the price of a service are likely to be in place. For example, the per diem rates for a hospital room may be determined based on different factors by two competing hospitals, thereby making comparisons meaningless.

Healthcare consumers are not just hampered by a lack of knowledge on the cost of care but on other issues as well. Few consumers are knowledgeable concerning the operation of the healthcare system or have direct experience with many aspects of its delivery mechanisms. There is typically no basis for evaluation of the quality of services provided by health facilities or practitioners, leaving the consumer with no means to make meaningful distinctions. Consumers must make judgments based on the provider's reputation or superficial factors such as the appearance of the facilities, available amenities, or tastiness of the hospital's food. The consumer has no means for comparing services, and the marketer has no real basis for differentiation.

Another factor that sets healthcare consumers apart from other consumers is the personal nature of the services involved (see Box 2.2). While few healthcare encounters involve matters of life or death, virtually all involve an emotional component absent in other consumer transactions. Every diagnostic test is fraught with the possibility of an adverse finding, and every surgery, no matter how minor, carries the potential for complications. Today's well-informed consumers are aware of the level of medical errors characterizing hospital care and the amount of system-induced morbidity associated with healthcare settings. Even if individuals remain stoic with regard to their own care, they are likely to exhibit an emotional dimension when the care concerns a parent, child, or some other loved one. Whether this emotionally charged and personal aspect of the healthcare episode prevents the affected individual from seeking care, colors the choice of provider or therapy, or leads to additional symptoms, the choices made by the patient or other decision makers are likely to be affected. The fact that many consumers cannot bring themselves to even say the word "cancer" supports this view; emotions like fear, pride, and vanity often come into play.

Why No Healthcare Marketing?

Given the pervasiveness of marketing in the United States, how can we explain the relative lack of marketing within an industry that accounts for 15 percent of the gross national product? A number of reasons can be cited to explain this situation, and most reflect characteristics noted in the earlier discussion of health industry attributes. The following factors can be seen as barriers to the incorporation of marketing within the healthcare arena.

No (Real or Perceived) Need

Until the 1980s most healthcare organizations felt they had no competitors. There were plenty of patients, and revenues were essentially guaranteed by third-party payers. Competition had been minimized through gentlemen's agreements among various healthcare providers. If providers did not overtly collude to carve up the patient market, they respected informal boundaries set to reduce competition. They maintained monopolies or oligopolies in their market areas and evinced a product orientation. Even

Box 2.2: Healthcare Consumers Versus Other Consumers	Consumers of Health Services	Consumers of Other Services
	Seldom determine their need for services	Usually determine their need for services
	Seldom the ultimate decision maker	Usually the ultimate decision maker
	Often have subjective basis for decision	Usually have objective basis for decision
	Seldom have knowledge of price	Always have knowledge of price
	Seldom make decision based on price	Usually make decision based on price
	Cost mostly covered by third party	Cost virtually never covered by third party
	Usually make nondiscretionary purchase	Usually make discretionary purchase
	Usually require professional referral	Almost never require professional referral
	Limited choice among available options	No limit to choice among available options
	Limited knowledge of service attributes	Significant knowledge of service attributes
	Limited ability to judge quality of service	Usually able to judge quality of service
	Limited ability to evaluate outcome	Able to evaluate outcome
	Little recourse for unfavorable outcome	Ample recourse for unfavorable outcome
	Seldom the ultimate target for marketing	Always the ultimate target for marketing
	Not susceptible to standard marketing techniques	Susceptible to standard marketing techniques

today many providers remain at the production stage of their development, expecting patients to seek them out because of the services they provide, whether they market them or not.

These factors contributed to the perception (and, in many cases, the reality) that marketing was an unnecessary activity for healthcare organizations. From the perspective of mainstream providers, physicians referred their patients to the hospital and insurance plans steered their enrollees to the facility. Why market to end users who were not going to make the decision anyway? This mind-set perpetuated the impression that marketing was not needed and overlooked the important marketing tasks of physician-relationship development and health plan contract negotiation.

No Knowledge of Marketing

Few healthcare administrators in the past were schooled in the business aspects of healthcare, and fewer still had training or experience in marketing. Many senior healthcare administrators had not received formal training in their field, and those trained prior to the 1980s were not likely to have received much exposure to healthcare marketing. The almost total absence of marketing within healthcare provided no exposure for healthcare executives, and the fact that their fellow administrators were similarly unenlightened with regard to marketing further underscored the lack of knowledge about marketing on the part of health professionals.

Even if a healthcare administrator had some interest in marketing, until recently few sources of information related to the topic existed. Unlike in other fields, there have been few texts on the topic and a limited number of models could be held up for emulation. Few administrators had an inclination to develop competency in marketing; as a result, few took the initiative to make themselves knowledgeable on the topic.

Resistance to "Business" Aspects

Much of the resistance to marketing reflected misconceptions with regard to the nature of *business* and *marketing*. For health professionals business practices carried an unfavorable connotation that implied the subjugation of clinical concerns to business needs. At the same time many of these health professionals were providing less-than-optimal care or suffering resource shortfalls because of a failure to incorporate business principles. A similar misperception existed with regard to the nature of marketing. Marketing as advertising was the dominant perception early in the history of healthcare marketing; even today many health professionals retain that narrow (and negative) perception of marketing. Case Study 2.1 demonstrates a situation in which a hospital departed from its core philosophy to pursue a business opportunity.

Concern over Marketing Costs

A number of concerns related to the cost of marketing played a role in the slow incorporation of marketing practices. Marketing (again, primarily advertising) was seen as an expensive proposition. While more commercial operations like pharmaceutical companies saw marketing expenses as a normal cost of doing business, hospitals and physicians with no previous experience in this regard suffered sticker shock from the marketing price tag.

Their lack of experience with marketing caused them to overlook numerous aspects of marketing that involved little or no expense.

There was, and still is, concern in healthcare over the return on investment that marketing can generate. While most industries have well-developed mechanisms for measuring the return on their marketing investments, healthcare does not. Healthcare organizations are seldom able to measure the cost of providing a specific service, making cost-benefit analyses extremely difficult. Furthermore, so many factors come into play (e.g., referral patterns, consumer attitudes) in determining the use of services that isolating the effect of marketing activities is difficult.

Given a chronic shortage of resources, many health professionals question the appropriateness of expending scarce resources on an activity perceived to have limited benefit. These concerns have been reinforced by disgruntled patients who linked their high hospital bills to excessive spending on expensive advertising. Even if the spending does not affect the patient's bill, the negative fallout from highly visible marketing has affected the public image of many healthcare organizations.

Unlike other industries, healthcare has viewed marketing as an expense, not an investment. The lack of knowledge of marketing, and its potential impact, has led health professionals to consider marketing at best a necessary evil. Furthermore, there is widespread concern that marketing can do little to alter practice patterns, market shares, or any other indicator of importance to the provider.

Ethical and Legal Constraints

A major barrier to the incorporation of marketing into healthcare has been the ethical and legal constraints that have characterized the industry. Until recently it was considered unethical for physicians and many other clinicians to advertise. While other types of marketing were generally accepted, overt advertising initiatives were discouraged, if not prohibited. Physicians were restrained by professional considerations, and hospitals often imposed internal constraints on their marketing activities.

In some cases legal restraints have prohibited advertising and other overt forms of marketing. The Federal Trade Commission, for example, has placed limits on the types and content of advertising that pharmaceutical companies and other healthcare consumer products companies can provide. Congressional legislation has been enacted to limit the marketing activities of providers being reimbursed under the Medicare and Medicaid programs. The nature of health-related goods and services had made them the target of restrictions not found in other industries. Box 2.3 presents additional issues related to the ethics of healthcare marketing.

Why Healthcare Marketing Is Different

After considering the barriers to healthcare marketing outlined above, it becomes obvious that, to the extent that marketing does exist in healthcare, it is going to be different from marketing in other industries. As many marketers who enter healthcare from other industries have found, marketing philosophies and techniques cannot readily be transferred from other industries to healthcare. For this reason healthcare marketing requires its own unique approach and takes on characteristics unlike those in any other sector of the economy.

One factor that makes healthcare marketing different is the nature of the demand for health services. While the demand for health services has a certain elasticity overall, and elective procedures for which demand can actually be generated exist, most major healthcare episodes occur relatively rarely and almost always unpredictably. Such major events as a heart attack, a stroke, or the onset of cancer are likely to arise unexpectedly

---

**Box 2.3:
Ethical Issues
in Healthcare
Marketing**

Ever since the advent of the marketing era in the United States, ethical issues related to marketing have nagged the healthcare industry. Even before marketing was incorporated by healthcare providers as a standard business practice, ethical issues were being raised in regard to the marketing of healthcare goods and services. Concerns over the marketing practices of various medical remedies can be traced back 200 years—to the days of patent medicines sold on street corners, at carnivals, and through traveling salesmen. Eventually, government regulations were put into place to control the claims of purveyors of such products and, with the support of the American Medical Association (AMA), the first medicine labeling laws were passed in 1938. Today the federal Food and Drug Administration and Federal Trade Commission serve as watchdogs over health-related products.

In the post–World War II period, physicians commonly endorsed various products in exchange for payment from the product's producer. Physicians were paid to endorse various pharmaceutical products, for example, indicating that one drug was superior to its competitors. During this period, physicians sometimes strayed from their areas of expertise and endorsed other products as well. The most controversial of these actions involved the endorsement of various cigarette brands. Doctors were paid to attest that Brand X was healthier for the consumer to smoke than Brand Y. The influence of the AMA and other forces were eventually brought to bear, and such practices were eliminated.

These experiences led to a virtual prohibition, enforced by the AMA, of marketing on the part of physicians. The AMA's 1947 prohibition on physician advertising contin-

and affect a small segment of the population. The marketing of such services represents a particular challenge for marketers who are faced with a disconnect between the service and the anticipated need.

A second factor is the fact that the end user may not be the target for the marketing campaign. In virtually every other industry the end user is responsible for the purchase decision, and the decision maker actually consumes the good or service. This is often not the case in healthcare, where the end user of the service (i.e., the patient) does not make the decision to purchase the service. Thus, a physician is likely to determine the what, where, when, and how much of the service provided. The decision maker may be a provider, a health plan, or a family member, not the party who eventually consumes the service. The marketer is faced with the challenge of determining where to place the promotional emphasis under these circumstances.

Healthcare is also different in that the product may be highly complex and not lend itself to easy conceptualization. This issue was raised

ued through 1957, when it was modified to only restrict physicians from soliciting patients. These restrictions did not affect such traditional marketing activities as networking and entertaining would-be referring physicians, and it was even customary at that time for doctors to provide kickbacks (in the form of "fee splitting") to referring physicians. The AMA eventually backpedaled from its strong stance against physician advertising, and in the 1990s many physicians initiated aggressive marketing campaigns.

While hospitals were not constrained to the same extent, many hospital administrators also had ethical qualms concerning marketing (or at least the advertising dimension of marketing). These qualms did not restrict marketing activities such as public relations, educational activities, and communication strategies, but they did discourage many hospitals from overt media advertising. Ultimately, practical considerations on the part of hospitals and health systems overcame any lingering reluctance related to marketing.

Much of the controversy surrounding marketing in healthcare has involved the pharmaceutical industry. The marketing of over-the-counter drugs is covered by federal regulations that control the claims that can be made with regard to their efficacy. The marketing of prescription drugs directly to consumers is tightly controlled by federal regulation; until the end of the twentieth century pharmaceutical companies were prohibited from marketing directly to consumers. Even today, there are strict limits on the claims that can be made in the advertising.

Drug manufacturers have focused their marketing activities almost exclusively on the physicians who prescribe drugs to their patients, and this area has created the most controversy. Pharmaceutical companies spend up to 25 percent of their budgets on marketing and sales activities, and the bulk of this has historically been allocated to adver-tisements in medical journals, support of educational programs, and direct sales to physi-cians. Pharmaceutical companies' longstanding practice of providing free samples of drugs to physicians eventually came under fire and is facing restrictions. More controversial, however, have been the blatant attempts to "buy" physician support for particular phar-maceuticals by providing gifts, trips, and other incentives designed to encourage physi-cians to endorse a particular drug through their prescribing practices. Legislation was eventually enacted to severely limit the ability of drug companies to provide incentives to physicians.

Pharmaceutical companies have been particularly aggressive in their attempts to define new health conditions that could benefit from one of their products and to sub-sequently promote that product to both consumers and those writing prescriptions.

Ostensibly engaged in raising public awareness concerning underdiagnosed and undertreated problems, pharmaceutical companies may attempt to promote a view of a particular condition as widespread, serious, and treatable. Demand is created by classify-ing ordinary processes or ailments of life as medical problems, portraying mild symptoms as portents of a serious disease, defining personal or social problems as medical ones, con-ceptualizing risks as diseases, or maximizing disease prevalence estimates to enhance the perceived size of a medical problem. Once a seed has been planted concerning the exis-tence of a health condition, the "solution" is aggressively promoted to consumers and prescribers. While such activities are not illegal, they do raise serious ethical questions related to the creation of anxiety (and subsequent drug sales) in individuals who may not actually be sick.

While the marketing activities of health professionals will continue to be guided by self-imposed ethical standards, external controls are likely to be maintained and strength-ened. Because of the nature of healthcare products and services, continued oversight on the part of various regulatory agencies can be expected. As marketing activities expand in healthcare, they will continue to be affected by a combination of ethical restraints and legal regulations.

earlier when the nature of healthcare products was discussed. Many health-care procedures, especially those that rely on technology, are complex and difficult to explain to a layperson. Marketing such procedures to an audi-ence that is already somewhat intimidated by the status of the physician and his or her medical jargon represents a particular challenge. Complexity aside, many health services are difficult to conceptualize—just ask a spe-cialist what service he or she provides. While it would be convenient to be able to market heart care, senior care, or women's health, these terms do not lend themselves to conceptual clarity and specificity. The challenge for the healthcare marketer is to package these fuzzy concepts in understand-able terms without resorting to overly detailed descriptions.

Another challenge peculiar to healthcare, specifically in the case of healthcare providers, is the situation in which not all potential customers for a certain health service are considered desirable. While healthcare providers are bound to a certain extent to provide services to anyone who presents with a problem, regardless of that person's ability to pay, the marketer may not want to encourage certain categories of patients to appear for services. For example, there may be cases in which the Medicaid program reimburses at a very low rate for a particular service, or there may be services for which individuals without insurance (or other resources) are likely to present themselves for care. The marketer is faced with the challenge of attracting customers to the healthcare organization without over-attracting those likely to represent economic liabilities.

Healthcare marketing is also different from other forms of marketing in terms of the measurement of outcome. In most industries the objective of a marketing initiative is clear, and the outcome can be measured in terms of the initiative's contribution to the bottom line. The results can be quantified in terms of increases in customer volume, amount of sales, and profits. While the benefits of marketing can be measured in such concrete terms for some health services, the results are often much fuzzier in healthcare. Indeed, it is often difficult to separate profitable from unprofitable services in healthcare. Furthermore, a public hospital may measure the success of its promotions in terms of how many patients it *prevents* from using its emergency room. An academic medical center may measure the success of its marketing initiatives in terms of the volume of research grants it receives, innovative techniques it develops, or number of subjects it can attract for clinical trials.

Quantifying the differences that exist between healthcare providers in any meaningful way is difficult, particularly with hospitals and physician groups. It is often not possible to compare the level of technology, quality of the medical staff, or even price differentials for such organizations. Information that would allow quantitative comparisons between organizations may not be available; even when it is available (e.g., comparative hospital pricing), it may not be very meaningful because of varying approaches in calculating patient fees. As the healthcare system has become more complex, it has increasingly become the case that virtually all hospitals are characterized by some minimal level of services, personnel, and equipment; the same is likely to be true of large specialty practices. If all organizations have comparable attributes, making a case for a comparative advantage of one over another is difficult.

Healthcare marketing, to a great extent, shares a problem with certain other industries—the challenge of marketing services rather than goods. For our purposes, *products* can be either goods or services. Relative to goods, services are intangible and much more difficult to conceptualize. The purchase of goods tends to be a one-shot process, whereas services may be ongoing. It is more difficult to quantify services, and consumers evaluate them differently from more tangible products. Because services are often more personal (especially in the case of healthcare), they are likely to be assessed in subjective rather than objective terms.

Services are distinguished from goods in that they are generally produced as they are consumed, and they cannot be stored or taken away. Services are further characterized by (1) intangibility, (2) variability, (3) inseparability, (4) perishability, and (5) ownership considerations.

Services (e.g., physical examinations) are intangible in that they do not take on the concrete form of goods (e.g., drugs). They are variable in that they cannot be subjected to the quality controls placed on goods but rather reflect the variations that characterize the human beings who provide the services. Thus, we find substantial differences in the effectiveness of various surgical procedures from hospital to hospital. Services are inseparable from the producer in that they are dispensed on the spot, without any separation from the provider. Services are perishable in that they cannot be stored; once provided, they have no residual value. Finally, services defy ownership rules in that, unlike goods, they do not involve transfer of tangible property from the seller to the buyer.

The marketing of services is further complicated by the multidimensional nature of the service. Unlike a good, a service can be thought of as having three components: (1) the people who dispense it, (2) the physical conditions under which it is dispensed, and (3) the processes involved in its provision. Market researchers evaluating the level of patient satisfaction for a provider invariably find that customers rate the experience in terms of their treatment by the staff, the physical circumstances (e.g., the comfort of the waiting room, the quality of the hospital food), and the processes to which they are subjected (e.g., ability to get an appointment, length of time in the waiting room). While marketers of packaged goods must consider a number of aspects of the process, they generally are able to focus on the product. They do not have to be concerned with the characteristics of those dispensing the product, nor with the processes involved in the customer obtaining the product. For this reason marketers of health services must consider a wider range of issues.

Developments Encouraging Healthcare Marketing

Despite the barriers to the incorporation of marketing into healthcare noted above, significant progress was made during the last decades of the twentieth century in establishing marketing as an integral function of healthcare organizations. However, the lack of knowledge concerning marketing and the level of resistance were such that it took some significant developments for marketing to be considered a legitimate healthcare function. These developments reflect changes in society overall, trends within the healthcare industry, and changes in the nature of consumers. Some of the important developments are summarized below.

Introduction of Competition

Until the 1980s true competition was unknown in healthcare. Most healthcare organizations had operated since the 1960s in monopolistic or oligopolistic environments. Suddenly, healthcare organizations were faced with competition from many sources for what had become a shrinking market in many ways.

Overcapacity in the Hospital Industry

The hospital-building binge that spanned three decades, coupled with the trend toward a reduction in admission rates, created an oversupply of hospital beds. Suddenly, hospitals that had scrambled to find beds were faced with the prospect of closing nursing units. Given an essentially flat market for hospital services, additional patients were going to have to be acquired from competitors.

Rise of the Consumer

The traditional customers (i.e., patients) of healthcare organizations had historically had little say in the care they received and their choice of providers. Healthcare providers, especially hospitals, paid little attention to the characteristics of their patients. Surges of consumerism appeared in the 1970s, 1980s, and 1990s (bleeding over into this century), and healthcare organizations were forced to research the characteristics of customers and potential customers and determine the nature of their needs and wants.

Introduction of New Services

From the 1960s on, the healthcare industry witnessed the continuous creation of new services and programs. Innovative services were introduced, and existing services were repackaged. New boutique initiatives such as seniors' and women's programs were being developed. The public had to be educated about these new services and encouraged to obtain them from a particular provider.

Growth in Elective Procedures

Healthcare had always been characterized by certain procedures not considered medically necessary. Procedures to improve quality of life or enhance appearance were offered by a relatively small number of providers to patients who could pay for these procedures out of pocket. As consumer wants became as important as consumer needs, the variety of elective procedures increased dramatically and heated competition developed in many cases among practitioners providing these procedures.

Introduction of a Retail Component

By the late 1980s the healthcare industry had witnessed the emergence of a strong retail component. While different observers may view this development in different ways, a variety of services (mostly elective) and goods were added to the inventories of healthcare organizations. Fitness centers, weight-management programs, and hair-replacement services were among the retail-type services offered. Nutritional supplements, cosmeceuticals, and self-help products found their way into practitioners' offices.

Entry of Entrepreneurs

One reason for the surge in competition noted earlier was the entry into healthcare of entrepreneurs from other industries. By the 1970s the healthcare industry was seen as a lucrative field for business interests with no healthcare background. These new entrants were used to competing, observed sound business principles, and were accustomed to marketing. Not only did they set an example with regard to marketing, they also helped create an environment in which marketing became a factor in survival.

Service-Line Development

During the 1980s some hospitals adopted an approach from other industries that emphasized vertical service lines within the health system. Service lines were established around cardiology, oncology, women's services, orthopedics, and other clinical areas. These service lines were established as essentially self-contained business units that had to survive based on the resources available. It became common to organize marketing at the service-line level, as this was in effect the operational unit, with each service line having its own target market.

Mergers and Acquisitions

By the 1980s consolidation was well underway in the healthcare industry. Both for-profit and not-for-profit chains of hospitals, specialty facilities, and nursing homes were emerging and building regional or national networks through aggressive acquisitions. Physician practices were being consolidated by means of the short-lived surge in physician practice management organizations. Each merger and acquisition not only provided more resources for marketing, but the image issues that resulted from such actions led to an increased need for the marketing of corporate identities.

Need for Social Marketing

Public-sector organizations were faced with a need to get their messages to the consumer but had limited means to do so. The concept of social marketing emerged as public health agencies developed campaigns to inform the public about the dangers of smoking and drinking, methods of reducing the spread of sexually transmitted diseases, and importance of prenatal care. Marketing provided a channel for disseminating information that had not been successfully promoted in a wholesale fashion in the past.

The above developments do not exhaust the list of factors that contributed to a marketing-friendly healthcare environment. Perhaps the most important concept to develop during the 1970s was that of *healthcare consumer*. The shift from patient to consumer, with all that implies, encouraged healthcare organizations to not only attempt to understand the consumer for the first time but also to find ways of connecting with customers and prospective customers. A more informed consumer was demanding ever-increasing amounts of information, and the development of health-education material became a big business. Interest in establishing ties with the community also grew. These considerations caused many organizations to look to marketing, beginning with market research, to cultivate their service areas.

Reasons to Do Healthcare Marketing

By the late 1970s the arguments against investing in marketing were being stripped away one by one. While marketing was still a long way from being enthusiastically embraced, the reasons for incorporating marketing as a corporate function were beginning to mount up. Not all reasons were conceded by all healthcare organizations at the same time, but different reasons were cited under varying circumstances. The following justifications below began to be put forth to support marketing efforts during this period.

Building Awareness

With the introduction of new products and the emergence of an informed consumer, healthcare organizations were required to build awareness of their services and expose target audiences to their capabilities.

Enhancing Visibility or Image

With the increasing standardization of healthcare services and a growing appreciation of reputation, healthcare organizations found it necessary to initiate marketing campaigns that would improve top-of-mind awareness and distinguish them from their competitors.

Improving Market Penetration

Healthcare organizations were faced with growing competition, and marketing represented a means for increasing patient volumes, revenues, and market share. With few new patients in many markets, marketing was critical for retaining existing customers and attracting customers from competitors.

Increasing Prestige

For many healthcare organizations, especially hospitals, it was felt that success hinged on being able to surpass competitors in terms of prestige. If prestige could be gained through having the best doctors, latest equipment, and nicest facilities, these factors needed to be conveyed to the general public.

Attracting Medical Staff and Employees

As the healthcare industry expanded, competition for skilled workers increased. Hospitals and other healthcare providers found it necessary to promote themselves to potential employees by marketing the superior benefits they offered to recruits.

Serving as an Information Resource

As healthcare became more complex and healthcare organizations began to offer a growing array of services, organizations needed to constantly inform the general public and medical community about the products they had to offer. Whether through press releases or recorded telephone announcements, there was growing pressure to "get the word out."

Influencing Consumer Decision Making

Once it was realized that the consumer had a role to play in healthcare decision making, the role of marketing in influencing this process was recognized. Whether it involved convincing consumers to decide on a particular organization's services or speed up the decision-making process, marketing was becoming increasingly important.

Offsetting Competitive Marketing

Once healthcare organizations realized that their competitors were adopting aggressive marketing approaches, they began to adopt a stance of defensive marketing. They felt compelled to respond to the gambits of competitors by outmarketing them.

Summary

The marketing of healthcare goods and services is not comparable to the marketing that takes place in any other industry, and in this regard healthcare marketing presents special challenges.

Healthcare is different from other industries in terms of characteristics inherent in the industry and the attributes of its buyers and sellers. Healthcare does not involve a "market" in the normal sense of the term, nor does it have the established patterns of financing that other industries possess. The goals of healthcare providers are often diffuse and, unlike other industries, they may provide services that do not, and even are not expected to, make a profit.

The variety of healthcare organizations and their various patterns of ownership set them apart from other organizations. The mix of private-sector healthcare and government-subsidized health services in the United States creates a perplexing situation for one seeking to understand the operation of the system and marketing's role in it. In many communities private-sector hospitals seek to attract the most desirable patients and are willing to allow the less-desirable patients (i.e., those without resources) to seek services at the area's public facilities. Thus, a challenge for healthcare marketers is attracting the "right" patients.

Healthcare is differentiated in terms of the distinctive goods and services it offers its clients. Health professionals have not traditionally thought in terms of "products," and it is often difficult for them to conceptualize the products that are being offered. Health professionals themselves are also different from professionals in other industries. They may not have an appreciation of standard business practices and invariably place clinical concerns over financial concerns.

The incorporation of marketing functions in healthcare has been further limited by the existence of a number of misconceptions (even myths) about marketing held by healthcare professionals and, to a lesser extent, healthcare consumers. The existence of these misconceptions resulted in the preclusion of marketing as even a topic of discussion in U.S. healthcare until the late 1970s. Despite dogged resistance, these myths surrounding healthcare marketing are slowly being put to rest.

Discussion Questions

- In what ways is healthcare different from other industries, and to what extent do these differences affect marketing?
- How has the fact that healthcare providers have historically operated under monopolistic or oligopolistic conditions affected their attitudes toward marketing?
- Why do health professionals view marketing differently from their counterparts in other industries?
- What legal and/or ethical constraints affect healthcare marketing but not marketing in other industries?
- Why can it be said that it may not be in the interest of healthcare providers to attract all potential consumers for a particular service?

2.1

MARKETING UP THE WRONG TREE

Protestant Memorial Hospital (PMH), a pseudonym, is a 600-bed facility located in a medium-sized city in the southeastern United States. The hospital had historically capitalized on its affiliation with a religious denomination and had developed a reputation for providing excellent care in a loving, Christian environment. During the 1980s, when it became obvious that the hospital was going to have to add marketing capabilities to counter its competition, PMH reluctantly sponsored tasteful, low-key media advertisements that fostered its image as an organization of caring health professionals dedicated to community service.

As the need to market became more intense, PMH sought outside resources to shore up its marketing capabilities. Because few marketers in the mid-1980s had experience in healthcare, the hospital brought in marketers from other industries. These outsiders were encouraged to buy into the PMH philosophy, and the initial marketing efforts were considered successful.

PMH, like many other hospitals in the 1980s, experienced a decline in revenues and a decrease in profit margins. Also, like many of these other hospitals, PMH began exploring nontraditional sources of revenue that might serve to offset losses experienced as a result of reduced reimbursement for inpatient services. One potential service identified by PMH was commercial blood banking. The demand for the blood components supplied by a few small organizations appeared to be increasing.

During this period, AIDS had begun to emerge as a national health issue. The disease was causing a great deal of anxiety among the populace because of its devastating effects and the fact that, at the time, little was known of its origin and transmission mechanisms. In an uncharacteristic move, PMH decided that an opportunity existed to capitalize on the apprehension of the population and capture a significant share of the blood-banking market in its service area.

To this end, PMH's marketers were instructed to develop full-page advertisements for the major daily newspaper to promote PMH's blood-banking services. While it is not clear who established the parameters for the campaign, these large-print ads trumpeted the spread of AIDS and other blood-borne diseases, warned potential patients of the dangers of infected blood, and reminded donors of the need to be tested for such diseases. In smaller print, the ads encouraged both blood donors and would-be patients to rely on PMH's blood bank as a safe source of blood components.

By the time the advertisement had run for a couple of weeks, an uproar was raised by the general public and PMH supporters alike. The hospital that claimed to be carrying on the healing ministry of Jesus was linking itself (in three-inch letters) to the AIDS epidemic, attempting to exploit the fears of area residents, and ultimately seeking to profit from the personal tragedy affecting many in the community.

The public outcry was such that PMH administrators not only canceled the advertisements but backed away from the commercial blood-banking initiative completely. This experience led the hospital's executive staff to redefine their marketing philosophy and rethink their headlong rush into the provision of nontraditional services that may not be in keeping with the mission of the hospital.

THE EVOLVING SOCIETAL AND HEALTHCARE CONTEXT

S everal developments in U.S. society and in healthcare over the last quarter century laid the foundation for the emergence of healthcare marketing, and current trends in healthcare are bringing marketing to center stage. Changes in demographic characteristics, lifestyles, and other population attributes are all contributing to the growing significance of healthcare marketing. Trends in the healthcare arena anticipated to continue for the foreseeable future, such as an increase in consumer choice and the growing demand for elective surgery, support a growing role for healthcare marketing in the future healthcare system. This chapter reviews recent developments within both U.S. society and its healthcare system and discusses their implications for healthcare marketing.

The Emergence of Healthcare as an Institution

The healthcare system of any society can only be understood within the sociocultural context of that society. No two healthcare delivery systems are exactly alike, with the differences primarily a function of the contexts within which they exist. The social structure of a society, along with its cultural values, establishes the parameters for the healthcare system. In this sense the form and function of the healthcare system reflect the form and function of the society in which it resides. Ultimately, the development of marketing in healthcare (or any industry) reflects the characteristics of both that industry and the society in which it exists.

Societal Context and Governance

U.S. society (or any society, for that matter) can be viewed as a system or an assemblage of parts combined in a complex whole. Each of the parts is interconnected either directly or indirectly; thus, all are interdependent with the others. These parts working in concert create a dynamic, self-sustaining system that maintains a state of equilibrium. The various parts perform their respective functions, and each component must work in synchronization with the others if the system is to function efficiently and, indeed, survive as a system. These major components can be thought of as *institutions;* rather than being tangible objects, they constitute patterns of behavior directed toward the accomplishment of certain societal goals.

The goals of society reflect the needs that every social system must address. Every society must perform the functions of reproducing new society members; socializing the new members; distributing resources; maintaining internal order; providing for defense; dealing with the supernatural; and, importantly, providing for the health and well-being of its population. Organizational structures (institutions) evolve to meet each of these needs. Some form of family evolves to manage reproduction; some form of educational system deals with socialization; some form of economic system deals with the allocation of resources; and so forth. A healthcare or social service system of some type evolves to ensure the health and welfare of the population.

These social institutions are gradually established through the repeated behavior of individuals attempting to address personal needs within the context of the societal framework. Some institutions, like healthcare, are dependent on a certain level of knowledge, and even technology, to be able to fully develop. Thus, healthcare was one of the slowest of U.S. institutions to be formally established, with many tracing its origins as a modern institution only to the post–World War II period.

The factors that influence the form a particular institution takes include the society's cultural history, environment, relationships with other societies, and demographic characteristics. Numerous forms can be taken by the family, political institution, and economic institution, with the particular form being uniquely tailored to the situation of that society. Similarly, the healthcare institution can take a variety of forms. Thus, one may speak in terms of traditional healthcare systems (e.g., shamanism among Native Americans), more complex traditional systems such as holistic Asian systems (e.g., ayurvedic healthcare in India), capitalistic systems (e.g., for-profit healthcare in the United States), socialized systems (e.g., the National Health Service in Great Britain), or communistic systems (e.g., the type of system that once existed in the Soviet Union—found today perhaps only in Cuba).

Like other institutions, healthcare establishes rules that guide the behavior of individuals within the institutional context. For example, guidelines are put forth for living a long, healthy life; if citizens do not follow these rules, they risk sickness and death. These guidelines are often codified in the form of "doctor's orders." Because individuals in a free society cannot be forced to live a healthy lifestyle, the healthcare institution invokes various legal and regulatory contrivances to enforce its requirements. Thus, all individuals are required to obtain certain childhood immunizations, addicts are forced to enter rehabilitation, and patients with contagious diseases are isolated from the rest of the population.

On another level, rules state that patients must have insurance before being treated by certain healthcare providers, receive annual checkups to maintain their low insurance premiums, and pay higher prices for insurance if they are involved in risky activities. While no systematic plan for encouraging or discouraging the behaviors that support the healthcare system exists, various parties, appearing to act in their own self-interest, work toward the goals of the healthcare institution through the promulgation of such rules.

Adaptability and Change

Despite the permanence that institutions achieve in society, they must also have the flexibility to adjust to changing conditions. As will be discussed later, no other institution has experienced such dramatic changes as healthcare during the twentieth century. At the start of that century, healthcare was a rudimentary institution with limited visibility and little credibility in society. Hospitals were considered to be places where people went to die, and doctors were to be avoided at all costs. Indeed, the doctor could do little for the patient anyway. There was no agreement on the nature of health and illness, and scientists were only beginning to document the effectiveness of medical care. Healthcare was not even on the national radar screen for the first half of the twentieth century and accounted for a negligible portion of the gross national product.

Contrast that situation to the healthcare institution at the end of the twentieth century. Not only had the institution become well-established in the United States, but it had come to play a dominant role in U.S. society. The importance of the institution had become such that sociologists often referred to the *medicalization* of American society. Indeed, few members of contemporary U.S. society are able to avoid some type of medical management. In the latter half of the twentieth century the institution came to be accorded high prestige and exert a major influence over other institutions. The healthcare institution today can claim 15 percent of the gross national product and 10 percent of the nation's workforce.

The significance placed on a particular institution varies from society to society. While all societies must address the same basic needs, the importance accorded these needs and the significance of the associated institution vary from system to system and from time period to time period. U.S. society at the beginning of the twenty-first century is dominated by the economic and educational institutions and, increasingly, by the health-care institution. Economic success is a driving motivation for the behavior of Americans, who spend an inordinate amount of time earning money, spending money, and planning how to invest their money. Indeed, many of the activities in other institutions serve to support the goal of economic success.

Formal Organization and Scope of Influence

The ascendancy of the healthcare institution in the twentieth century was given impetus by the growing dependence on formal organizations of all types. The industrialization and urbanization occurring in the United States reflected a transformation from a traditional, agrarian society to a complex, modern society in which change, not tradition, was the central theme. In such a society, formal solutions to societal needs take precedence over informal responses.

Healthcare provides possibly the best example of this emergent dependence on formal solutions because it is an institution whose very development was a result of this transformation. Our great-grandparents would have considered formal healthcare the last resort in the face of sickness and disability. Few of them ever entered a hospital, and not many more regularly used physicians. Today, in contrast, the healthcare system is often seen as the first resort, rather than a necessary evil, when health problems arise. Traditional, informal responses to health problems have given way to complex, institutionalized responses. Healthcare has become entrenched in the fabric of American life to the point that Americans turn to it not only for clear-cut health problems but also for a broad range of psychological, social, interpersonal, and spiritual problems.

By any measure, healthcare could be considered a dominant institution in contemporary U.S. society. Healthcare now accounts for a significant 15 percent of the gross national product, and its share is expected to grow. Other institutions—such as the political institution, the military, and the arts—receive comparatively fewer resources. Americans have become increasingly obsessed with their health. In public opinion polls respondents frequently site health as among their most pressing personal concerns and healthcare as a major societal issue.

The size of the healthcare institution has attracted substantial resources from other industrial sectors, and healthcare is an unavoidable issue in political contests. Indeed, the pharmaceutical industry, insurance industry, American Medical Association, and American Hospital Association are among the major political lobbying groups. Furthermore, much of our educational system is devoted to the training of health personnel. The fact that the federal government has become responsible for 60 percent of personal healthcare expenditures suggests the influence of healthcare on the central government.

Perhaps more telling has been the extent to which the healthcare institution has been successful in the medicalization of everyday life. During the golden age of medicine in the 1960s and 1970s the success of medicine resulted in an expansion of the scope of the field and led it to encompass various conditions that heretofore had not been considered medical matters. Thus, conditions like drug and alcohol abuse, homosexuality, child abuse, hyperactivity in children, and obesity came to be defined as medical problems. This served to widen the breadth of influence of the healthcare institution, increase the prestige accorded to its representatives, and garner grant funds and other sources of wealth for the institution's representatives.

Americans increasingly turned to the healthcare institution in the late twentieth century as the solution for a wide range of social, psychological, and even spiritual issues, and physicians came to be regarded as experts in regard to virtually any human problem. This expansion of scope is evidenced by the fact that fewer than half of the people in a general practitioner's waiting room suffer from a clear-cut medical problem; they are there because of emotional disorders, sexual dysfunction, social-adjustment issues, nutritional problems, or some other nonclinical threat to their well-being. Despite the fact that physicians are generally not trained to deal with these conditions, the healthcare system is seen as an appropriate place to seek solutions to these and other nonmedical maladies.

Media Coverage

Another measure of the healthcare institution's dominance in an age of media overkill may be reflected in the amount of airtime allocated to various aspects of society. Certainly, Americans continue to be deluged by advertisements for all manner of consumer goods. The most obvious change over the past decade or two is the explosion of advertisements and paid programming related to health, beauty, and fitness. A tally of television ads would indicate the extent to which health products and services have come to dominate advertising venues; paid programming featuring fitness training and cable television channels devoted solely to health issues indicate the extent to which the healthcare institution has gained ascendancy. Thus, healthcare marketing in the mass media has grown from a cottage industry in the postwar years to a major player.

The rise of healthcare marketing in the media has been accompanied by an explosion of healthcare information on the Internet. More web sites are purportedly devoted to healthcare than to any other topic. Increasing numbers of healthcare consumers are turning to the World Wide Web for their healthcare information, and the health content online is playing an increasing role in consumer decision making (see Box 3.1). Consumer interest in cyber information has been accompanied by an explosion of Internet-based marketing on the part of healthcare organizations. Once considered an important device for providing information on the part of hospitals, health plans, pharmaceutical companies, and consumer-products companies, the Internet has become a medium for aggressive marketing of healthcare goods and services.

Box 3.1: The "Wired" Healthcare Consumer

A number of recent studies have documented the fact that the U.S. healthcare consumer is becoming increasingly wired (see, for example, Fox and Fallows 2003). These studies have found that between 50 percent and 80 percent of all adults with access to the Internet use it to find information about healthcare. Although some researchers dispute these high figures, there is no question that the Internet has become an important source of health-related information and that many consumers are increasingly relying on it as their source of knowledge.

The Pew Internet & American Life Project, sponsored by the Pew Research Center for People and the Press, has been heavily involved in research on web access to health-related data. According to their most recent studies (based on data from surveys conducted in 2001 and 2002), 62 percent of Internet users, or 73 million people in the United States, have gone online in search of health information. Referred to as *health seekers,* a majority of these people go online at least once a month for health information. About six million Americans go online for medical advice on a typical day. That means more people go online for medical advice on any given day than actually visit health professionals, according to figures provided by the American Medical Association (Schanz 2004). Many health seekers say the resources they find on the web have a direct effect on the decisions they make about their healthcare and on their interactions with doctors.

Among the findings from the Pew Internet & American Life Project are as follows:

- 48 percent found advice that improved the way they take care of themselves
- 55 percent said the Internet has improved the way they get health information
- 92 percent found the information from their last online search useful
- 81 percent said they learned something new from their last search
- 47 percent said the retrieved information affected their health
- 50 percent said the information influenced the way they eat and exercise
- 36 percent said the information affected their decisions on behalf of someone else

For the 21 million health seekers who said they were swayed by what they read online the last time they sought health information, the impact included the following:

All things considered, healthcare was the up-and-coming institution of the second half of the twentieth century. The growing significance of health for our personal lives and healthcare's growing role in the public arena cannot be denied. Indeed, many corporations have indicated that health benefits are one of their single largest costs. The increasing involvement of U.S. citizens in the use of health services and the annual per capita expenditures on healthcare set the United States apart from other countries and have substantially contributed to the need for healthcare marketing.

- 70 percent said the web information influenced their decision about how to treat an illness or condition
- 50 percent said the web information led them to ask a doctor new questions or get a second opinion from another doctor
- 28 percent said the web information affected their decision about whether or not to visit a doctor

Interestingly, most users go to health web sites for research and reference purposes; few use the Internet to communicate with their caregivers or buy medicine. Most health seekers have been able to get the information they need without making any significant trade-offs by giving up personal information. Thus, it is not clear whether most Internet users will embrace a full range of healthcare activities online, such as filling prescriptions, filing claims, participating in support groups, and e-mailing doctors.

Many are using the web to gather information on behalf of family and friends. Those in excellent health often seek material to help someone else; those in less-than-excellent health are more likely to be hunting for information for themselves. Some 54 percent of health seekers say they sought information on behalf of someone else, including their children, parents, and other relatives, during their most recent online search. Another 43 percent of health seekers were looking for information for themselves during that most recent visit.

During their most recent Internet search for health information most health seekers focused on getting information about an immediate medical problem; the majority got information in conjunction with a doctor's visit. In fact, 70 percent of health seekers said they went online for information about a specific illness or condition the last time they consulted the web; 11 percent were checking out news related to healthcare; and 9 percent were seeking information about specific doctors, hospitals, or medicines. More often than not, health seekers consult web resources after they have been to a doctor, presumably after a diagnosis has been given. Women are much more likely than men to seek online health information; 72 percent of online women have gone on the Internet for health information, compared with 51 percent of online men. Some 71 percent of Internet users between 50 and 64 years old have gone online for health information, compared with 53 percent of those between 18 and 29 years old. Those with more education and more Internet experience are more likely to search for medical advice online.

Those accessing the Internet for health information appreciate the convenience of being able to seek information at any hour, the fact that they can get a wealth of information online, and the fact that they can do research anonymously. On the other hand, health seekers are anxious to have their privacy protected. They are worried about web sites selling or giving away information about them, insurance companies learning what they have done online and making coverage decisions based on that, and their employers learning what they have accessed online. Among the most sensitive to privacy violations are African Americans, parents, and Internet newcomers (those who first went online fewer than six months ago).

The credibility of health information and advice on the Internet is also a concern. One major reason is that most health seekers are doing general Internet searches for the material they need, rather than relying on recommendations about web sites from health providers or friends. Compared to other Internet users health seekers show greater vigilance in checking the source of online information. Health seekers are fairly evenly divided about whether or not the information they get online is credible.

The Cultural Revolution and Healthcare

The restructuring of U.S. institutions during the twentieth century was accompanied by a cultural revolution resulting in extensive value reorientation within U.S. society. The values associated with traditional societies that emphasized kinship, community, authority, and primary relationships became overshadowed by the values of modern industrialized societies, such as secularism, urbanism, and self-actualization. Ultimately, the restructuring of American values was instrumental in the emergence of healthcare as an important institution.

The modern values that emerged within the U.S. after World War II supported the development of a healthcare system that would support the archetype of modern Western medicine. These values shifted the emphasis in U.S. society to economic success, educational achievement, and scientific and technological advancement. These values also supported the ascendancy of healthcare as a dominant institution during the latter half of the twentieth century.

Implicit throughout the evolution of U.S. healthcare has been the importance of economic success, and the U.S. healthcare system emerged as the only for-profit system in the world. Today the profit motive remains strong, as for-profit national chains have absorbed much of the nation's health services delivery capacity. The free-enterprise aspect of healthcare is intrinsically linked to other American values such as freedom of choice and individualism.

Other values became important as American culture evolved in the twentieth century. For example, change became recognized as a value in its own right. Americans came to value change and frequently sought changes in residences, jobs, partners, and lifestyles. At the same time an activist orientation emerged that called for a proactive approach to all issues, including healthcare. The aggressive approach taken by Americans in the face of health problems reflects this activist orientation.

The conceptualization of health as a distinct value in U.S. society represented a major development in the emergence of the healthcare institution. Prior to World War II, health was generally not recognized as a value by Americans but rather was vaguely tied in with other notions of well-being. Public-opinion polls prior to the war did not identify personal health as an issue for the U.S. populace, nor was healthcare delivery considered a societal concern. By the 1960s, however, personal health had climbed to the top of the public-opinion polls as an issue, and the adequate provision of health services became an important concern in the mind of the American public. By the last third of the twentieth century, Americans had become obsessed with health as a value and with the importance of institutional solutions to health problems.

Once health became established as a value it was a short step to establishing a formal healthcare system as the institutional means for achieving that value. An environment was created that encouraged the emergence of a powerful institution that supported many other contemporary American values; some, like the value placed on human life, were considered immutable. The ethos promoted by the emerging scientific, technological, and research communities contributed to the growth of the industry. The value that Americans came to place on youth, beauty, and self-actualization further contributed to an expansion of the role of healthcare. The ability of the nascent healthcare system to address emerging U.S. values and garner support from the economic, political, and educational institutions ensured the ascendancy of this new institutional form.

Changing Societal Context

The twentieth century spawned a dependence on formal institutions of all types, creating a favorable environment for the emergence of a strong healthcare system. Just as Americans had turned to formal educational, political, and economic systems for meeting their needs, they began to turn to a formal healthcare system to meet their health-related needs. The transformation of U.S. society in the twentieth century clearly affected the provision of healthcare, as the traditional managers of sickness and death—the family and the church—gave way to more formal responses to health problems. The health of the population became in part the responsibility of the economic, educational, and political systems and, eventually, of a fully developed and powerful healthcare system. Traditional, informal responses to health problems gave way to complex, institutional responses. High-touch home remedies could not compete in an environment that valued high-tech (and subsequently high-status) responses to health problems.

Demographic Trends

The U.S. population experienced a number of dramatic demographic trends during the latter half of the twentieth century. These demographic trends are important in that they contributed to the composition of the U.S. population; this in turn influenced the morbidity profile of that population. The demographic transformation of the U.S. population in the twentieth century may be considered a major, if not *the* major, determinant of the needs to be addressed by the healthcare system. The impact did not end simply with a changed age structure or racial composition but came to be reflected in the radically changed attitudes held by healthcare consumers.

These demographic trends also triggered the epidemiologic transition that took place in the United States in the second half of the twentieth century. Throughout recorded history acute conditions had constituted the major health threat and the leading causes of death. Communicable, infectious, and parasitic conditions; accidents; complications of childbirth; and other acute conditions were a constant companion to human beings. At the beginning of the twentieth century the leading causes of death were tuberculosis, influenza, and other communicable diseases. As the mortality rate for the U.S. population declined during the twentieth century and life expectancy increased, a significant change occurred in the morbidity and mortality profile of the population (Omran 1971).

During the second half of the twentieth century the changing demographic profile led to a shift away from acute conditions and toward chronic conditions as the predominant form of health problem. Improved living conditions, better nutrition, and higher standards of living, accompanied by advances in medical science, reduced or eliminated the burden of disease from acute conditions. This void was filled, however, by the emergence of chronic conditions as the leading health problems and causes of death. The older population that came out of these developments was now plagued by hypertension, arthritis, and diabetes as well as numerous conditions that reflected the lifestyles that emerged within the U.S. population in the second half of the century.

This section cannot begin to address all of the demographic trends that have contributed to the changing healthcare environment; it focuses on the key demographic trends and notes their likely implications for healthcare marketing.

Changing Age Structure

The first, and perhaps most important, demographic trend in the United States is the population's changing age distribution. The aging of America has obviously been one of the most publicized demographic trends in history. The implications of this trend for health services demand have been well documented, with age arguably the single most important predictor of the demand for health services.

The internal restructuring of the age distribution of the population has particular significance for the demand for health services. Population growth within the older age cohorts (age 55 and older), particularly among the oldest old (age 85 and older), is currently faster than that in the younger cohorts. The total population increased by 13 percent between 1990 and 2000, whereas the population 85 and older increased by more than 36 percent. The movement of the baby boomers into middle age will make the 45- to 65-year-old age group the largest age cohort in the next decade. Several younger cohorts (i.e., those ages 25 to 34) actually experienced a net loss of population during the 1990s. A continued shortage of younger, working-age individuals (i.e., those ages 25 to 40) will persist throughout this decade, until the baby boom echo cohort enters this age group toward the end of the decade (U.S. Census Bureau 2003).

The factor with the most significant implications for future healthcare demand is the movement of the huge baby boom cohort into middle age. The first of some 77 million baby boomers turned 50 during the 1990s. This cohort grew up in affluence and comfort, and they are used to having things, including their health, in working order. When they have to contend with the onset of chronic disease and the natural deterioration that comes with aging, the healthcare system will be significantly affected. This cohort grew up during the marketing era and is more comfortable with healthcare marketing than any previous generation. As will be discussed later, this is also a very savvy consumer population that requires special consideration from healthcare marketers.

The nature of the future senior population will be determined to a great extent by the characteristics of the baby boomers. Nearly 78 million Americans were born between 1946 and 1964, and the oldest among them were in their 50s as the twentieth century ended. Boomers are determined to reinvent retirement, a process that appears to already be underway. Retirement is no longer seen as a type of default condition but as a context for new and different lifestyles. Boomers have already influenced the healthcare delivery system in significant ways. They were primarily responsible for the establishment of health maintenance organizations, birthing centers, urgent care centers, and outpatient surgery centers as features on the healthcare landscape. Now they are driving the demand for a wide range of new services such as laser eye surgery, skin rejuvenation, and menopause management.

An automatic accompaniment to the aging of America has been the feminization of its population. The changing age distribution has important implications for the population's male–female ratio. Generally the older the population, the greater the "excess" of females. Except for the very youngest ages, females outnumber males in every age cohort. Among seniors, females outnumber males two to one, and at the oldest ages there may be four times as many women as men. This results in an older age structure for women. In 2000 the median age for women was 38.0 years, compared to 36.5 years for men. Furthermore, 23.2 percent of the female population was 55 or older, compared to 18.9 percent of the male population. In 2000 the excess of females over males in the U.S. population amounted to more than five million.

These statistics on the female population have important implications for healthcare marketers. The female healthcare market is considerably larger than the male market. Furthermore, women are more aggressive users of health services than men. Perhaps even more important, women bear much of the burden for healthcare decision making, not only for themselves but for their families. They are also more likely to influence the health behavior of their peers. Thus, a growing body of healthcare marketing lore highlights women as both healthcare consumers and decision makers.

Growing Racial and Ethnic Diversity

Another demographic trend that characterized U.S. society during the latter half of the twentieth century was increasing racial and ethnic diversity. The United States has once again become a nation of immigrants, with the number of newcomers during the 1990s equaling historic highs. In addition, the populations of long-established ethnic and racial minorities are growing at faster rates than are native-born whites. The cumulative effect of the trends of the past several years has been a diminishing of the relative size of the white population (especially the non-Hispanic white population) and the growing significance of the African-American, Asian, and Hispanic components of the U.S. population. The 2000 census revealed an America that was becoming less "white," with increases noted in the African-American, Asian-American and Pacific-Islander, and Native-American percentages of the population. More important, the census documented the rapid growth of the Hispanic population; by 2001 Hispanics had surpassed African Americans as a percentage of the U.S. population. Because most of the population growth during the next two decades will be a function of immigration, the proportion of non-Hispanic whites within the population will continue to decline. (A telling statistic is the fact that in 2000 minorities accounted for more than 46 percent of the children under age five but only 37 percent of the total population.)

Given the fact that the U.S. healthcare system has historically been geared to the needs of the mainstream white population, the trend toward greater racial and ethnic diversity cannot help but have major implications for the nature of the system. Any marketing activities must take into consideration the changing racial and ethnic characteristics of the population and the demands these changes will make on the system. Indeed, a subfield of healthcare marketing devoted to marketing to ethnic groups and minorities has developed.

Changing Household and Family Structure

Another demographic development characterizing U.S. society is its changing household and family structure. This trend is no surprise to demographers, although it has seldom been linked to health issues. For decades the family has been undergoing change; first it was high divorce rates, then fewer people marrying (those who did marry did so at a later age), then fewer people having children (those who did have children had fewer of them, at a later age).

The 2000 census reported that 54.4 percent of the U.S. population over 15 was married, a low figure by historical standards. Some 27.1 percent had never married, 11.9 percent were separated or divorced, and 6.6 percent were widowed; these figures for the nonmarried all represent record highs. Given that health status and health behavior differ considerably according to marital status, the current and future array of statuses should be a concern for the healthcare marketer (U.S. Census Bureau 2003).

These changes in marital status have had major implications for U.S. household structure; what is popularly considered the typical American family (two parents and x number of children) has become a rarity, accounting for only 24 percent of the households in 2000. Today married couples (without children) have become the most common household form, but this type of household accounts for fewer than 28 percent of the total. Nontraditional households have become the norm, and an unprecedented proportion of households consists of one person.

As with marital status, the changing household structure has important implications for both health status and health behavior. The demands placed on the healthcare system by two-parent families, single-parent families, and elderly people living alone are significantly different from one another and require different responses on the part of the healthcare system. The continued diversification of U.S. household types for the foreseeable future is likely to require commensurate modifications in the healthcare delivery system. To a great extent health services have been historically geared to the needs of traditional households involving two parents and one or more children. This has been encouraged by the extensive provision of employer-sponsored insurance that focused on the wage-earning head of household. In addition, traditional marketing approaches in other industries have focused on the family life cycle as a guide for the appropriate marketing approach. In 2000 fewer than 30 percent of U.S. households fell into the married-with-children category, indicating that marketing initiatives must take into consideration the complexity of the U.S. household structure.

Consumer Attitudes

Although patterns of consumer attitudes in U.S. society tend to be complex, a new orientation toward healthcare clearly emerged during the second half of the twentieth century. The patient was transformed into a customer, creating a new being with the combined expectations of a traditional patient and a contemporary customer. This consumer is much more knowledgeable about the healthcare system; open to innovative approaches; and intent on playing an active role in the diagnostic, therapeutic, and health maintenance processes than any previous generation.

These new attitudes are concentrated among the under-50 population and among certain demographically distinct groups. The movement toward gaining control of one's health has been spearheaded by the baby boom cohort that is now beginning to face the chronic conditions associated with middle age. This group has been influential in limiting the discretion and control of physicians and hospitals. This cohort has also provided the impetus for the rise of alternative therapies as a competitor for mainstream allopathic medicine.

The approach to healthcare favored by the baby boom population is more patient centered than the traditional approach and is more likely to emphasize the nonmedical aspects of healthcare. In general, baby boomers are less trusting of professionals and institutions and are control oriented to the point of stubbornness. This group is more self-reliant than previous generations and places greater value on self-care and home care. It is both outcomes oriented and cost sensitive. The generation prides itself on getting results and extracting value for its expenditures. While this cohort began influencing the healthcare system by "voting with its feet" during the 1980s, its members are increasingly in the positions of power that allow them to influence the reshaping of the healthcare landscape.

To a certain extent these new attitudes toward healthcare reflect the rise of consumerism affecting all segments of society. Seeing themselves as customers rather than patients, people expect to receive adequate information, demand to participate in healthcare decisions that directly affect them, and insist that the healthcare they receive be of the highest possible quality. Customers want to receive their healthcare close to their homes, with minimal disruption to their family life and work schedules. They also want to maximize the value they receive for their healthcare expenditures. The transformation of baby boomers from patients to customers clearly has significant implications for healthcare marketing.

Healthcare Developments

The trends affecting U.S. society during the second half of the twentieth century were accompanied by a number of significant healthcare developments. During the last two decades, Americans experienced a major transformation in the delivery and financing of care. A new generation of therapeutic techniques was introduced along with a new generation of pharmaceuticals; the delivery of care shifted from primarily an inpatient setting to an outpatient setting; and the manner of financing care was modified as managed care became a dominant feature of the healthcare landscape.

At the same time the healthcare institution experienced shifting power relationships as the unfettered influence of the physician was challenged by other competing providers and as third-party payers began to increasingly set the parameters for reimbursement, and hence the delivery of care. Employers, who were bearing most of the cost of private insurance, began to play a more active role, bringing about numerous changes in the delivery of care.

The high and unassailable status of the physician came into question during the last years of the twentieth century, as the fallibility and limitations of medical care were documented. The introduction of increasing numbers of female and foreign-trained physicians into the medical fraternity also led to a changing image of the physician. Baby boomers, armed with information from the Internet, influenced the shift away from the dependent patient to an aggressive consumer patient demanding a role in the therapeutic process.

The changes that have taken place in healthcare over the last two decades or so have been numerous and dramatic. These changes have served to transform the healthcare industry of the early 1980s into a quite different creature. These changes have also had significant implications for healthcare marketing. Lack of space in this book does not allow a review of all of the changes that occurred during the last decade and a half, but some of the more important ones are listed below, along with their significance for healthcare marketing.

Providers Faced Growing Competition

During the 1980s healthcare providers were exposed to unprecedented competition on a number of fronts. For the first time healthcare providers were forced to profile their customers and be able to determine their needs. They also had to understand their competition and develop a level of market intelligence never dreamed of in the past. Most observers would agree that the emergence of competition has been a major driver of healthcare marketing.

Emphasis Shifted from Inpatient to Outpatient Care

Until the last decade or so, medical care was synonymous with inpatient care. Hospitalization was often a prerequisite for the activation of insurance coverage. By the 1980s, almost every industry force was discouraging the use of inpatient care. Hospitals had to rapidly understand the changing market conditions and position themselves to capture the growing outpatient market. Hospitals had to think in terms of a different approach to marketing as the traditional patterns of physician referral for inpatient care were de-emphasized and consumerism emerged as a factor in the system.

Emphasis Shifted from Specialty to Primary Care

Hospitals have historically relied on the medical specialists on their staffs to admit patients and generate their revenue. By the late 1980s, industry forces were encouraging the use of primary care physicians rather than specialists. Hospital systems had to examine their referral patterns and revise their thinking with regard to primary care physicians. For the first time, hospitals had to actively court family practitioners, internists, and pediatricians and marketers had to develop means for showcasing their primary care capabilities to both consumers and health plans.

Employers Emerged as Major Players in the Industry

After World War II, employers began offering health insurance to their employees and passively footed the bill for their medical expenses. By the mid-1980s, however, employers were taking a more active role in the management of their employees' health benefits. Suddenly, healthcare providers found they had a new customer with a different set of needs from their traditional customers. Business coalitions emerged to negotiate with healthcare providers from a position of strength.

The Industry Became Increasingly Market Driven

Until the healthcare industry became market driven in the 1980s the opinions of patients were seldom considered important. Suddenly, healthcare providers needed to know what the patient liked and did not like about the services provided. Patient satisfaction surveys became common, and providers and health plans started being graded with report cards on their performance. Marketers were called on not only to identify the wants and needs of the market but also to assist in maintaining a high level of customer satisfaction.

Managed Care Emerged as a Dominant Force

The emergence of managed care as a major force essentially changed the ground rules for healthcare providers. The patient was transformed into an enrollee. Instead of searching for sick patients who would require health services, the marketer was directed to identify healthy persons who would not consume many services. Healthcare providers participating in managed care plans (particularly capitated plans) had to shift their focus from treatment and cure to health maintenance. Managed care plans had to develop marketing expertise to capture the employer market, and managed care negotiations came to be considered a marketing function by many health systems.

The Nature of the Decision Maker Changed

Before the marketing era in healthcare, virtually all decisions were made by physicians and consumers had limited control over their medical episodes. Later, health plans began exercising inordinate influence over the use of health services as their enrollees were directed to specific provider networks. During the 1990s consumers began to wield considerable influence as consumer choice began to characterize the industry, and the prospect of *defined contributions* brought a new perspective to healthcare marketing. Each of these developments had implications for marketers, with the focus shifting from physician to health plan to consumer. Pharmaceutical companies and health plans, which had traditionally marketed to middlemen, were now focusing on the consumer.

Medical Care Was Redefined as Healthcare

Most observers of the healthcare scene contend that the overarching development in healthcare of the late twentieth century was the paradigm shift from an emphasis on medical care to an emphasis on healthcare (see Box 3.2). *Medical care* is narrowly defined in terms of the formal services provided by the healthcare system. It refers primarily to those functions of the system under the influence of medical doctors. This concept focuses on the clinical aspects of care—diagnosis and treatment—and excludes consideration of the nonmedical aspects of care. *Healthcare* is more broadly defined and refers to any activity that directly or indirectly contributes to preserving, maintaining, or enhancing health status. Healthcare includes not only formal health-seeking activities (e.g., visiting a health professional) but also involvement in oral hygiene, exercise, and healthy eating habits. As acute conditions waned in importance and chronic and degenerative conditions came to predominate, the medical model began to lose some of its salience. Once the cause of most health conditions ceased to be microorganisms within the environment and became aspects of lifestyle, a new model of health and illness was required. The chronic conditions that had come to account for the majority of health problems did not respond well to the treatment-and-cure approach of the medical model. Chronic conditions could not be cured but had to be managed over a lifetime, calling for a quite different approach.

The Patient Was Redefined

Of all of the developments in healthcare of the past two or three decades, perhaps the one with the most implications for healthcare marketing is the redefining of the patient. By the end of the twentieth century fewer health professionals were using the term patient, primarily because of its narrow connotation. The term patient was being replaced by *client, customer, consumer,* or *enrollee,* depending on the situation. The major consideration regardless of the label applied was the fact that clients, customers, consumers, and enrollees all had different characteristics than did patients. While the term "patient" implies a dependent, submissive status, each of these other terms implies that the party so labeled is more proactively involved in the provision of his or her care. Healthcare consumers (i.e., patients with the attitudes of customers) were spawned by the baby boom generation and are used to a higher level of service than that typically offered through the healthcare system. They are demanding more attention from practitioners and more of a partnership in the therapeutic process. Ultimately, this development moved healthcare marketing closer to the marketing activities of other industries, as the consumer of the product became, essentially for the first time, the focus of the healthcare marketer. Case Study 3.1 illustrates a marketing approach to the "new" patient.

Summary

Changes in demographic characteristics, lifestyles, and other population attributes are all contributing to the growing significance of healthcare marketing. A number of trends in the healthcare arena, which are anticipated to continue in the foreseeable future, portend a growing role for this

| **Box 3.2: From Medical Care to Healthcare** | Since the 1970s the healthcare field has steadily moved away from medical care toward healthcare. The growing awareness of the connection between health status and lifestyle and the realization that medical care is limited in its ability to control the disorders of modern society have |

prompted a move away from a strictly medical model of health and illness to one that incorporates more of a social and psychological perspective (Engle 1977). By the late 1990s a true paradigm shift was occurring within the healthcare industry, involving a redefinition of medical care as healthcare.

Since the beginning of the twentieth century, the dominant paradigm in Western medical science has been the medical model of disease. Built on the germ theory formulated late in the nineteenth century, the medical model provided an appropriate framework within which to address and respond to the acute health conditions prevalent well into the twentieth century. During the later years of the twentieth century, enough anomalies had been identified to bring the prevailing paradigm into question. Despite the ever-increasing sophistication of medical technology, the nonmedical aspects of care were increasingly coming to the fore.

Clearly, the epidemiologic transition, through which acute conditions have been displaced by chronic disorders, has played a major role. Independent of this trend, patients had been expressing growing dissatisfaction with the operation of the healthcare system. The traditional approach to care is not a comfortable fit with the attitudes baby boomers bring to the doctor's office. This cohort emphasizes convenience, value, responsiveness, patient participation, and other attributes not traditionally incorporated into the medical model. Furthermore, the runaway costs of the system have led observers of all persuasions to question the wisdom of pursuing the one-size-fits-all approach to solving health problems traditional in medical care.

The transition from medical care to healthcare has affected every aspect of care, from the standard definitions of health and illness to the manner in which healthcare is delivered. Health status is now defined as a continuous process rather than in terms of a specific episode of care. The causes of ill health are now sought in the environment, and the social context of the individual as often as they are sought under the microscope. The importance of the nonmedical component of therapy has come to be recognized; now, fathers are allowed to participate in childbirth and families are encouraged to contribute to the treatment of cancer patients. Perhaps the most significant indicator of the paradigm shift is the fact that the term "patient" is increasingly being replaced with terms like "consumer" (see Chapter 4 for a further discussion of this phenomenon). This calls for a significant change in the manner in which healthcare organizations structure their marketing activities.

endeavor. Just as the form and function of the healthcare system reflect the form and function of the society in which it resides, the attributes of marketing in healthcare reflect those of both the industry and the society in which it exists.

Healthcare, like any other institution, has evolved to meet certain needs of society. Mechanisms are put into place by the institution for ensuring the health and well-being of the members of society. Over time, healthcare has come to be one of the dominant institutions in U.S. society, a society that has become increasingly medicalized. Healthcare now accounts for a significant 15 percent of the gross national product, reflecting the fact that Americans have become increasingly obsessed with their health.

The cultural revolution that occurred in the twentieth century resulted in extensive value reorientation within U.S. society and laid the groundwork for the emergence of a powerful healthcare institution. The rise of values such as economic success, educational achievement, and scientific and technological advancement all contributed to the development of a modern healthcare system. These new values supplemented the emphasis traditionally placed on human life, humanitarian efforts, and personal autonomy. The increasing emphasis on youth and beauty also did much to spur the development of an expansive healthcare system.

The nature of the U.S. healthcare system has been shaped by both broad societal trends and developments within healthcare itself. Demographic trends characterizing American society during the last quarter of the twentieth century had both direct and indirect implications for healthcare, perhaps none greater than the dramatic impact of the epidemiologic transition. Changing demographics has contributed to changing attitudes among healthcare consumers, and the proliferation of widely varying lifestyles has served to further segment the healthcare market.

Within healthcare, developments such as growing competition, the shift from inpatient care to outpatient care, the growing influence of employers, and the emergence of managed care have led to a major transformation of the industry. An appreciation of the role of the market in driving the demand for health and the growing importance of the consumer have been important factors in the emergence of marketing as a core function for healthcare organizations. Not only has medical care been redefined as healthcare, but the very nature of the patient himself has been transformed in recent years.

Discussion Questions

- Prior to World War II, what factors constrained the development of healthcare as a distinct institution?
- What were some of the contributions of World War II to the emergence of healthcare as an institution?
- What postwar developments facilitated the growth of healthcare as an institution?
- What are some of the implications of the emergence of *health* as a distinct value in U.S. society?
- How can we account for the rapid increase in the prestige of physicians and hospitals during the "golden age" of healthcare?
- What evidence can be offered for the *medicalization* of American society?
- How has the *epidemiologic transition* contributed to change in the U.S. healthcare system?
- What factors led to the redefinition of the *patient* as *consumer* during the late twentieth century?
- What factors within the healthcare system itself fueled the rapid change that has taken place in healthcare?
- How can we explain the paradigm shift that has led to a deemphasis of the medical model and an emphasis of the healthcare model?

References

Engle, G. L. 1977. "The Need for a New Medical Model: A Challenge for Biomedicine." Science 196: 129–35.

Fox, S., and D. Fallows. 2003. *Internet Health Resources*. Washington, DC: Pew Internet & American Life Project.

Omran, A. R. 1971. "The Epidemiologic Transition: A Theory of the Epidemiology of Population Change." *Milbank Memorial Fund Quarterly* 49: 515ff.

Schanz, S. 2004. *Using the Internet for Health Information*. Chicago: American Medical Association.

U.S. Census Bureau, Department of Commerce. 2003. American Factfinder [Online material; retrieved 04/15/03]. http://www.census.gov.

3.1

CAPTURING AN EMERGING MARKET

The growing racial and ethnic diversity of the U.S. population has seemed to overwhelm some healthcare providers. A system that is used to providing one-size-fits-all care is now faced with an increasingly heterogeneous patient population whose members often have different perspectives on healthcare than do the providers of care. However, if a provider can adapt to the needs of this growing market, a lot of opportunities will present themselves.

The challenge of engaging the community in the opening of a birthing center is always significant, and it becomes even more daunting when community members speak 40 different languages. One urban, community hospital in the midwest not only took on this challenge but turned it into one of its greatest marketing success stories.

Thirteen hospitals within a ten-mile radius of the primary service area provided obstetrical services. An estimated 24,274 childbearing-age women lived in the primary service area. Another 134,055 childbearing-age women lived in the secondary service area. A service-area analysis identified the following ethnic populations: 72.2 percent non-Hispanic white, 7.0 percent African American or black, 0.5 percent Native American, 11.2 percent Asian or Pacific Islander, and 9.1 percent other. Some 18.9 percent of the population was classified as Hispanic. The percentage of Asians in the service area was quadruple the state and national averages, and the percentage of Hispanics in the service area was double the state and national figures. The basic racial and ethnic breakdown of the service-area population failed to convey the unique features of the service-area. Among the white population, recent immigrants from the Middle East and Eastern Europe predominated. The Asian immigrants came predominantly from Korea, Pakistan, India, and the Philippines.

To narrow the ethnic childbearing market, obstetrics discharge data were reviewed and physicians were asked to identify the major ethnic and cultural groups among their patients. The following major groups using obstetrics services were identified using this technique: Korean

(23 percent); Indian, Pakistani, and Middle Eastern (29 percent); Assyrian (6 percent); and Hispanic (13 percent). Research into cultural considerations for these groups identified a significant subgroup of Indian, Pakistani, and Middle Eastern patients who were Muslim. Based on this information four target ethnic markets were defined: Korean, non-Muslim Middle Eastern, and Hispanic (Mexican, Puerto Rican, and Cuban).

In an effort to increase market share for obstetrical services at the hospital, marketing strategies were developed to increase awareness of the new family birthing center in these ethnic communities. To achieve this goal in a highly competitive market the following objectives were adopted:

- Differentiating services from those of competitors by means of the following:

  a. Graphic images and color coding for directional signage within the facility
  b. Multilingual and multicultural physicians (male and female), nursing staff, cultural liaisons, and interpreters
  c. Culturally diverse artwork throughout the facility
  d. Large, state-of-the-art labor-delivery-recovery-postpartum rooms with hot tubs and room for family members
  e. Ethnic menus, microwaves, and refrigerators for patient use
  f. Childbirth-preparation classes taught by native language speakers in Spanish, Korean, Arabic, and Hindi
  g. Family-centered program of care
  h. Superior quality measures (low Cesarean-section rates and successful post-Cesarean-section vaginal-birth initiatives)

- Enhancing the hospital's marketing presence through the following:

  a. Creating a new maternity-services "brand" for the hospital (the graphic image of infant footprints was chosen)
  b. Aggressively marketing and promoting the new features and benefits of the hospital's maternity services
  c. Reinforcing the unique positioning by the hospital based on its culturally sensitive family-centered maternity care

Based on these objectives the following marketing initiatives were identified for the hospital:

- Targeted market research to build knowledge and understanding of each ethnic group

- Implementation of culturally appropriate advertising campaigns for each targeted group, including native-language posters/fliers, newspaper and radio ads, and billboards
- Development of a comprehensive "Guide to Hospital Services" in Spanish, Arabic, Hindi, and Korean
- Aggressive media-relations efforts to promote the hospital's unique commitment to meet the needs of its "neighborhood of nations"
- Implementation of a comprehensive community-relations programs
- A series of grand-opening events tailored to each ethnic market, with ethnic menus, appropriate dignitaries, and entertainment
- Development of a strong community presence for customized ethnic maternity services, including photos of the physical space and amenities in the hospital newsletter distributed to 125,000 households in the primary and secondary service areas
- Distribution of fliers in the religious institutions of the target market

Events planned for the grand opening included a series of receptions for the Korean, Middle Eastern, and Muslim populations. Korean physicians and nurses planned the Korean reception with the assistance of the marketing staff. On the evening of the reception five Korean obstetrical and neonatal nurses dressed in traditional Korean gowns and led Korean-language tours of the facility. Korean food was served, and gifts were distributed to the more than 400 guests. A program of dance and chamber music provided by Korean dancers and musicians followed the reception. The uniqueness of the event captured extensive Korean television coverage.

The Middle Eastern, Muslim, and Hispanic receptions were similar in structure. Each event was planned with the help of bicultural and bilingual nurses and physicians and included facility tours, ethnic foods, and culturally appropriate gifts and entertainment. In total, 2,700 individuals attended the events.

As a result of these marketing efforts the family birthing center experienced 25 percent growth per year over the three years following its opening. Patient satisfaction has improved consistently, and quality measures have remained above national averages. This hospital found that serving ethnic markets appropriately is an excellent business development strategy.

Source: Noonan, M. D., and R. Savolaine. 2001. "A Neighborhood of Nations." *Marketing Health Services* 21 (4): 40–43.

BASIC MARKETING CONCEPTS

This chapter introduces the basic marketing concepts used in health-care and other industries. Standard marketing terminology is presented, and the relationships between the various concepts are outlined. Because many of these concepts are foreign to healthcare, some have different implications for the industry; other established marketing notions are actually problematic in the healthcare setting. Most concepts considered in this chapter are addressed in more detail in later chapters.

Marketing Concepts

Far too often, textbooks dive straight into the intricacies of their subject matter without clearly defining the concepts with which they are working. They assume that the reader already has an appreciation of the basic concepts; for those approaching healthcare marketing for the first time this is not likely to be the case. For that reason the basic concepts that are the central concern of this text are presented here, along with relevant applications from the healthcare arena.

Marketing

Marketing can be defined in a variety of ways. According to the American Marketing Association marketing is "the process of planning and executing the conception, pricing, promotion, and distribution of ideas, goods, and services to create exchanges that satisfy individual and organizational objectives" (Bennett 1995). Another definition depicts marketing as a management process that identifies, anticipates, and supplies customer requirements efficiently and profitably. Philip Kotler (1999), one of the early proponents of marketing in healthcare, defines marketing as a social and managerial process by which individuals and groups obtain what they need and want through creating and exchanging products and value with others.

A parsing of the first definition provides some important information about marketing. First, marketing involves a process, implying that the marketing operation involves several systematic steps. The definition specifies planning as part of the process, indicating that marketing should not be done impulsively, but the execution of a marketing campaign should be well thought out. It notes four components of the marketing process (elsewhere referred to as the four Ps) to include product conception, pricing, promotion, and distribution channels (or the place) through which the products are distributed.

These products are the ideas, goods, or services being promoted by the organization. Ideas may involve concepts such as the image of a hospital or the notion that pregnant women should receive prenatal care. Goods and services combined are thought of as products, and in healthcare these would include tangible goods such as crutches, hospital beds, and Band-Aids and intangible services such as physical examinations, immunizations, and cardiac catheterizations.

The economic aspect of the marketing transaction is demonstrated by the fact that an exchange is seen as the end result of the process. Thus, a physician offers medical services in exchange for money (directly from the patient or from a third party), a hospital offers a physician staff privileges in exchange for his or her admissions, and an insurance plan offers healthcare coverage in exchange for the insured's premiums. All of these exchanges are facilitated through marketing at some level.

Ultimately, the intent of marketing is to meet the goals of the organization (as seller) while at the same time meeting the needs of the customer (as buyer). Unless the goals of both parties are met the marketing process would be considered unsuccessful. A recognition of the importance of these mutually beneficial relationships has spawned almost universal efforts to measure customer satisfaction in healthcare.

From the perspective of this text, marketing is seen in the broadest possible terms. Marketing is not limited to press releases, advertising, or direct mail, for example, but involves a comprehensive process that affects all dimensions of the organization and should be intertwined with all aspects of its operation. As an umbrella term, marketing refers to any means of promotion devoted to the ends indicated in the definition. These means of promotion range from phone-book listings to networking with colleagues, sales calls, and advertising in print and electronic media.

Healthcare Marketing

Healthcare marketing would be defined by extending the initial definition of marketing to the healthcare field. However, not all components of the definition are comfortable fits for all players in the healthcare environment, requiring that the process often be modified for application to healthcare. For example, providers may have limited ability to use pricing as a marketing tool in the sense that third-party payers are willing to pay a specified amount regardless of the provider's fee. Hospitals may be limited in their ability to change their locations in response to consumer demand. Thus, much of the challenge for the healthcare marketer is in the accommodation of marketing principles to the unique characteristics of the healthcare industry.

Market

The existence of marketing implies the availability of a *market*. In its original premarketing form, a market referred to a real or virtual setting in which potential buyers and sellers of a good or service came together for the purpose of exchange. The notion of a market *place* has been modified to refer to the individuals or organizations in that market that are potential customers. Thus, to marketers a market is the set of all people (or organizations) who have an actual or potential interest in a good or service or, according to Kotler (1999), the set of actual and potential buyers of a product. Alternatively, a market is defined as a group of consumers who share a particular characteristic that affects their needs or wants and makes them potential buyers of a product.

Markets are often thought of in terms of a *market area*—a geographic area containing the customers of a particular organization for specific goods or services. Markets may also be defined in nongeographic terms and refer to segments within the population independent of geography. The market, however defined, is thought to be characterized by a measurable level of *market demand*—the total volume of a product or service likely to be consumed by specific groups of customers in a specified market area during a specified period. (*Demand* is a problematic concept in healthcare, and Chapter 9 is devoted to this topic.)

Components of Marketing

A number of different aspects of marketing derivative of the above definitions may be introduced at this point. In actual practice, health professionals are not likely to deal with marketing in the abstract but are involved with concrete marketing activities. These concepts will recur repeatedly throughout the text, and it is worthwhile to pin down their definitions at this point.

Public Relations

Public relations (PR) is a form of communication management that seeks to make use of publicity and other nonpaid forms of promotion and information to influence feelings, opinions, or beliefs about the organization and its offerings. PR includes press releases, press conferences, distribution of feature stories to the media, public-service announcements, and other publicity-oriented activities.

In the past, healthcare organizations often used PR for crisis management, particularly for damage control, justifying questionable actions, explaining negative events, and so forth. Over time, however, PR has been cast in a more proactive light as healthcare organizations have come to appreciate the benefits of a strong PR program.

Communications

Large healthcare organizations typically establish mechanisms for communicating with their various publics (both internal and external). Communications staff develop materials for dissemination to the public and employees of the organization. Internal newsletters and publications geared to relevant customer groups (e.g., patients, enrollees) are generated, and patient education materials are frequently developed by communications staff. Separate communications departments may be established, or this function may overlap with the PR or community-outreach functions.

Implicit in all aspects of the marketing process is the act of communicating. Indeed, marketers have expended a great deal of effort in the examination of various models of communication (see Box 4.1).

Community Outreach

Community outreach is a form of marketing that seeks to present the programs of the organization to the community and establish relationships with community organizations. Community outreach may involve episodic activities such as health fairs or educational programs for community residents. This function may also include ongoing initiatives involving outreach workers who are visible within the community on a recurring basis. This aspect of marketing emphasizes the organization's commitment to the community and its support of community organizations. While the benefits of community-outreach activities are not as easily measured as some more direct marketing activities, the organization often gains customers as a result of its health-screening activities, follow-up from educational seminars, or outreach-worker referrals.

One objective of community-outreach initiatives is to generate word-of-mouth communication concerning the organization or its services. Word-of-mouth communication occurs when people share information about products or promotions with friends. Efforts to generate positive word-of-mouth support are important, as word-of-mouth communication often tends to be negative.

Students of marketing have expended considerable effort in specifying models of communication that relate to the marketing process. *Communication* refers to the transmission or exchange of information and implies the sharing of meaning among those who are communicating. Communication in marketing may be directed at (1) initiating actions; (2) making known needs and requirements; (3) exchanging information, ideas, attitudes, and beliefs; (4) establishing understanding; or (5) establishing and maintaining relations.

Communication in marketing can occur in a variety of ways. *Face-to-face communication* can involve formal meetings, interviews, and informal contact. *Oral communication* can involve telephone contact, public-address systems, and video-conferencing systems. *Written communication* can include letters (external), memoranda (internal), e-mails, reports, forms, notice boards, journals, bulletins, newsletters, and organization manuals. *Visual communication* can include charts, films and slides, and video and video-conferencing. *Electronic communication* can include Internet chat, voicemail, and electronic data interchange.

A number of communication models have been developed for application to marketing. The one described has been adopted for healthcare. This marketing communication model has the following eight components in healthcare. An understanding of each is important for effective marketing communication.

1. The *sender* is the party sending the message to another party. Also referred to as the communicator or the source, the sender is the "who" of the process and takes the form of a person, company, or spokesperson for someone else.
2. *Message* refers to the combination of symbols and words the sender wishes to transmit to the receiver. This would be considered the "what" of the process and indicates the content the sender wants to convey.
3. *Encoding* refers to the process of translating the meaning to be transmitted into symbolic form (e.g., words, signs, sounds). At this point a concept is converted into something transmittable.
4. *Channel* refers to the means used to deliver a marketing message from sender to receiver. This indicates the "how" of the process or what connects the sender to the receiver.
5. The *receiver* is the party who receives the message, also known as the audience or the destination. The marketing effort is directed toward the receiver.
6. *Decoding* refers to the process carried out by the receiver when he or she converts the symbols transmitted by the sender into a form that makes sense to him or her. This process assumes that the receiver is using the same basis for decoding that the sender used for encoding.

7. *Response* refers to the reaction of the receiver to the message. This is the point at which the effect of the message and its meaning to the receiver are gauged, and it relates to the meaning the receiver attaches to it.

8. *Feedback* refers to the aspect of the receiver's response that the receiver communicates back to the sender. The type of feedback will depend on the channel, and the effectiveness of the effort is gauged in terms of the feedback.

Communication experts indicate that effective communication requires certain attributes. The communication must contain value for the receiver and be meaningful, relevant, understandable, and capable of being transmitted in a few seconds. Furthermore, the communication must lend itself to visual presentation if possible, be relevant to the lives of real people, and stimulate the receiver emotionally. The marketing communication should also be interesting and entertaining.

Source: Berkowitz, E. N. 1996. *Essentials of Health Care Marketing.* Gaithersburg, MD: Aspen.

Government Relations

Long before most healthcare organizations considered the incorporation of a formal marketing function they were involved in government relations activities. Healthcare organizations are typically regulated by organizations within their state and for some purposes by federal regulations. The reimbursement available to healthcare providers may be controlled by government agencies, and not-for-profit organizations must continuously demonstrate to government agencies that they deserve their tax-exempt status. For these reasons healthcare organizations often must maintain discourse with a variety of government agencies, cultivate relationships with politicians and other policymakers, and initiate lobbying activities directed toward various levels of government.

Networking

Networking involves developing and nurturing relationships with individuals and organizations with which mutually beneficial transactions may be carried out. Physicians and other clinicians, who until recently would never deign to advertise, do actively network among their colleagues. This may involve a specialist casually running into potential referring physicians at the country club or attending meetings that may involve potential clients, partners, or referral agents. Arranging activities (e.g., golf tournaments) that would bring together various parties with whom one might want to interact is another form of networking. Networking is particularly effective when dealing with parties with whom it is difficult to get "face time" or when one desires an informal setting involving personal interaction.

Sales Promotion

Sales promotion refers to any benefit (tangible or intangible) that offers a direct inducement to purchasers or an incentive for resellers, salespersons, or consumers. Sales promotions are more likely to be associated with the sale of consumer-health products (e.g., rebates) or business-to-business healthcare sales (e.g., low-interest financing) than with the provision of health services. The sales-promotion mix could include health fairs and trade shows, exhibits, demonstrations, contests and games, premiums and gifts, rebates, low-interest financing, and trade-in allowances. Sales promotion is separate from, but often adjunct to, personal sales.

Advertising

Advertising refers to any paid form of nonpersonal presentation and promotion of ideas, goods, or services by an identifiable sponsor that is transmitted via mass media for purposes of achieving marketing objectives. The advertising mix could include print advertising, electronic advertising, mailings, catalogs, brochures, posters, directories, outdoor ads, and displays. These activities are organized in the form of an advertising campaign that involves a series of ads placed in various advertising media to reach a particular target market.

Personal Sales

Personal sales involves the oral presentation of promotional material in a conversation with one or more prospective purchasers for the purpose of making sales. The process attempts to achieve mutually profitable economic exchanges between buyer and seller based on interpersonal contact and the seller's persuasive communication of his or her product's/service's qualities and the benefits for the buyer. The personal selling mix could include sales presentations, sales meetings, incentive programs, distribution of samples, and fairs and trade shows.

Database Marketing

Database marketing involves the establishment and exploitation of data on past and current customers, along with future prospects, structured to allow for implementation of effective marketing strategies. Database marketing can be used for any purpose that can benefit from access to customer information. These functions may include evaluating new prospects, cross-selling related products, launching new products to existing customers, identifying new distribution channels, building customer loyalty, converting occasional users to regular users, generating inquiries and follow-up sales, and establishing niche marketing initiatives. The database established for this purpose often provides the basis for customer relationship management and may be an integral part of an organization's call center.

Direct Marketing

Direct marketing is a form of marketing that targets specific groups or individuals with specific characteristics and subsequently transmits promotional messages directly to them. These promotional activities may take the form of direct mail or telemarketing as well as other approaches aimed at specific individuals. Increasingly, the Internet is being used for direct marketing. An advantage of direct marketing is that the message can be customized to meet the needs of target populations.

Target Marketing

Target marketing refers to marketing initiatives that focus on a market segment to which an organization desires to offer goods or services. Target marketing stands in contrast to mass marketing, in which the promotional efforts are aimed at the total market. Whereas mass marketing involves a shotgun approach, target marketing is more of a rifle approach. Target markets in healthcare may be defined based on geography, demographics, lifestyles, insurance coverage, usage rates, or other customer attributes. Thus, target marketing is likely to involve the use of customer-segmentation systems.

Micromarketing

Micromarketing is a form of target marketing in which companies tailor their marketing programs to the needs and wants of narrowly defined geographic, demographic, psychographic, or benefit segments. Customers and potential customers are identified at the household or individual level to promote goods or services directly to selected targets. Micromarketing is most effective when consumers with a narrow range of attributes must be reached.

Customer Relationship Management

Customer relationship management is a business strategy designed to optimize profitability, revenue, and customer satisfaction by focusing on customer relationships rather than transactions. While long used in other industries, customer relationship management is relatively new to healthcare; the industry's lack of focus on customer characteristics and limited data-management capabilities have retarded this strategy's acceptance in healthcare.

However, the new market-driven environment is encouraging the development of customer databases and their use by healthcare organizations.

Healthcare Products and Customers

Healthcare Products

The definition of marketing offered early in this chapter refers to the promotion of ideas, goods, or services. (The term *product,* as is seen throughout the text, is often used interchangeably with healthcare *service.*) In contrast to other industries, in healthcare it is often difficult to precisely specify the product to be marketed. Most of what is offered by healthcare organizations takes the form of services, which unlike goods tend to be more nebulous when it comes to description.

In addition, the nature of the product in healthcare has changed dramatically over the past couple of decades. Twenty years ago one could define the product simply as a medical procedure, orthotic device to correct a physical disability, or consumer health product. In today's climate healthcare products include not only these traditional products but also goods and services such as prepaid health insurance plans offered by health maintenance organizations and group purchasing contracts offered by provider networks. (The nature of healthcare products is discussed further in Chapter 8.)

Many healthcare organizations offer a variety of products to their customers. Certainly, the hospital is an example of an organization that offers a wide range of goods and services. Indeed, a major hospital will offer hundreds, if not thousands, of different procedures. In addition, hospitals offer a variety of goods (in the form of drug doses, supplies, and equipment) that are charged to the customer. We can speak of an organization's product mix as it relates to the combination of services, goods, and even ideas it offers.

Ideas

Much of what healthcare organizations promote takes the form of ideas—intangible concepts that are intended to convey a perception to the consumer. The organization's image is an idea likely to be conveyed through marketing activities. The organization may want to promote the perception of quality care, professionalism, value, or some other subjective attribute. The development of a brand, for example, would involve the marketing of an idea. The intent, of course, is to establish a mind-set that places the organization at the top of the consumer's mind, on the assumption that familiarity will breed utilization.

When advertising was first incorporated by healthcare organizations most of the attention was accorded to the promotion of ideas. In particular, early marketers attempted to promote the organization's image and establish it as the preferred provider in its market. While the trend has been away from image advertising and toward service advertising, many healthcare organizations continue to market ideas to their target audiences.

Goods

For our purposes products can refer to either goods or services. A *good* refers to a tangible product typically purchased in an impersonal setting on a one-at-a-time basis. The purchase of goods tends to be a one-shot episode, whereas services may represent an ongoing process. While we generally think of healthcare in terms of a service, the sale of goods is ubiquitous in the industry. Consumer-health products (e.g., Band-Aids, condoms, toothpaste) are household items. Pharmaceuticals—whether prescription or over the counter—are purchased by virtually everyone at some point. Home-testing kits and therapeutic equipment are increasingly being acquired by consumers, and the sale and rental of durable medical equipment is a major industry. Even in a hospital setting, the bill for care is likely to include a number of goods among the itemized charges.

Services

Relative to goods, *services* are difficult to conceptualize. Services (e.g., physical examinations) are intangible in that they do not take on the concrete form of goods (e.g., drugs). It is more difficult to quantify services, and consumers evaluate them differently from tangible products. Because services are often more personal (especially in the case of healthcare), they are likely to be assessed in subjective rather than objective terms. Services are variable in that they cannot be subjected to the quality controls placed on goods but rather reflect the variations that characterize the human beings who provide them. Services are inseparable from the producer because they are dispensed on the spot, without any separation from the provider. Services are perishable, as they cannot be stored and once provided have no residual value. Finally, services defy ownership rules in that, unlike goods, they do not involve transfer of tangible property from the seller to the buyer.

Healthcare Customers

A marketing activity must be directed at someone or something, and a number of terms are used to refer to the target for marketing. After having answered the question "What are we marketing?" the next question becomes "To whom are we marketing it?" Just as the healthcare product has been undergoing change, so has the healthcare customer. While health-care organizations not involved in patient care have long used business ter-minology for their customers, healthcare providers are now undergoing a redefinition of the parties who use their services. Producers of consumer-health products have always had their *purchasers* and insurance plans their *members,* but now the customer for healthcare providers is being trans-formed from a *patient* into a *consumer, customer, client,* or some other manifestation more in keeping with the current healthcare environment. Some of the terms used for those consuming healthcare are defined below (see Box 4.2).

Consumers

Consumer, as usually used in healthcare, refers to any individual or organi-zation that is a potential purchaser of a healthcare product. (This differs from the more economics-based notion of consumer as the entity that actually *consumes* the product.) Theoretically, everyone is a potential con-sumer of health services, and consumer research, for example, is generally aimed at the public at large. The consumer is often the end user of a good or service but may not necessarily be the purchaser. *Consumer behavior* refers to the utilization patterns and purchasing practices of the popula-tion of a market area.

Customers

The *customer* is typically thought of in healthcare as the actual purchaser of a good or service. While a patient may be a customer for certain goods and services, the end user (e.g., the patient) often may not be the customer; someone else may make the purchase on behalf of the patient. Furthermore, treatment decisions may be made by someone other than the patient. For this reason hospitals and other complex healthcare organizations are likely to serve a range of customers, including patients, referral agents, admit-ting physicians, employers, and a variety of other parties who purchase goods or services from the organization. For this reason the customer-identification process in healthcare is more complicated than in other industries.

Clients

A *client* is a type of customer who consumes services rather than goods. A client relationship implies personal (rather than impersonal) interaction and an ongoing relationship (rather than an episodic one). Professionals typi-cally have clients, whereas retailers, for example, would have customers or purchasers. Clients are likely to have a more symmetrical relationship with the service provider than do patients, who are typically dependent and

Box 4.2: What's in a Name? Implications of Redefining the Patient

One of the developments in healthcare over the past couple of decades that has significant implications for marketing is the redefinition of the user of health services. Historically referred to as a *patient,* this term is coming to be replaced by *consumer, client,* and *customer.* While part of the changed nomenclature reflects the different parties who deal with the patient, this redefinition involves something of a paradigm shift in the orientation toward the health services user.

Patient technically refers to an individual who is formally under the care of a physician. While other clinicians may also refer to their charges as patients, the term implies that the symptomatic individual has been formally diagnosed as sick and now takes on a new set of attributes. The patient role (also referred to as the sick role), like any social role, involves certain characteristics. Someone performing this role is considered to be "abnormal" and thus different in important ways from other individuals. The patient role implies a degree of helplessness and a state of dependence on clinicians and health facilities. It also implies a condition of relative powerlessness and an inability to take an active part in the therapeutic process. The patient is also typically characterized by a relative lack of knowledge concerning the situation in question. The patient remains in this role until officially discharged by a physician.

A *client* is similar to a patient in many ways. In the healthcare context a client is a patient of a nonphysician. Outside healthcare a client is someone who uses the services of a professional; certain health professionals may refer to their customers as clients. These providers include mental health professionals, social workers, and other nonmedical personnel. The difference between patient and client goes well beyond the different professionals involved. Being a client involves a more symmetrical balance of power than that involved in the doctor-patient relationship. Clients are typically not thought of as being dependent to the extent that patients are; in fact, clients can fire their providers much more readily than patients can fire their doctors. Thus, a client is theoretically less dependent, more involved in the decision-making process, and more knowledgeable concerning the issue at hand than a patient.

powerless relative to the service provider. Many also feel that the term "client" implies more respect than "patient."

Patients

While *patient* is used rather loosely in informal discussion, a patient is technically someone who has been defined as sick by a physician. This almost always implies formal contact with a clinical facility (e.g., physician's office, hospital). Technically, a symptomatic individual does not become a patient until a physician officially designates the individual as such, even if he or

As healthcare became more marketing oriented, terms like *consumer* and *customer* were introduced. While some purists may consider this sacrilege, the fact is that patients are steadily taking on the characteristics of consumers and customers, not because of redefinition by marketers but because of the dramatic changes that have occurred in healthcare. In other industries the consumer is often thought of as the end user of the product, but this is not necessarily a comfortable conception in healthcare. From a marketing perspective essentially anyone in the population could be considered a consumer, as virtually everyone is a potential user of health services. Whereas patients or clients are effectively under the direction, if not control, of health professionals, consumers are thought to be independently determining what choices they will make with regard to the consumption of health services. Unlike the typical patient, the healthcare consumer evaluates options and makes choices in the same manner as any other consumer.

A *customer* for our purposes is a consumer who is currently consuming a good or service. The customer has chosen to purchase a healthcare product or use a healthcare service. Unlike a patient (even if he or she is the same person), a customer is considered someone who is knowledgeable about the available options and has made a rational choice with regard to the consumption of goods or services. A customer is considered to be more independent and assertive than a patient. Importantly, customers are likely to have different expectations than patients. Whereas a patient might be concerned about humane treatment and effective outcomes, a customer is likely to expect (in addition to these benefits) fast, efficient service; convenient locations; respectful treatment by practitioners; value for his money; and a meaningful role in the process.

This new patient-cum-customer is having a major effect on the healthcare system, and the baby boom generation now coming to dominate the patient pool epitomizes this new manifestation. These individuals want the outcomes of the healthcare system as patients and the benefits incurred by customers. This development not only has implications for the delivery of care but is particularly important from a marketing perspective. Customers are solicited by marketers in a much different manner from patients, bring different traits to the examination room, and use different criteria for measuring their satisfaction with the services.

she has consumed over-the-counter drugs and taken other measures for self-care. Under this scenario an individual remains a patient until he or she is discharged from medical care.

While nonphysician clinicians may treat "patients," it is often not considered appropriate for them to use that term. For example, mental health therapists are likely to refer to their patients as clients. Those dependent practitioners who work under the supervision of physicians (e.g., physical therapists), however, are likely to define their charges as patients.

Enrollees

Although health insurance plans have historically conceptualized their customers as enrollees, this concept has only recently become common among healthcare providers. However, with the ascendancy of managed care as a major force in healthcare, other healthcare organizations began to adopt this term. Thus, providers who contracted to provide services for members of a health plan began to think in terms of enrollees. This represents a significant shift in nomenclature, as an enrollee has different attributes from a patient. Enrollees may be variously referred to as members, insureds, or covered lives.

The Four Ps of Marketing

The marketing mix is the set of controllable variables that an organization involved in marketing uses to influence the target market. The mix includes product, price, place, and promotion. The four Ps have long been the basis for marketing strategy in other industries and are increasingly being considered by healthcare organizations. However, as discussed here, these aspects of the marketing mix do not necessarily have the same meaning for health professionals as they do for marketers in other contexts.

Product

The first P—the *product* of healthcare—represents what healthcare providers are marketing. The product represents goods, services, or ideas offered by a healthcare organization. The product is difficult to precisely define in healthcare, creating a challenge for healthcare marketers.

As noted, products can refer to either goods or services. A good refers to a tangible product typically purchased in an impersonal setting on a one-at-a-time basis. Relative to goods, services are difficult to conceptualize. It is more difficult to quantify services, and consumers evaluate them differently from more tangible products. For health plans, for example, the product may be thought of as the sense of security and protection against financial hardship or catastrophe that could arise from a serious illness or injury and the assurance that personal finances will not stand in the way of getting needed care.

Healthcare providers have seldom given much thought to the product concept in the past. A surgical procedure was considered just that, not something that had to be packaged. Today, however, the design of the product, its perceived attributes, and its packaging are all becoming more important concerns for both healthcare providers and marketers.

Price

The flip side of product benefits is product costs to the purchaser. *Price* refers to the amount charged for a product, including the fees, charges, premium contributions, deductibles, copayments, and other out-of-pocket costs to consumers for health services. In economics, the price is thought of in terms of exchanges—that is, a healthcare provider offers a service in exchange for its customers' dollars. An employee paying an annual premium to a health plan, an insurance company reimbursing a physician's fee, and a consumer purchasing over-the-counter drugs are all exchanges involving a specified price. These costs could also include the pain, discomfort, embarrassment, anxiety, frustration, and other emotional costs of dealing with providers, plans, and the disease or injury that prompts the experience. That these costs must be at least perceived to be worth the investment, considering the benefits available from the relationship, reflects the reality of marketing and the definition of the value of the product for the price.

The issue of pricing for health services is becoming a growing concern for marketers as the healthcare environment changes, and a number of factors are contributing to the greater role of the pricing variable in developing marketing strategy. For marketers the challenge is in developing (1) an understanding of what a customer is willing to exchange for some want-satisfying good or service and (2) a pricing approach compatible with the goals of the organization and its cost constraints.

Place

The third P—*place*—represents the manner in which goods or services are distributed for use by consumers. Place may refer to the location or the hours a health service can be accessed. Increasingly, as more healthcare organizations establish relationships with managed care plans, the place variable assumes a more critical role. Companies offering health plans must consider location and primary-care access for potential enrollees. While in past years a physician could establish an office in a location convenient for him or her, today the consumer increasingly dictates the role of place in the marketing mix.

Place relates to all factors of the transaction or relationship experience that make it easy rather than difficult for consumers to obtain an organization's products. While the obvious factors of location and layout are included, so are hours, access procedures, obstacles, waits for appointments, claims payment, and so on. In most cases the negative place aspects of the encounter impose costs such as lost time, frustration in finding the service site, parking fees, boredom, or other emotional burdens. Positive place aspects minimize such costs, as when a physician who offers early morning or evening hours enables patients to obtain care on the way to or from work and thus avoid time off from work, travel costs, and lost wages.

In some cases place factors may enhance perceptions of the quality of the product, as when the physician's office or hospital is in a trendy location or on a campus that facilitates efficiency of care. Doctors who make house calls may be the only way that homebound patients can get routine care. Systems or health plans may speed up or hinder the setting of appointments by making them available through online communications, for example. Offering health-plan sign-up and status access and benefit-change capacity online at a worksite kiosk or home computer adds place value. The ability to have one's medical record available online has added a different dimension to the concept of place.

Promotion

Promotion is the fourth P of the marketing mix. For many people this has historically meant advertising. Promotion represents any way of informing the marketplace that the organization has developed a response to meet its needs and includes the mechanisms available for facilitating the hoped-for exchange. Promotion involves a range of tactics involving publicity, advertising, and personal selling (Berkowitz 1996). The *promotional mix* refers to the various communication techniques such as advertising, personal selling, sales promotion, and PR or product publicity available to the marketer to achieve specific goals.

Because promotion covers all forms of marketing communication, it includes communications that deliver value in addition to those that entice transactions. For example, health plans can devise communications that enable new members to better understand their coverage and rules for accessing care, enabling them to avoid frustration and get better use of their coverage in addition to promoting member satisfaction and retention. Providers can advise new patients on how to avoid place frustrations and costs and address symptoms and concerns online prior to appointments to improve quality and patient satisfaction.

The application of the traditional four Ps of the marketing mix to healthcare is considered problematic by many observers. Some consider these dimensions of marketing inappropriate for a service-oriented institution like healthcare. The uncomfortable fit between the four Ps of marketing and healthcare has even led some to pronounce the death of the four Ps and suggest their replacement with some other, more appropriate model in healthcare (see Box 4.3).

**Box 4.3:
The Death and
Resurrection
of the Four Ps
in Healthcare** Some observers of healthcare have suggested that the traditional marketing mix may not be appropriate for the contemporary healthcare
environment (see, in particular, *Marketing Health Services* [Summer
2000]). Some have announced the death of marketing's traditional
four Ps, often calling for some other conceptualization of the marketing mix to replace them.

Citing these pillars of the marketing mix as anachronisms in healthcare, English
(2000) has argued for their replacement with a more contemporary set of letters—the
four Rs:

• *Relevance*—getting to know consumers, acting and speaking in their interests, listening to and understanding them, creating and using databases about them
• *Response*—creating and fulfilling brand expectations, orchestrating service experiences that profitably meet the needs and wants of consumers
• *Relationships*—forging formal links between the organization and targeted consumers
• *Results*—gaining market share and share of customers

There is no need to argue over the usefulness of the four Rs championed by English.
Who could argue against getting to know consumers better, responding to the needs
identified for the market, building relationships with customers, and focusing on the
results produced through the organization's programs? However, none of the four Rs
represent a cause of death for the four Ps. They remain distinct factors still appropriate
for application to healthcare marketing. Relevance and response are valid emphases for
marketing, with both relationships and results essential outcomes for them. Nevertheless,
the four Ps are still the attributes we work with to achieve marketing outcomes, with the
four Rs involving a somewhat different perspective on these attributes. The sections that
follow reflect an updated conceptualization of the four Ps.

Product

The first P, the *product* of healthcare, still represents what healthcare providers are marketing—the benefits to consumers of using particular services in specific contexts. One
of the Rs, relationships, does significantly alter marketing, although not in the ways
described by English. If a lasting, loyal relationship is the aim of healthcare marketing, it
makes sense for the product to be the *lasting benefit* to consumers that the relationship
offers and delivers.

Price

The flip side of product benefits is product costs to the purchaser, which may well be
reduced through more efficient and responsive staff and systems but are rarely eliminated
altogether.

Effort costs are likely in relationships, where long-term benefits are involved. The benefits of health promotion and risk reduction typically require significant lifestyle changes and additional efforts by consumers and often their families as well in supporting or enabling such changes. Gym workouts, changes in diet, and even change of jobs to reduce stress may impose financial burdens, although quitting smoking or obtaining treatment for alcohol or drug abuse should improve finances. Considering the often lasting and significant benefits available through healthcare and the coverage that makes it feasible, compared to the typical one-time costs thereof, the value of long-term relationships is likely to be perceived more positively than the typical encounter.

Place

The third P relates to all factors of the transaction or relationship experience that make it easy to obtain their benefits. In some cases *place* factors may enhance perceptions of the quality of the product. Enabling communications with providers between visits online, for example, can add value of its own and eliminate the need for some face-to-face visits and their place costs. Knowing that one's personal physician, or at least an on-call surrogate, is always available can add a lasting sense of security for parents with a new baby or those with life-threatening conditions. Having one's medical record available online for emergency or for out-of-area physicians to use can improve both quality and convenience for patients and give them confidence when traveling.

Promotion

This fourth marketing P—*promotion*—is hardly on the way out either. All forms of marketing communications in healthcare seem to be increasing, particularly direct-to-consumer advertising by pharmaceutical firms. Advertising alone is estimated as a $1 billion annual expenditure for healthcare providers and a $2 billion annual expenditure for phar-

Other Marketing Processes

A variety of other marketing concepts could be introduced at this point. The following sections present selected concepts that are likely to be useful to reader in later chapters. Each concept will be addressed in greater detail later in the book.

Marketing Planning

Marketing planning may be defined as the development of a systematic process for promoting an organization, service, or product. This straightforward definition masks the wide variety of activities and potential complexity that characterize marketing planning. Marketing planning can be limited to a short-term promotional project or comprise a component of

maceutical companies. While most of these expenditures are devoted to attracting new transactions, a considerable portion is devoted to maintaining relationships.

Promotion, which covers all forms of marketing communication, has entirely new applications in relationship marketing. While communications discussions are often limited to the use of databases about consumers to improve the efficiency and effectiveness of healthcare organization advertising, the potential benefit to consumers, plans, and providers is far greater. Communications can be used, for example, to prompt consumers to obtain needed immunizations and screenings, initiate or persist in beneficial lifestyle changes, and make or keep appointments that will deliver value.

Conclusion

MacStravic (2000) argues that the four Ps are alive and well and indeed essential to marketing until something truly replaces them. The latest set of recommended letters adds to the list of functions that marketing can and must perform but is far from displacing the old set. When it comes to the most important components of the new set—relationships and results—they should be supplemented to include new possibilities: a fifth P, prompting consumers to adopt changes in behavior and make contacts with providers that will enhance their health and quality of life, and a fifth R, reminding consumers of the differences that plans and providers (as well as their own efforts) have made and can continue to make in their lives as perhaps the best reason for maintaining such efforts and existing relationships.

Sources: English, J. 2000. "The Four 'P's of Marketing Are Dead." *Marketing Health Services* 20 (2): 21–23; MacStravic, S. 2000. "The Death of the Four Ps: A Premature Obituary." *Marketing Health Services* 20 (4): 16–20.

a long-term strategic plan. It can focus alternatively on a product, service, program, or organization. The marketing plan should summarize a company's marketing strategy and serve as a guideline for all those involved in the company's marketing activities.

Of the various types of planning that could be carried out by a healthcare organization, marketing planning is the most directly related to the customer. Marketing plans are by definition market driven, and they are single minded in their focus on the customer. Whether the targeted customer is the patient, referring physician, employer, health plan, or any number of other possibilities, the marketing plan is built around someone's needs. Although a consideration of internal factors is often pertinent (and internal marketing may be a component of many marketing plans), the marketing plan focuses on the characteristics of the external market with the objective of influencing change in one or more of these characteristics.

Marketing Management

Marketing management refers to the analysis, planning, implementation, and control of programs designed to create, build, and maintain beneficial exchanges with target buyers for the purpose of achieving organizational objectives. The steps involved in the marketing management process include (1) analyzing marketing opportunities, (2) selecting target markets, (3) developing the marketing mix, and (4) managing the marketing effort.

While marketing management is a well-defined function in most industries, it is still in its infancy in healthcare. The fragmented approach to much of the marketing that has taken place and the immature status of marketing in healthcare reflect the slow development of marketing-management skills.

Marketing Research

Marketing research is the function that links the consumer, customer, and public to the marketer through information used to identify and define marketing opportunities and problems; generate, refine, and evaluate marketing actions; monitor marketing performance; and improve understanding of the marketing process. Often used interchangeably with *market research*, marketing research is usually thought to encompass market, product, pricing, promotional, and distribution research. The marketing-research process serves to identify the nature of the product or service, characteristics of consumers, size of the potential market, nature of competitors, and any number of other essential pieces of the marketing puzzle.

Branding

Branding refers to the process of creating a brand for a company, service, or product. A brand consists of a name, term, design, symbol, or any other feature that identifies one seller's product(s) as distinct from those of other sellers. A brand may identify one item, a family of items, or all items offered by a seller. *Brand identity* refers to the range of visual features that assist in stimulating demand. Branding incorporates values, image, awareness, recognition, quality, features, benefits, and name, among others (Mangini 2002).

The limited use of branding in healthcare reflects the historical monopoly many healthcare organizations have maintained—a belief that services cannot be branded to the same extent as products, and perhaps a misunderstanding of the nature of branding. Some major exceptions (e.g.,

Mayo Clinic, HealthSouth) have emphasized their brand and focused on promoting a brand image. For the most part, however, the use of branding among healthcare organizations has been limited. (Case Study 10.2 in Chapter 10 presents an example of the branding of a health service.)

Summary

As the industry has come to accept marketing as a legitimate function for healthcare organizations, health professionals have had to learn the language of the marketing field. This has meant the incorporation of a whole new vocabulary for healthcare providers and the use of terms previously foreign to the healthcare field. Many of these terms and concepts could be adopted wholesale by healthcare, while others required modification to fit the special circumstances of the healthcare endeavor.

The peculiarities of the healthcare industry present a challenge in the application of even some of the most basic concepts from marketing. The notion of a "market" does not exist in healthcare in the same sense that it does in other industries. Health professionals have seldom thought in terms of products in the past, and redefining patients as customers requires quite a leap for health workers. The use of such terms involves more than just a new vocabulary but a totally different way of looking at the world.

The healthcare field differs from other industries in the nature of its traditional constituent—the patient—and in the variety of other types of customers that have emerged. In most industries a customer is just that—a customer, but in healthcare the customer may be a patient, a client, a consumer, or an enrollee. Each of these terms carries different connotations, and the circumstances determine what category a customer falls into and the approach to marketing that is most appropriate.

The traditional four Ps of marketing—product, price, place, and promotion—have been adapted to healthcare, although not without some limitations. All four of them are somewhat problematic when applied to healthcare because of the peculiar characteristics of the industry. As a result, various attempts have been made to modify these components of the marketing mix for healthcare or even replace them with concepts that are more suitable for the field.

Discussion Questions

- Why is it difficult to adopt the marketing approaches of other industries and apply them directly to healthcare?

- How do we distinguish between goods and services, and what are the implications of the differences for marketing?
- Which components of marketing have healthcare providers been most comfortable with in the past, and which are becoming more accepted today?
- What are some ideas that healthcare organizations have tried to market, and why are these more difficult to market than specific goods or services?
- What factors have contributed to the metamorphosis of the patient into a consumer, customer, or client?
- Why is it not possible to apply the four Ps of marketing to healthcare in the same manner it is done in other industries?

References

Bennett, P. D. (ed.) 1995. *Dictionary of Marketing Terms, 2nd ed.* Chicago: American Marketing Association.

Berkowitz, E. N. 1996. *Essentials of Health Care Marketing.* Gaithersburg, MD: Aspen.

Kotler, P. 1999. *Marketing Management: Analysis, Planning, Implementation, and Control.* Upper Englewood Cliffs, NJ: Prentice Hall.

Mangini, M. K. 2002. "Branding 101." *Marketing Health Services* 22 (3): 20–23.

Additional Resources

American Marketing Association. http://www.marketingpower.com.

MarketProfs.com. http://www.MarketProfs.com.

5

MARKETING AND THE HEALTHCARE ORGANIZATION

The incorporation of marketing as a corporate function on the part of healthcare organizations has occurred at different times and different rates for various healthcare organizations, and different organizations are at different stages in the marketing progression. The role of marketing for various organizations is reviewed in this chapter, along with the perspective of healthcare toward marketing as a profession and as a component of the healthcare delivery system. The evolving relationship between the marketing profession and the various types of healthcare organizations is described. The challenge of integrating marketing with more traditional healthcare functions is considered.

Factors Affecting the Adoption of Marketing

For-profit commercial businesses in consumer or industrial settings have historically led the way in terms of formal marketing activities. From the start of the marketing era traditional businesses, including those in healthcare, employed the full range of marketing techniques, including advertising. The types of organizations in healthcare that come to mind are consumer-product companies and retail-oriented healthcare organizations. Indeed, as early as the 1950s numerous healthcare brands had become household names as a result of aggressive marketing.

Marketers of consumer-health products typically used the same techniques as companies marketing other types of consumer products. However, some approaches unique to healthcare emerged. Insurance companies pioneered the concept of group sales, for example, and pharmaceutical companies developed physician-oriented sales approaches.

Despite these applications of marketing techniques to healthcare, the primarily not-for-profit nature of the industry slowed the widespread acceptance of marketing. Healthcare purists considered marketing—often equated with advertising—antithetical to the philosophy of charitable organizations. These organizations were inherently conservative and often viewed the allocation of resources to marketing as in bad taste at best and unethical at worst. Despite the revelations of various academic marketing experts (see, for example, Kotler 1975) that marketing was both common and acceptable among not-for-profit organizations, health professionals as a group continued to resist the intrusion of formal marketing techniques. Furthermore, as a practical matter marketing was not a reimbursable expense for hospitals within the context of Medicare participation. Box 5.1 addresses the changing characteristics of not-for-profit healthcare organizations.

The scope and nature of healthcare marketing had broadened considerably by the mid-1980s. While distinct aspects within any industry require the modification of marketing principles to fit particular needs, the core of marketing and the marketing mix are relevant for almost every organization. Yet, few marketing techniques could be applied unchanged by healthcare; with appropriate modifications, however, many techniques could be adopted. At the same time, novel approaches were required in the face of some of the unique attributes of the healthcare industry.

The attributes that complicate the marketing function include, for example, the fact that most healthcare organizations have multiple markets or customer types to whom they must be attentive. While a traditional busi-

Box 5.1:
Putting the
Profit into
Not-for-Profit
Organizations

Not-for-profit organizations (NFPs) are typically conservative in their actions, particularly regarding expenditure of funds. They tend to restrict their spending to activities that directly relate to their mission. Historically, NFPs have marketing activities not considered worthy uses for scarce organizational resources.

Furthermore, the "noble" pursuits of NFPs were thought to set them apart from their more avaricious for-profit kin. Indeed, a certain snobbishness in healthcare has been associated with not-for-profit status (even on the part of executives who draw salaries larger than their counterparts in for-profit organizations). Some NFPs have overtly eschewed the pursuit of profit as an activity that is beneath them. Even the general public wants to believe that NFPs are just that—not for profit—and expresses surprise when a hospital reports a "profit."

The downside of this attitude among many NFPs has been a disdain for basic business practices. Indeed, many have historically argued that they are *not* in business but rather in a noble calling; as a result, standard business practices have often been ignored.

During the 1980s many NFPs in healthcare, particularly provider organizations, found that their world was changing and that their disdain for profit needed rethinking.

ness can focus on the prospective customers within the general population, healthcare organizations may have to consider physicians, nurses, patients, referral physicians, employee assistance personnel, managed care plans, and regulators. An organization offering a mental health or substance abuse program for adolescents might have to accommodate the needs of judges, probation officers, or social workers. Organizations marketing a sports medicine program would have to consider employers, schools, and health plans among their potential customers, in addition to individual consumers.

An increasingly important market includes employers. For many years this segment was considered of secondary importance, even though companies paid the bulk of insurance premiums for their labor force. Now, however, major employers are attempting to control rising healthcare costs by dealing directly with providers to meet their employees' healthcare needs.

The situation for healthcare providers is also unique in that the health plans in which consumers are enrolled are likely to exert inordinate influence on the choice of medical facilities. Most health plans specify which facilities and practitioners can be used by the insured. While there may be allowances for use of out-of-network practitioners or the option of paying more out of pocket for the privilege, as a practical matter the patient's insurance plan exerts a great deal of influence over the choice of facility or practitioner.

While the phrase may not have been coined by these organizations, the notion of "no margin, no mission" came to be frequently heard during this period.

Most NFPs came to realize that profit was not necessarily a bad thing; indeed, many boards of directors during this period started focusing on the bottom line. Although health professionals are still loath to use the "p" word, the pursuit of profit or net revenue under some other moniker came to be accepted. This meant that NFPs had to adopt many of the practices standard to other industries and for-profit organizations that had come to be prominent in healthcare during this period. They particularly had to focus on the financial aspects of the operation, developing cost-accounting methods and formulating business plans.

Marketing was one of the business practices that came to be accepted by NFPs. The margin necessary to support ongoing operations and continued development of the organization needed to be nurtured, and the role of marketing in this process came to be recognized. If revenue was to flow to the bottom line, increases in customer traffic, sales volumes, market share, and all of the other indicators normally used by the industry were required. Marketing was recognized as the key to the augmentation of these processes, which would ultimately contribute to the bottom line. NFPs came to recognize the necessity for turning a profit and the importance of marketing for this process.

Healthcare Organizations and Marketing

It is impossible to generalize about healthcare organizations when talking about marketing. The variety of organizations is endless; as a practical matter distinctions must be made between the various types. This discussion, for example, addresses healthcare organizations in the form of providers, suppliers, consumer-product companies, pharmaceutical companies, insurance companies, and vendors of support services. The marketing experience of various categories of healthcare organizations are discussed in turn.

Healthcare Providers

When most people think of healthcare marketing they think of the campaigns initiated by healthcare providers. These tend to be the marketing efforts most geared to consumers and are the ones most recognized by the general public. This perception is supported by the statistics on the growth of marketing expenditures on the part of healthcare providers during the 1980s and 1990s. Hospitals have accounted for the lion's share of health services marketing among providers, although many other types of healthcare organizations have made contributions.

Hospitals are perhaps the most visible of healthcare organizations, and their marketing activities in a particular market are likely to be significant. Marketing by general hospitals is usually traced back to the late 1970s. A few hospitals had hired marketers or established fledgling marketing departments by 1980, but the real surge in marketing occurred in the early to mid-1980s. As noted, hospitals became enamored with advertising, and many embarked on multimillion-dollar spending sprees. The print and electronic media were awash with advertisements for hospitals and their services, and some hospitals employed billboards to get in front of the public. Although the ultimate benefit of these expenditures was hard to determine, increased competition among providers fueled the growing advertising fires.

By 1990 hospital administrators had begun to rethink a marketing strategy that focused primarily on advertising. Advertising budgets, and in some cases marketing departments and personnel, were cut back. Hospitals began to adopt a much more balanced approach to marketing, integrating advertising with public relations (PR) and communications activities and adding direct-sales capabilities. Hospitals also began adopting more contemporary forms of marketing through the establishment of marketing databases and call centers. New approaches like customer relationship marketing and direct-to-consumer marketing were adopted in the 1990s, and the ultimate contemporary approach—Internet marketing—was widely adopted by hospitals. Much of this trend reflected movement toward a relationship management approach rather than a sales approach.

Marketing on the part of specialty hospitals may have actually emerged sooner than that for general hospitals, as some types of specialty hospitals (e.g., psychiatric hospitals) were early targets of for-profit chains seeking to expand their markets and gain some economies of scale. Even independent specialty hospitals became involved in aggressive marketing before general hospitals did, as they had a much more targeted consumer pool than general hospitals. As for-profit organizations came to dominate the specialty hospital field, marketing became more widespread.

Media advertising was the approach of choice with regard to the general public, and specialty hospitals have attempted to maintain high visibility within their communities. National chains often conducted national advertising campaigns supplemented by more customized advertising in the local community. Many of these hospitals employed sales forces that called on potential referrers of psychiatric or substance abuse patients. PR approaches, including open houses and dissemination of feature stories, have also been common. As with other facilities, a compelling Internet site has become de rigueur for specialty hospitals.

The marketing approach employed by nursing homes has been somewhat different from that of other inpatient facilities. The target for nursing home services is much more limited than that for general hospital services, and the marketing has been less visible and more low key. Nursing homes do not need the volume of patients other facilities require because of their patients' long stays. Because someone other than the patient may be involved in the admission decision, nursing homes must consider both prospective patients and their caregivers. They tend to emphasize advertising as a means of remaining top of mind and, where appropriate, maintaining relationships with referral agencies. Word of mouth is an important means of promoting nursing homes (see Box 5.2).

Assisted-living facilities are more like nursing homes than hospitals in their approaches to the market. They do not require a large volume of patients but rather a small number of qualified prospects. Someone other than the residents may be involved in the decision to enter an assisted-living facility, so marketing must be geared to both potential residents and their caregivers. While few nursing homes are being built, assisted-living facilities in their various forms continue to spring up around the country. Marketing research plays an important role in the siting of assisted-living facilities and in the development of subsequent marketing programs. Print and electronic advertising is important, as is ongoing positive publicity. Like nursing homes, word-of-mouth endorsement is important for assisted-living facilities.

Box 5.2:
Nursing Home
Marketing:
What Are
Customers
Looking For?

Customers for nursing home services include not only residents but also third-party payers, employees, doctors and hospitals as well as caregivers. In this era of the "graying of America," with an enormous potential market for senior services of all sorts, keeping current nursing home customers satisfied is vital for establishing positive word of mouth. It also is vital for nursing homes to recognize family and friends as customers who may generate a large proportion of the word-of- mouth notoriety—either positive or negative. Because both the resident and these proxies may be considered customers for nursing home services, it is important to understand the needs and evaluations of both groups. Meeting the needs of the resident is the mission of the organization; meeting the needs of their relatives may ensure that the business continues to get referrals.

Data obtained from 2,709 residents living in 26 different nursing homes across the nation provide some insights into these marketing issues. Some 71 percent of the residents in this study were women; the average age of men was 75, whereas the average age of women was 80. Many of the residents were relatively new to their facility—43 percent of the men had lived in the facility for less than one month, compared to 30 percent of the women. Furthermore, 21 percent of the female residents had been in the facility for more than three years, whereas only 12 percent of the male residents had been there that long. The reported health status of the residents (as measured on a five-point scale anchored by "very poor" and "very good") did not vary by gender. Fifty-six percent of the residents were identified as having less than good health (fair, poor, or very poor ratings).

Survey administrators found that only 31 percent of the questionnaires were completed by the resident. The others were completed by a spouse (12 percent), friend (3 percent), family member other than the spouse (40 percent), legal guardian (4 percent), or some other person (10 percent); completion of a questionnaire by a proxy was strongly associated with the health of the resident. The questionnaire covered 39 service issues related to the nursing home experience. It also contained a question to assess "positive word of mouth," which was operationalized as the "likelihood of your recommending the (facility) to others."

Respondents reported that the nursing homes did well in the areas of courtesy and friendliness but not as well with noise, food, and responsiveness. Fortunately for the facilities the individual items with the lowest scores are not among those with the highest correlation to likelihood to recommend. The single items with the highest correlation with a recommendation dealt with being treated with respect and dignity, technical skill of nurses, nurses' explanations of care, and friendliness of nurses—domains in which nursing facilities tended to score relatively well. Less closely related with propensity to recommend were noise level and quality of the laundry service. The service variables with the lowest scores were noise level in and around the room, followed by variety of food selections and quality of the food. The highest marks were given to courtesy of the admitting staff, friendliness of nurses, and courtesy of the housekeeping staff.

When the relative score and the relative correlation are compared using a priority index, the issues that need the greatest attention are those dealing with services provided by the aides (e.g., information from aides, assistance with meals, aides' response to the call button). Among the service domains identified through the factor analysis, scores were highest for the admission and nursing domains but lower for meals, room, and aides. Interestingly, however, ratings differed depending on who was doing the rating. For example, residents were more positive about the aides and the facility than were family and friends. In fact, when the overall satisfaction scores are compared for each type of respondent, the residents gave the highest scores. Friends, family, and guardians generated lower scores than residents, although the difference in scores between residents and other respondents was significant only in the case of friends. It is interesting to note, however, that the likelihood of recommending a nursing home was higher among family members than among residents and was significantly higher than the ratings given by friends.

The relationships between the eight service domains and "likelihood to recommend the facility" are reflected in standardized beta coefficients obtained from regressions done for each type of respondent. The most consistently related service domain was nursing. The experiences with dining and aides also were important predictors of recommendations. Admission issues, not surprisingly, influenced recommendations by the family and resident but not other respondents. Finance issues, similarly, were strongly related to recommendations only for the residents and their legal guardians. Taken together the service domains explained about 60 percent of the variation in likelihood to recommend.

When the residents responded, they tended to give higher ratings than did proxies. This difference may reflect some acquiescence bias from residents who are reluctant to criticize staff or service-delivery processes on which they continue to depend. Again, consistent with that concern, family members' responses, compared to those of residents, were particularly critical of the aides and housekeeping.

On the other hand, some of the differences in score may stem from anxiety or guilt associated with placing a loved one in a nursing home. The family member may believe that "Father should be treated the way family would treat him" or that "The aides aren't giving Mom all of the attention she deserves." Clearly, quality of care has many components, of which patient and family assessments represent just one element. Nevertheless, these ratings can help the organization identify the perceived strengths and weaknesses in service delivery and make corrective action to both meet customer needs and manage word of mouth in the community.

The difficulty in identifying the customer for nursing home services creates special challenges in determining and meeting customer requirements. Should the facility operate with an eye to the ratings of the residents or those of the family?

One could argue that whoever responds to the questionnaire is the customer. Some facilities with a relatively healthy patient base must manage to the residents' expectations, as these residents will complete questionnaires of this sort and are capable of offering word-of-mouth exposure. Other facilities that treat patients whose health is poor or whose mental state precludes them from completing a questionnaire must manage to the expectations of some proxy.

Nursing homes would be wise to collect data from all the identified customers—patient or family—and make efforts to satisfy each. By directly polling the family member, nursing homes may be able to get a better response rate from the healthy residents whose questionnaires would not otherwise be completed by the family. The net result is not only more data from other consumers but potentially more data from the healthy residents whose voices previously have been lost to the proxy.

Irrespective of customer segment, the data suggest that nursing homes can maintain positive word of mouth by ensuring that nursing, aide service, and dining needs are met. Because the scores for nursing already are relatively high, the greatest opportunity appears to rest in improving scores for the aides and food. The pressure on the nursing home industry is just starting to heat up. The baby boom generation is approaching retirement age; it is time to get the service right before the market explodes.

Source: Becker, B. W., and D. O. Kaldenberg. 2000. "Factors Influencing the Recommendation of Nursing Homes." *Marketing Health Services* 20 (4): 22–28.

Residential treatment centers have historically operated in a manner similar to specialty hospitals when it comes to marketing. They tend to focus on advertisements for the general public and relationship building for potential referral agents. They often employ sales forces and may be very aggressive in seeking out prospective customers.

Taken as a group, inpatient facilities have historically employed PR, advertising, and community outreach as their primary marketing tools. Many have used direct sales. More recently, more contemporary approaches such as customer relationship marketing, database marketing, and Internet marketing have become common. The trend among health facilities, especially hospitals, has been toward more relationship development and more sophisticated information technology (IT)–oriented approaches. However, a reaction of sorts has resulted in a turn toward a more low-cost/high-exposure type of marketing (see Case Study 5.1).

Marketing by healthcare providers is influenced by some peculiar characteristics of the healthcare industry. Chief among these is the referral relationship. Hospitals do not generally attract patients directly but must depend on their medical staff to refer patients for admission. Similarly, many medical specialists do not accept patients directly but rely on referrals from primary care physicians and other specialists. Given that most patients are not going to walk into a specialist's office off the street, advertising to the end user has limited value for many medical practices.

Marketing activities among healthcare providers are also constrained by ethical and regulatory considerations. For the most part it is inappropriate for healthcare providers to offer the incentives to potential sources of business normally offered in other industries. For example, incentives that hospitals may offer physicians to encourage them to admit patients to their facility (either inappropriately or in lieu of a competitor) are either unethical or illegal.

Clinicians have for the most part lagged behind hospitals and other healthcare organizations in their marketing efforts. Many physicians did not face the same competitive situations that hospitals began facing in the 1980s. In addition, ethical constraints limited the amount of advertising that was acceptable for physicians. Individual physicians and professional medical associations were overtly hostile to what they thought of as marketing.

Most physicians have long engaged in various forms of marketing to promote their practices, although most were loath to advertise. However, increasing numbers of physicians and physician practices are using advertising to gain visibility and attract patients. These are often specialty groups trying to distinguish themselves from other specialists in their field. More often, physicians involved heavily in advertising are those who offer elective procedures. Thus, ophthalmic surgeons performing laser eye surgery and cosmetic surgeons are more likely to advertise their services directly to consumers than are specialists offering more traditional services. Because these services are typically not covered by insurance, these practitioners depend less on referrals from colleagues and more on direct solicitation of potential customers.

Physicians have historically been involved in networking (both formal and informal) and relationship development. More recently some have ventured into advertising, although many of the hard-sell advertisements have been initiated by physicians involved in the more retail or elective aspects of healthcare, and some practices use billboards for promotional purposes. Physicians may use direct mail to reach selected audiences or announce changes in the practice, and they are increasingly using the Internet as a means of promoting the practice and maintaining contact with their patients. In some markets larger groups are using managed care and health plan contracting as a means of market development.

The level of marketing and the approach used by other clinicians vary from profession to profession and market to market. Independent practitioners such as dentists, podiatrists, and chiropractors may use low-key advertising to attract patients and maintain their visibility. They may also rely on referral relationships in some cases. Direct mail may be occasionally used to contact prospects directly, but Internet marketing has not become widespread among these providers.

Various types of alternative therapists employ a wide range of marketing techniques. Many advertise for their services, often targeting select populations thought to be better prospects. An outreach approach is often important for alternative therapists in that they may have to educate the public concerning their forms of therapy.

Certain types of health programs face unique challenges when it comes to marketing their services. Behavioral health programs designed for psychiatric or substance abuse patients have to display a certain sensitivity to their prospective patients. Advertising for such programs tends to be subtler than for some other programs, and particular care has to be taken in formulating the message conveyed. Much of the marketing related to these types of programs, especially for private-pay patients, is carried out via behind-the-scenes relationship building.

The marketing approach for services such as HIV/AIDS programs is particularly problematic, and challenges exist on a number of fronts. For various reasons affected individuals may be difficult to identify and contact. There may be resistance to receiving unwanted information and concerns about confidentiality related to such a controversial condition. AIDS service agencies need to attract the attention of those in need of services without attracting undue attention to their organizations.

Some public health activities relate to the public health infrastructure or to health and safety issues that do not directly involve healthcare consumers. Thus, activities aimed at maintaining clear air and water and ensuring a safe food supply typically involve activities unrelated to healthcare consumers.

On the other hand, public health agencies deal with a range of issues that do involve interface with the public. Some activities, such as child immunizations and nutritional counseling, may be noncontroversial and promoted through traditional information and referral channels and word of mouth. Other, more controversial programs, such as those dealing with family planning, teen pregnancy, sexually transmitted diseases, and HIV/AIDS, require both more aggressive and more sensitive approaches. Many public health agencies also provide basic patient care services, and these programs must be promoted as well.

Public health agencies have relied on information and referral approaches and standard PR approaches in the past to publicize their services. They have also made use of community outreach programs to promote their services. However, given the increasing significance of certain problems considered to be in the public health domain, such agencies have become much more aggressive in terms of marketing. A variety of social marketing initiatives have been launched, many coordinated by the Centers for Disease Control and Prevention or some other federal agency. Initiatives aimed at sexually transmitted diseases, HIV/AIDS, and tuberculosis, as well as nonclinical programs such as nutritional counseling and family planning, have begun to use social marketing approaches. Various forms of health communication have been added to the stable of marketing approaches for public health agencies.

Healthcare Suppliers

This component of the healthcare industry includes a wide range of organizations that supply a myriad of goods and equipment. Healthcare organizations use an extensive range of supplies, from office supplies (e.g., computer forms) to cloth products (e.g., uniforms, linens) to disposables (e.g., gloves, syringes). Indeed, a large physician practice may have a vendor list of dozens of suppliers, and a hospital may have a list of hundreds.

Healthcare organizations also use a wide range of equipment and deal with a variety of vendors for these products. The equipment used includes a variety of standard office machines as well as equipment related to clinical activities, including sterilizers, blood pressure cuffs, stethoscopes, x-ray machines and other imaging equipment, monitors of various types, and laboratory equipment. They also use a considerable amount of durable medical equipment, including examination tables, hospital beds, wheelchairs, and other items used for extended periods. (IT is addressed below.)

Supplies and equipment may be obtained directly from producers, but more often they are obtained from distributors who handle a range of supplies or equipment. In either case, supply and equipment vendors are likely to use trade advertising aimed at business customers through publications targeted to hospitals, physicians, or some other type of facility or personnel. They also use sales representatives who employ direct sales approaches to facilities and health professionals. Supply and equipment vendors also use sales promotion in the form of appearances at professional meetings and exhibitions, where representatives of health facilities and health professionals are likely to be in attendance.

Unlike the patient care side of healthcare, organizations marketing medical supplies, biomedical equipment, and durable medical equipment can operate in much the same manner as their corollary organizations in other industries. Perhaps the primary difference is related to the logistics involved in being able to get in front of a physician or the right person at a hospital to make a presentation. The decision makers in other industries are often much more clearly identified and available.

The types of marketing generally used by healthcare suppliers include direct sales, business-to-business marketing, advertising, and sales promotion. Suppliers are increasingly using the Internet for online marketing and promotions.

Consumer-Product Companies

While marketing on the part of healthcare providers is still evolving, the marketing of consumer goods in healthcare is a well-established phenomenon. Consumer-health products have long been marketed to the U.S. public, and arguably some of the best known among the early consumer brands were associated with health-related products. Brand names like Bayer, Johnson & Johnson, and Ex-Lax were household terms long before the emergence of the modern healthcare system in the United States.

Today, pharmacy shelves are filled with consumer-health products. Every household is supplied with headache remedies, cold medicine, Band-Aids, heating pads, and a variety of other products used for personal health needs. Feminine hygiene products and goods for baby care are likely to be common. These household inventories may also include products for foot care, dental care, and eye care. Recent advances in home diagnosis and treatment abilities have added new lines of products and equipment to the options available to the household. (Over-the-counter drugs will also be discussed below.)

The traditional over-the-counter medical remedies and personal health products have been supplemented by a wide range of nutritional products as well as a growing plethora of cosmeceuticals and nutriceuticals (see Box 5.3). There has been an explosion of products that bridge the gap between cosmetics and drugs and that promise younger skin or hair regrowth. Products that combine nutritional benefits with medicinal benefits are now common.

Another factor in the rapid growth of personal health products has been the emergence of alternative therapies as a preference for many U.S. healthcare consumers. A variety of "natural" products have entered the market as alternatives for or supplements to more conventional health products or treatments. The increasing interest on the part of the U.S. consumer in alternative medicine and holistic health has fueled the growth of a major industry in alternative therapies.

The market for consumer-health products continues to grow dramatically as the U.S. population continues to become more health conscious, new products are developed, and a do-it-yourself attitude becomes more pervasive among healthcare consumers. The variety of products and level of competition ensure the continued high level of marketing among producers of consumer-health products.

Box 5.3: Marketing Vanity Products: The Case of Cosmeceuticals

One of the growing retail markets in healthcare involves *cosmeceuticals*, the term used by the cosmetic industry to refer to cosmetic products that have medicinal or drug-like benefits. The term was coined by Albert Kligman, the University of Pennsylvania researcher credited with discovering the effectiveness of Retin-A, a form of vitamin A, in smoothing aging skin. Cosmeceutical products bridge the gap between cosmetic products that simply cleanse and beautify and pharmaceuticals that cure and heal. Generally, cosmeceuticals are products sold over the counter that provide a health benefit in addition to traditional cosmetic qualities. Healthy growth in the cosmeceuticals market worldwide is primarily attributed to the aging baby boomer generation in the United States and an increase in disposable income in Asia and South America.

The Food, Drug, and Cosmetic Act defines drugs as those products that cure, treat, mitigate, or prevent disease or that affect the structure or function of the human body. While drugs are subject to a review-and-approval process by the FDA, cosmetics are not approved by the FDA prior to sale. If a product has drug properties, it must be approved as a drug.

The explosion in popularity of products formulated with cosmeceuticals has been driving growth in the global skin-care market since the late 1980s. Products with visible antiaging effects continue to be extremely popular across categories in skin care. The cosmeceuticals market, including skin-, hair-, and sun-care products, is highly diversified, with products coming from both major manufacturers and small, local companies around the world.

Cosmeceutical products are marketed by mass-market and direct-marketing retailers as well as prestige retailers, including increasingly popular spas, plastic surgeons, and dermatologists. The cosmeceutical consumer is becoming more sophisticated, demanding exceptional qualities from these products, and technological innovations will have to keep up with this demand. As the nutrition and natural personal-care industries have grown and evolved throughout the last decade, they have taken on new definitions to bridge the gap between pharmaceuticals and cosmetics.

When the FDA created the Food, Drug, and Cosmetic Act in 1939, it defined cosmetics and drugs separately. By 1998, as both industries continued to cross over their defined lines and the barrier between the two blurred, the industry was forced to create a new definition—cosmeceuticals. The definition initially included only skin-care products that claimed therapeutic benefits through the inclusion of alpha hydroxy acids; beta hydroxy acids; or vitamins A, C, and E. Just as the cosmetics industry continued to evolve and transcend its original boundaries, so too has the cosmeceuticals industry. It has now come to mean much more: functional cosmetic products that produce physiological changes in appearance, feature improvement of function, and offer specific therapeutic benefits for skin and hair.

Depending on the definition, the size of the total health-and-beauty category can range from $25.2 billion to $52.9 billion. From a global perspective the natural personal-care and cosmeceutical markets are reaching in excess of $13 billion, with growth in the United States and Europe exceeding all other areas of the global marketplace. The United States saw growth of 17 percent to 20 percent, and Europe experienced slightly lower growth at about 15 percent to 17 percent.

With largely premium-priced items in the cosmeceutical segment—even products from mainstream companies, not just department store counters—the attraction for marketers is easily understood. With no regulation on how much of an ingredient is needed to create the desired effect, many manufacturers include only trace amounts of an expensive ingredient. Even those companies that are truthful to their claims are receiving huge price premiums for their products. Consumers have had to carefully wade through the profusion of new product introductions, trying to determine which ones deliver the promised benefit.

Even so, consumers have yet to understand the difference between the cosmetics market and the cosmeceutical market. Consumers see only an abundance of new products that offer added benefits being put on their neighborhood shelves. However, the fact that they are being drawn to these new products is a result of the changing consumer attitude. A growing focus on wellness and the connection between health and diet coupled with the availability of information are leading consumers to make more educated choices. Cosmeceutical and natural personal-care companies are also educating consumers about what to avoid, including such ingredients as imidazolidinyl urea and diazolidinyl urea (preservatives), methyl/propyl/butyl/ethyl parabens (microbial inhibitors), stearalkonium chloride, triethanolamine, and synthetic colors and fragrances. Demographics are also a factor. The pool of aging women, as well as ethnic and affluent consumers, is growing and driving demand for products that promise real results. Not only are they in need of such products, but they can afford to pay a premium. For example, the aging woman offers both skin-care and hair-care companies the ideal consumer. Antiaging creams have been the hot new products introduced by nearly every cosmetic company, and many manufacturers now offer shampoos that promise to thicken thinning hair.

Both women and men are enjoying the benefits of these new products. Interestingly, according to Datamonitor, men are typically more brand loyal, less price sensitive, and increasingly self-indulgent, making them a high-priority target for cosmeceutical manufacturers. Still, cosmeceuticals represent only about 6 percent to 7 percent of the entire

These products tend to be marketed in a similar manner to other types of consumer products. Producers of personal health products heavily employ media advertising (both print and electronic), along with advertising inserts, to promote their products. They also employ sales promotion techniques such as discount coupons, rebates, and contests. Marketers of

health-and-beauty industry. Whether they have become dedicated cosmeceutical consumers or not, one thing is clear to consumers: Something has changed—cosmetics are no longer made up of ingredients that they cannot pronounce or read and instead include familiar plants and ingredients they have been told to consume for centuries, like soy, zinc, or antioxidants.

Marketers are constantly blurring the boundaries of the cosmeceutical market for the consumer by leveraging this connection with food. They are stretching the definition of cosmetics to include an angle of nutrition. For instance, ads by companies like Unilever, which markets the soap product Dove, are stretching the line between food nutrition bars and cosmetic nutrition bars. In ads the company calls its soap bar a "nutrition bar" that includes a combination of ingredients it calls Nutrium skin nourishment. Most cosmeceutical products leverage the benefits of ingredients most commonly found in our food, leaving many consumers to wonder about the connection.

Other companies are staying away from the term *cosmeceutical* and are choosing to use the term *natural* as a marketing tool to draw attention. Marketers will continue to leverage the term natural when it affects purchasing behavior. Consumers generally believe their self-esteem can be enhanced through improved physical condition and personal appearance, so brands have used "natural" and "bonus benefits" to appeal to that belief.

Although these types of high-quality products were once reserved for department store cosmetic counters, the tides have changed. Large mainstream players are tweaking their products to fit into the high-growth cosmeceutical market. One reason these players are breaking down the walls between cosmetics and drugs is that they have the financial resources to conduct studies to prove the positive effects of their products. Those leading the pack in the mainstream channel are Nivea, with its leg-firming and CoQ10 creams, and Neutrogena, with its copper-containing eye-firming creams. Companies like Procter & Gamble, Johnson & Johnson, and Revlon are together spending nearly $100 million on a flurry of antiaging products.

The cosmeceutical industry, like the nutraceutical industry, no longer fits within the boundaries of its original definition. It has outgrown itself. Society is evolving, and soon creams with vitamin E or aloe will become market standard, just as orange juice with calcium has become the standard in the food market. Such products will no longer require the differentiating label that cosmeceutical implies. Industry insiders hurry to label new product categories, spurred by sizing up the market and comparing growth trends, but from the eyes of the consumer this is merely the evolution of an industry.

personal health products also emphasize in-store advertising, and highly visible shelf space is pursued.

Perhaps the most important development in the marketing of these products has been the emergence of the Internet as a new marketplace. While mainstream brands typically use traditional retail marketing approaches, producers of marginal products and newcomers to the market have latched onto the Internet as their primary channel for distribution. To a certain extent, many of these products are shut out of the mainstream market (e.g., because of lack of access to retail shelf space); at the same time, these products often cater to a market that is innovative and prefers to take advantage of the Internet for accessing goods and services.

Pharmaceutical Companies

The manufacturing of pharmaceuticals in the United States is an enormous and highly profitable industry. Sales of prescription drugs in 2002 approximated $140 billion. Profits often reach 15 percent or more of sales, an extraordinarily high figure. Despite the huge potential profits, the drug industry is highly risky and competitive. Research and development costs average more than 20 percent of revenue, the highest share of any U.S. industry. After approval a new drug often faces stiff competition from numerous similar drugs already on the market. As a result, no single corporation holds a substantial share of the market.

Over the past 25 years prescription drug use has grown significantly as the increased availability of better and cost-effective medicines has changed healthcare practice to address prevention and treatment with pharmaceuticals. Patients today spend less time in the hospital and more time at the prescription counter. As a result U.S. healthcare expenditures, including expenditures on prescription drugs, are rising, with drug expenditures increasing 16.9 percent from 2000 to 2001.

Because of the competitive nature of the industry and the pressure to recoup investments in research and development, the drug industry has developed sophisticated, aggressive, and expensive marketing strategies. More than $12.7 billion per year was spent on pharmaceutical marketing in 1998. Marketing expenditures account for 20 percent or more of sales.

Print advertisements in medical publications are the oldest and best-established form of drug marketing. Despite a decrease of 30 percent in the early 1990s, spending on print advertisements is still substantial. Since the 1960s drug advertisements that make any mention of the drug's uses or effectiveness have had to contain information on contraindications, side effects, and interactions with other drugs. In addition, the Food and Drug Administration (FDA), which regulates drug advertisements, requires that they not be "false or misleading," mention only approved uses of the drug, and present a "fair balance" between beneficial and detrimental effects.

As the volume of published medical information has mushroomed, drug companies have provided doctors with alternatives to tedious forays into the medical literature. By acting as intermediary in providing information to doctors, drug companies save time and expense for the doctors while maintaining some control over what they see and hear. These services have historically taken print form but are increasingly being produced in television format or disseminated via the Internet.

Continuing medical education (CME) is one area of medical communication that is massively subsidized by the drug industry. In the late 1970s regulations that required physicians to obtain a minimum amount of accredited training each year to maintain their hospital privileges and some categories of professional certification were established. CME conferences, thousands of which are held each year, grew out of these requirements. In exchange for financial support for CME meetings drug companies are often given the privilege of selecting speakers and sending representatives to the meetings to promote their products. A majority of CME courses now have industry support; much of the continuing professional education is largely paid for by the drug companies, and they select expert speakers with predictably favorable views on their products.

Field representatives are a crucial link in the information chain between clinicians and drug companies. More than 30,000 pharmaceutical company representatives or detailers—one for every 15 U.S. doctors—make tens of millions visits to doctors' office annually. Drug representatives dispense promotional brochures, medical literature, and verbal information about their products as well as free samples.

Gifts to physicians were a cornerstone of pharmaceutical marketing for many years. The most abundant category of gifts includes reminder items, such as pens or pads of paper, that prominently display the name of a drug. Gifts are often offered to physicians in exchange for attention to promotional material or presentations. Drug lunches in large hospitals and clinics are an example, with pizza or sandwiches provided to an audience, often medical students and junior physicians, who hear a sales presentation from a pharmaceutical company representative while they eat. Pharmaceutical companies also sponsor dinner meetings that feature speakers who promote the company's products. The doctors in attendance are typically paid $100 to $200 honoraria for their time. Exorbitant gifts and cash payments of any amount were banned by the American Medical Association in 1990 and have been replaced in many cases with gifts of medical textbooks or instruments of comparable value.

Current trends in the healthcare system are changing the way prescription drugs are chosen, and marketing techniques have rapidly adapted to the new environment. The growth of managed care in the United States has had a profound effect on drug prescribing, mostly through the growing role of formularies. A *formulary* is a healthcare organization's list of allowed medications and usually includes a limited number of drugs in any given therapeutic class.

Managed care organizations account for an increasing share of drug sales. The managers of both private and public health plans are now, through formulary decisions, in a position to control billions of dollars of drug purchases a year. Health professionals are no longer their customers, replaced by those who pay for healthcare. One unique aspect of this change is the opportunity it presents for drug companies to obtain a market for otherwise uncompetitive drugs.

Another growing target for drug company marketing is pharmacists, who are increasingly induced to convince both doctors and patients to change medications. At least one pharmaceutical company was criticized in recent years for offering cash payments to pharmacists for each patient they managed to switch.

During the late 1970s and 1980s the relatively small industry of mail-order pharmacy houses grew dramatically, fueled by the greater pharmaceutical needs of an aging population and the cost advantages these discount businesses provided. Because they offer drugs at lower cost than many retail pharmacies, these companies have obtained exclusive contracts to supply prescriptions for many managed care organizations. Because they provide an opportunity to influence which drugs are used by millions of people, they have become targets for acquisition by drug companies. By controlling the mail-order pharmacies a pharmaceutical company can influence prescribing patterns.

The major development of the end of the twentieth century was the emergence of direct-to-consumer marketing on behalf of the pharmaceutical industry. Direct-to-consumer advertising helps prompt treatment of more patients for previously untreated conditions and improve patient compliance with physician-prescribed treatment.

An additional wrinkle has been added to pharmaceutical marketing in the past few years with the introduction of a growing number of generic drugs. These unbranded drugs are comparable to the highly advertised brands (although not identical) and sell for a much lower price. Pharmacies can reduce prescription drug costs substantially through the substitution of generics. Pharmacists who counsel and educate patients at the point of care are primarily responsible for this phenomenon.

Over-the-counter drugs are marketed in a manner similar to other consumer-health products, but they often have the power of pharmaceutical marketing behind them. Growth in the sales of over-the-counter drugs has been boosted by the introduction of a wide range of alternative therapies and natural products that may not face the same advertising restrictions as pharmaceuticals.

Health Insurance Companies

Health insurance companies were among the earliest of healthcare organizations to use marketing techniques. In the early days of health insurance, policies were generally sold to individuals or families, and health insurance plans were marketed in the same manner as other types of insurance. Health plans advertised their programs and through their agents used direct sales to promote the company's plans. Because health insurance was a somewhat novel phenomenon until the 1960s, the marketing approach often involved educating the prospect.

By the 1960s, health insurance was predominantly sold in wholesale fashion through employers on behalf of their employees. Group plans came to be the norm, and individual policies became less common. The spread and entrenchment of employer-based insurance was abetted by a substantially unionized workforce for whom health benefits became an almost inalienable right. While insurance companies might advertise group plans (e.g., through print and electronic media or billboards), they were primarily sold through sales representatives who called on benefits managers. Exhibitions by insurance plans at trade shows are also vehicles for exposing potential purchasers of group plans to insurance programs.

The major development in health insurance during the last quarter of the twentieth century was the emergence of alternative forms of financing healthcare coverage to compete with traditional indemnity insurance. During the 1970s, health maintenance organizations emerged as a form of prepaid insurance that minimized the fee-for-service aspect of reimbursement.

Although a certain level of competition had always existed among health plans, the competition for enrollees was typically low key. The emergence of managed care resulted in much more intense competition for clients as managed care plans competed with existing indemnity plans and with each other. The marketing of managed care plans involved the approaches used for both group and individual plans. Legislation that required employers to offer their employees an option of managed care had been passed. This meant that employees were likely to have a choice of two or more plans at their work sites. Thus, the first task of managed care marketers was to convince employers to offer their plans to employees. Subsequently, marketers had to encourage employees to choose their plan over any others offered. This encouraged managed care plans to offer special benefits to encourage enrollment and retain employees once they were enrolled.

During the late 1990s managed care enrollment leveled off, with at least half of the insured enrolled in some type of managed care plan. This decade also saw the emergence of the *defined contributions* approach to health insurance benefits. Traditional insurance and managed care plans alike offered *defined benefits*—that is, the provisions of the plan were established a priori and all enrollees received the same benefits regardless of their circumstances or preferences. Under the defined contributions approach employees are given credit for a certain amount of insurance resources and can disburse these funds in the manner they see fit by choosing options from a menu of benefits. This added a new wrinkle to marketing, as plans could now be customized for individual enrollees. The standardized approach to benefits that had become common gave way to a tailored approach. This development was aided by the Internet, as health plans offered access to information on benefits via the World Wide Web.

By the end of the 1990s the conventional approach to group insurance began losing ground for various reasons. A growing number of employers no longer offered insurance as a benefit, and many others cut back their coverage. A growing number of Americans were becoming uninsured, and they were no longer strictly marginal participants in the economy but increasingly working-class and middle-class individuals who did not have access to group insurance. This led to a revival of the individual insurance policy, a development that has been greatly aided by Internet marketing and distribution. Insurers are offering health plans via the Internet and advertising them through print and electronic media. By virtue of being national plans they can enroll millions of individuals, thereby creating a viable pool of enrollees.

One other aspect of health insurance marketing that should be noted involves government-sponsored insurance programs. Medicare and Medicaid are entitlement programs with respective criteria for enrollment. As a rule no competition for such enrollees exists, as seniors are automatically enrolled in Medicare when they reach the specified age and Medicaid enrollees are signed up by their respective states. Social marketing campaigns have been initiated to ensure that eligible individuals know about these programs and the services they offer. This has been particularly the case with supplemental insurance programs, such as those for children, that are new and require promotion to those who can benefit from them.

During the 1990s managed care options were offered to Medicare beneficiaries and, to a lesser extent, Medicaid enrollees. Although the enrollees would remain part of a group plan, they were essentially solicited as individuals. Thus, insurers offering managed care plans to seniors had to aggressively market their option to encourage seniors to switch to these new programs. In many states several Medicare managed care plans may have been competing for senior citizens, and in certain states Medicaid managed care plans competed for enrollees within that population. Organizations promoting Medicare or Medicaid managed care plans used a wide range of marketing techniques, including advertising, publicity (e.g., sponsorship of events), community outreach, direct mail, telemarketing, direct sales, and Internet marketing.

Support-Services Vendors

Much of the growth in the size of the healthcare workforce has occurred among organizations providing support services to healthcare organizations. While hospitals and other facilities may provide for many types of support services in-house, there have always been services that are not appropriate for internal management. Since the 1980s healthcare organizations have increasingly outsourced many services to other organizations. Physicians and other clinicians have many of the same needs as health facilities, and much of the practice's time is spent in dealing with external service providers.

Among the support services required by hospitals are transcription, billing and collections, utilization review, recruitment and staffing, hazardous waste disposal, laboratory services, and IT. IT services have become particularly important as healthcare has become increasingly technology dependent.

Many of these services are unique to healthcare and do not have corollaries in other industries. These services are typically marketed via direct sales, with sales representatives soliciting business from the healthcare organizations. Vendors may also advertise in print or electronic media and often sponsor community events. Direct mail may also be used to maintain visibility for the vendor. The Internet has increasingly become a vehicle for the marketing of support services. (Physicians are particularly difficult to market support services to. Box 5.4 reviews the challenges involved in selling IT to physicians.)

Stages of Healthcare Marketing

Discounting the more retail aspects of healthcare, a review of the evolution of marketing among healthcare provider organizations is worthwhile. These are the organizations that come to mind when we think of healthcare, and these are the organizations with which most consumers are likely to interface.

The role of marketing within provider organizations has evolved through a number of stages, which have occurred for different organizations at different times, and the progression has not been at all smooth. Indeed, some backsliding has occurred. Nevertheless, certain stages in the evolutionary process can be identified.

Physicians represent a major market for a variety of goods and services, and anyone who has tried to market to physician practices realizes what a challenge it presents. The challenge is particularly great when a vendor is seeking to market IT to a medical practice. Research continues to indicate that physicians (and healthcare in general) are well behind the curve in applying IT to their practices, and a number of factors have contributed to slow adaptation of innovations in this area.

Despite their presumed scientific orientation and interest in advancing their practices, many physicians are reluctant to even consider new technology. Physicians tend to be risk averse in this regard and resistant to anything that requires a change in practice operations. Because they already feel sensory overload, the thought of a major new initiative is overwhelming for most of them. Furthermore, a surprising number of physicians, especially older ones, suffer from computer phobia. They did not grow up with computers; even if they concede the potential, they are aware of horror stories from other practices that had negative experiences with IT.

Physicians also typically take a hands-on approach to their patients—that is, they want to have their medical records in hand when addressing patient needs. The thought of interjecting a computer between doctor and patient is alien to many of them. There are also concerns over the confidentiality of electronic patient records; these concerns have only been heightened by recent enactment of HIPAA (Health Insurance Portability and Accountability Act) regulations. Physicians are also put off by the cost of IT, especially when they virtually never budget any funds for such expenditures. Even though most technology purchases could be financed on reasonable terms, the sticker shock experienced by physicians deters many from thoughtful pursuit of possible solutions.

Even if a physician is interested in new technology, physicians are deluged with marketing and promotional materials from a wide range of organizations that provide legitimate services to physician practices. They are also swamped with materials from any marketer who sees physicians as a prospect for their goods and services, most of which have nothing to do with healthcare but are seeking to tap into this presumed source of revenue. For this reason every physician's desk becomes piled with stacks of mail, faxes, and other documents, most of which are never opened, much less read. Many physicians use their nurses, administrative assistants, or front-office personnel as screening agents to eliminate all but the most important correspondence. As a result, physicians typically read only a fraction of the material sent to them.

Vendors of information systems will typically need to meet with physicians (or their designees) face to face and, if possible, present a demonstration of their software. Scheduling such a meeting represents a major hurdle in its own right for a variety of reasons. Most physicians are already swamped with the demands of their practices and must spend some of their spare time with pharmaceutical representatives, medical supplies salespersons, and other parties whose products are considered critical for practice operation. Scheduling additional appointments, especially those that may require an hour or more of time, is extremely difficult.

Even if a physician has expressed an interest in adopting new IT, most practices use gatekeepers to shield the physician from presumed unwanted intrusions. This gatekeeper is likely to be instructed to be selective in terms of who gains access to the physician. Not only are these gatekeepers usually zealous in shielding the physician from unwanted intrusions, they may also be threatened by the prospect of an innovation that transforms the practice's operations. Concerns for their future well-being cause many practice managers, for example, to deflect any initiatives that may threaten their position with the practice.

Ultimately, traditional marketing approaches do not work well with physicians when it comes to IT. Physicians are not likely to respond to direct mail, faxes, or any type of unsolicited promotional materials. They may have their awareness raised by articles in medical journals or other publications they consider legitimate. They may look to their specialty associations for guidance with regard to new products or services. They may also be willing to attend (or at least send a representative to) a workshop or conference on the technology, but any follow-up depends on the vendor's ability to get through to the physician for subsequent discussions.

Vendors may benefit from offering demonstrations of their products at professional meetings for physicians, practice managers, or other clinic personnel. Trade shows, conferences, and other meetings provide the opportunity for face-to-face interaction with physicians or their representatives. Although it is important to be sensitive to pricing considerations, marketing efforts should focus on the attributes, not the costs. They should also focus on the ease of installation and use, as these are likely to be important considerations for physicians adopting technology. The challenge of following up with prospects after the meeting remains, however.

Electronic means of communication are becoming more useful, and maintaining an informative web site is critical. Once a physician becomes interested in a form of technology, he or she is likely to want to find information right away, making easy electronic access essential.

Perhaps the only approach to marketing IT that invariably works with physicians is word-of-mouth promotions. For an initiative that promises to substantially change practice operations most physicians are followers, and they want a product to be given legitimacy by their colleagues before they express an interest. To the extent that a vendor is able to secure some installations of the application, it becomes possible to leverage these successes into additional physician contacts. Few physicians will commit to an initiative of this type unless it has been granted acceptance by their peers.

Source: David K. Rea, M.H.A., FACMPE, president, David Rea & Associates, Memphis, Tennessee.

Public Relations, Communications, and Government Relations

One of the ways to view this progression is in terms of the types of marketing approaches that have been used at various points in time. For most provider organizations this progression starts with PR. Even in the earliest days of modern healthcare, hospitals maintained PR staff and sought publicity in a manner accepted by the industry. The main purpose of PR was information dissemination and, when necessary, damage control.

Over time the PR function expanded to include communication and government-relations activities. The communications department advanced the cause of information dissemination by providing more detailed information on the organization's activities to employees, key constituents, and the general public. The government-relations function became necessary as provider organizations faced interaction with various regulatory agencies, federal funding agencies, and other governmental and quasigovernmental entities. The publicity function was expanded beyond information dissemination to include image development, referral development, and lobbying.

Advertising

Advertising was introduced in the 1980s, and the addition of this form of marketing represented a major shift in the approach taken by provider organizations. The low-key approach used by PR and communications staff was replaced by a much more aggressive approach to the market. While some of the same objectives were preserved from earlier approaches (e.g., information dissemination and image building), much of the advertising effort was aimed at attracting new business.

The acceptance of advertising was accompanied by an increase in sales-promotions activities. Providers participated in health fairs and community events and offered incentives for patients to use their services. As providers realized that many aspects of their businesses were retail in nature, sales promotions played an increasingly prominent role. The objective here was not only to attract the attention of prospective customers but also to provide incentives to encourage their business and ensure their continued loyalty.

Customized Approaches

These developments were accompanied by a realization that many of the relationships required by provider organizations were with other organizations. Business-to-business marketing became important, and provider organizations established sales forces to deal with employers, health plans, and other groups of purchasers. These corporate representatives used direct sales to take the provider's message to prospective clients. While the intent was the same as previous forms of marketing, this approach emphasized the wholesale nature of the business.

As the nature of healthcare changed and providers became more sophisticated at marketing, advertising became less important as new, often technology-oriented, approaches emerged. Database marketing was established to operate in conjunction with call centers, and customer relationship marketing programs were developed. While the intent was still to attract business, the effort was much more focused as hospitals ceased to be all things to all people. These approaches allowed the provider not only to micromanage the marketing effort but also to customize the approach for specific target audiences. The ability to cross-sell, up-sell, and induce repeat sales offered a significant advantage over standard advertising approaches. These approaches also ensured ongoing communication with customers and prospective customers and kept customers involved with the organization.

Internet Marketing

The most recent stage in the evolution of marketing on the part of provider organizations is Internet marketing. This development in itself reflects a number of stages. While initially serving an information-and-referral function, provider-sponsored web sites have evolved beyond an inventory of services to offer a range of interactive functions that encourage two-way communication between the provider and its customers. Not only does the Internet serve as a mechanism for attracting attention to the provider, but it also offers a means of keeping customers engaged once they become a part of the system.

Marketing's Intent

The process described above could also be looked at in terms of the intent of the marketing effort and the progression it followed. Early on, the intent of marketing on the part of provider organizations was to provide general information on the organization, report new developments, maintain visibility among the general public, and generally establish awareness of the organization and its services. This low-key, blanket approach to marketing was broad in nature. As marketing became more aggressive, the intent was to induce referrals to the organization's services and solicit customers from the general population. This process was much more specific in terms of its approach, message, and targets. Like the previous stage, however, this approach still involved one-way communication and provided no opportunities for formal feedback.

Through the development of customer databases, call centers, and web sites, healthcare marketing entered a new phase. These marketing tools offered opportunities for interaction and input on the part of customers. With the two-way communication these tools afforded, it became possible to develop relationships with existing or prospective customers. Web sites in particular became a draw for patients and other customers who were seeking general information or dealing with their own particular health conditions. The ability to schedule appointments, check on laboratory results, and interact with providers served to create a bond not afforded by other forms of marketing.

The intent of marketing shifted to relationship maintenance or management as the progression unfolded. With industry maturity and a situation of limited patient growth, it becomes important for providers to retain existing customers. The techniques to capture patients described above can also be used to retain them. Thus, an important function of web sites and other electronic communications is to hook the customer on the provider's services. When additional care is required, the provider hopes to benefit from a relationship that has already been established.

Marketing's Role

One other way of looking at this progression is in terms of the role played by marketing within the provider organization. In the early stages the activities directed toward marketing ends were not thought of as marketing. Indeed, the term itself was avoided by many provider organizations. As the need to market more aggressively developed, a more formal marketing function emerged. This typically began through an expansion of publicity and communication activities, with these tasks becoming more formal. As the need to advertise was realized, providers were likely to contract with consultants for marketing know-how and engage outside agencies to develop creative materials and purchase advertising space.

As marketing became more important, many providers established marketing departments. This may have begun with a single individual and developed over time to include a strong marketing staff. Marketing may have initially been subsumed under PR, planning, business development, or some other department but was eventually carved out as a stand-alone function. Marketing was accorded its own budget and figured increasingly prominently in the corporate organizational chart.

As provider organizations became more sophisticated at marketing, the marketing department took on an increasingly important role. Many organizations established a vice president for marketing or otherwise elevated the marketing staff within the organization. The movement of marketing from a function external to the organization to an internal one was an important development. Marketing was also redefined—from a necessary evil to an important contributor to the success of the organization, from an unnecessary expense to a direct contributor to the bottom line. Through all of this marketing personnel were being moved closer to the center of the organizational structure. The marketer was no longer called in after all of the decisions were made but now emerged as a major contributor to corporate decision making.

Summary

The incorporation of marketing as a corporate function on the part of healthcare organizations has occurred at different times and different rates for various healthcare organizations, and different organizations are at different stages in the marketing progression. For-profit commercial businesses in consumer or industrial settings have historically led the way in terms of formal marketing activities. Despite these applications of marketing techniques to healthcare, the primarily not-for-profit nature of the industry slowed the widespread acceptance of marketing.

While the scope and nature of healthcare marketing had broadened considerably by the mid-1980s, few marketing techniques could be applied unchanged by healthcare. Most healthcare organizations have multiple markets or customer types to whom they must be attentive. While a traditional business can focus on the prospective customers within the general population, healthcare organizations may have to consider physicians, nurses, patients, referral physicians, employee assistance personnel, managed care plans, and regulators. Novel approaches were required in the face of some of the unique attributes of the healthcare industry.

It is impossible to generalize about healthcare organizations when talking about marketing. The variety of organizations is endless; as a practical matter, distinctions must be made between the various types. Healthcare providers tend to sponsor the marketing efforts most geared to consumers and are the ones most recognized by the general public. Hospitals have accounted for the lion's share of health services marketing among providers, although many other types of healthcare organizations have made contributions.

Hospitals are perhaps the most visible of healthcare organizations, and their marketing activities in a particular market are likely to be significant. Specialty hospitals have been particularly active in marketing, and nursing homes, assisted living facilities, and other residential facilities face their own peculiar marketing challenges. Most physicians have long engaged in various forms of marketing to promote their practices, although most were loath to advertise. However, increasing numbers of physicians and physician practices are using advertising to gain visibility and attract patients.

Public health agencies promote activities—such as child immunizations and nutritional counseling—through traditional information and referral channels and word of mouth. Other, more controversial programs—such as those dealing with family planning, teen pregnancy, sexually transmitted diseases, and HIV/AIDS—require both more aggressive and more sensitive approaches.

Organizations marketing medical supplies, biomedical equipment, and durable medical equipment typically operate in much the same manner as their corollary organizations in other industries. Consumer-health products have long been marketed to the U.S. public, and arguably some of the best known among the early consumer brands were associated with health-related products. The pharmaceutical industry has developed sophisticated, aggressive, and expensive marketing strategies and spends more on marketing than any other component of healthcare.

Health insurance companies were among the earliest of healthcare organizations to use marketing techniques. In the early days of health insurance, policies were generally sold to individuals or families, and health insurance plans were marketed in the same manner as other types of insurance. By the 1960s health insurance was predominantly sold in wholesale fashion through employers on behalf of their employees. By the end of the 1990s the conventional approach to group insurance began losing ground for various reasons. This led to a revival of the individual insurance policy, a development that has been greatly aided by Internet marketing and distribution.

The role of marketing within provider organizations has evolved through a number of stages, which have occurred for different organizations at different times. This progression has carried the marketing in healthcare from its origins in public relations and communications to advertising and direct-marketing techniques to technology-based techniques—such as Internet marketing and customer relationship management—in use today.

As the field has evolved, the role of the marketer has shifted from that of an outside resource to full participation in the organization's decision-making process.

Discussion Questions

- What are some of the factors that account for the different rates at which healthcare organizations have adopted marketing techniques?
- What types of organizations were the fastest (and slowest) to adopt marketing?

- Why did healthcare organizations (particularly hospitals) emphasize advertising early in their marketing experience, and what lessons did they learn from an overdependence on advertising?
- How does the development and marketing of "cosmeceuticals" illustrate an attempt to identify and meet a felt need within the consumer population?
- How is the approach used by pharmaceutical companies in the sale of prescription drugs unique in healthcare?
- How would the approach of insurance companies selling to individuals differ from that for selling group plans to employers or other organizations?
- What types of marketing were initially adopted by healthcare organizations?
- What role is technology playing in the evolution of marketing in healthcare?
- Describe how the healthcare industry has transitioned from an emphasis on "the sale" to an emphasis on long-term relationships.

Reference

Kotler, P. 1975. *Marketing for Nonprofit Organizations*. Englewood Cliffs, NJ: Prentice Hall.

Additional Resources

Baum, N., and G. Henkel. 2000. *Marketing Your Clinical Practice*. Gaithersburg, MD: Aspen.

Joseph, S. R. 2000. *Marketing the Physician Practice*. Chicago: American Medical Association.

Rose, E. 2003. "Pharmaceutical Marketing in the United States: A Critical Analysis." [Online article; retrieved 10/30/03.] http://faculty.washington.edu/momus/pharm.htm.

Smith, M. C., E. M. Kolassa, G. Perkins, B. Siecker, and B. Highsmith Taylor (eds.). 2002. *Pharmaceutical Marketing: Principles, Environment, and Practice*. Binghampton, NY: Pharmaceutical Products Press.

5.1

LOW-INTENSITY MARKETING

L ike many other healthcare organizations Yale–New Haven Hospital (YNHH) is being asked to do more with less when it comes to marketing. Given its moderate advertising budget and the area's high media costs, YNHH had focused its advertising in the past on billboards, newspapers, and Yellow Pages. Radio, television, and magazines had proven to be too expensive. From 1995 to 1999 the bulk of YNHH's advertising dollars went into three-quarter-page newspaper display ads in daily newspapers across Connecticut. These ads were developed through a lengthy review process with a traditional advertising agency. The ads were only somewhat effective in increasing awareness because the limited budget prevented consistent exposure to the public.

In an effort to find a more effective yet inexpensive means of advertising, YNHH considered banner ads. Banner ads in newspapers are defined as small strip ads ranging from 2-3 inches tall and from 5-12 inches long. These are comparable to 15-second spots on television. Usually one topic is covered per ad, and artwork may or may not be included. Banner ads are designed to pop out through use of color and regular placement at the same spot in the newspaper. In newspapers they generally are run on a daily basis and placed at the top and bottom of the front page. The cost of the banner ad depends on the size and location. Most banner ads include a *call to action*. (YNHH also used television banner ads, but this discussion will focus on the newspaper variety.)

As an experiment in early 1999 a $\frac{1}{2}$ inch by 12-inch strip ad was placed at the bottom of the front page of the local newspaper twice a week. After monitoring the impact of the strips for a few months it became clear that there was no noticeable increase in calls to YNHH's call center for information or to find a physician. A meeting was scheduled with the local paper's sales executives, and the unfavorable results were shared. The newspaper was asked to find a better approach, or the hospital would cease running the strip ads. The paper came back with a novel approach that required discussions with and approval of the editorial side of the newspaper and a major redesign of the front page of the paper to develop space for a bigger ad at no additional cost.

YNHH expanded its banner-ad initiative in the fall of 2000; since then more than 350 newspaper ads have been developed. The largest number of ads promoted specific clinical programs, such as heart, cancer, maternity, and diabetes, as well as ongoing clinical trials. Other ads were call-center specific and promoted the physician-referral program, health information library, nurse advice line, and women's heart line. A third group of ads promoted consumer-oriented services such as web-based services, the baby press conference, and support groups. The final category of ads promoted general awareness of YNHH programs and announced special events such as Nurses Day.

Follow-up research indicated that the banner-ad campaign was highly successful. Between the fall of 2000 and 2002 consumer awareness of YNHH in the southern Connecticut market increased from 29 percent to 49 percent. The proportion of consumers associating YNHH with state-of-the-art care increased from 22 percent to 40 percent. Because the hospital's marketing budget had declined 30 percent between 2000 and 2002 and there had been no increases in other marketing activity, the bulk of the change in consumers' attitudes and behaviors was attributed to the banner ads. In addition, it was found that 49 percent of the calls routed to the call center were generated by the banner ads during this period, and a large portion of follow-up calls for other services were stimulated by the banner ads. There was also evidence that callers who found YNHH through the Yellow Pages were often encouraged to seek them out after seeing the banner ads.

Although banner ads are not a panacea for marketing challenges, they have been generally beneficial to YNHH. They have generated considerable inquiries and allowed the organization to spread its marketing budget much further than traditional advertising would have allowed. The volume of consumer interaction with the hospital has grown dramatically, and most of the increase in admissions during this period has been attributed to the campaign. Furthermore, the banner ad campaign has contributed substantially to the development of the YNHH customer database, with 40,000 names added since the ads began running.

There is little downside to the use of banner ads as the focal point of a marketing campaign. It is necessary, however, to have the capability to respond to responses and maintain a wide range of publications and other resource materials to make available in response to inquiries.

Source: Gombeski, W. R., J. Taylor, K. Krauss, and C. Medeiros. Forthcoming. "Cost Effective Advertising Through TG and Newspaper Banner Ads." *Health Marketing Quarterly* 20 (3): 37–54.

UNDERSTANDING HEALTHCARE MARKETS

All marketing initiatives begin with an effort to understand the market. In healthcare, this is a particular challenge given that the healthcare "market" is so different from that in any other industry. Defining customers, products, and marketing targets are all critical issues in healthcare and require an in-depth understanding of the industry and its customers. The bewildering combination of consumers, providers, and payers creates special challenges for the healthcare marketer.

An understanding of the unique characteristics of healthcare markets is necessary for the development of effective marketing initiatives. Marketers must appreciate who the "sellers," the "buyers," and the "middlemen" are and be able to identify the distribution channels for healthcare products and services. Furthermore, an understanding of consumer decision making and the sources of information that consumers use is important.

Chapter 6 describes the context within which healthcare marketing takes place. Marketing activities do not take place in a vacuum but emerge out of the sociocultural environment in which they reside. Societal factors influence the nature of marketing in general, and these same factors influence the role of marketing in healthcare. To understand the intersection between healthcare and marketing, it is necessary to understand the societal framework in which they exist.

Chapter 7 introduces the reader to the healthcare consumer and the factors that influence consumer behavior in the healthcare arena. All marketing starts with an understanding of the consumer for the marketed goods and services, and such an understanding is particularly important in healthcare because of the unique characteristics of healthcare consumers. Similarly, the decision-making process for the consumption of health services is different from that in other industries, and marketers must have an appreciation for the unique aspects of consumer behavior in healthcare.

Chapter 8 describes healthcare products—the ideas, goods, and services that the marketer markets. Health professionals are not accustomed to thinking in terms of "products," and marketers often face a significant challenge when conceptualizing the products that the healthcare organization is promoting. The unique characteristics of healthcare goods and services must be appreciated for successful marketing to occur.

Chapter 9 addresses the factors that contribute to the demand for health services and healthcare products and describes the manner in which demand is converted to "sales" (utilization). Demand can be measured in various ways, and a number of indicators of utilization must be understood by the marketer. The factors that determine the demand for, and the ultimate consumption of, health services are numerous and their interplay is complex.

THE NATURE OF HEALTHCARE MARKETS

An understanding of the market to be served is a critical requirement for marketing professionals in any industry. This is a particularly important issue in healthcare because of the unique nature and variety of its markets. This chapter describes the nature of markets available to healthcare organizations and reviews the various means of defining markets and delineating market areas. The unique characteristics of healthcare markets are discussed, and the variety of markets addressed by different types of healthcare organizations are described.

Marketing's Context

Marketing activities do not take place in a vacuum but are products of the sociocultural environment in which they occur. To understand the intersection between healthcare and marketing, it is necessary to understand the societal framework in which both enterprises exist. For effective marketing to occur, marketers must first fully understand the nature of the existing system within which they are marketing, including background information on how the system evolved to its current state. For healthcare organizations to be successful in today's environment, they must develop an appreciation for the markets their organizations serve and the salient characteristics of those markets.

This appreciation begins with an in-depth comprehension of the population being cultivated. The social, political, and economic characteristics of the target population must be thoroughly understood, along with its lifestyles, attitudes, and other traits. (These factors are discussed in more detail in Chapter 7.)

While it is not possible to describe all of the social and health system dimensions important for developing marketing initiatives, the important issues are addressed in the following sections. Previous chapters have addressed the characteristics of U.S. society and their implications for healthcare marketing. This chapter focuses on the nature of the markets for health-care goods and services that have emerged.

Although in the past physicians and most not-for-profit healthcare organizations have resisted the use of the term *marketing* in regard to any of their activities, they have nevertheless been concerned with markets on a daily basis. Physicians must consider the characteristics of the population they serve, and specialists must be cognizant of the market composed of physician referrers. Hospitals must appreciate the market constituted by their medical staffs, and health plans must develop an understanding of the individual or corporate entities that constitute the market for health insurance. While some of these target audiences may not constitute markets in the traditional sense—say, of retailers—they are real markets for the health professionals who deal with them.

The establishment of a marketing function implies the existence of a market. Prior to the marketing era the term "market" referred to a real or virtual setting in which buyers and sellers of goods or services came together for the purpose of exchange. The notion of a market as a physical location—a market *place*—has been modified in healthcare to refer to the individuals or organizations in that market that are potential customers. Thus, to contemporary marketers a market is the set of all people (or organizations) that has an actual or potential interest in a good or service. Although a strict definition of marketing would refer to the set of actual buyers of a product, this notion of a market has been expanded in healthcare. Increasingly, for healthcare marketers a market is defined as a group of consumers who share a particular characteristic that affects their needs or wants and makes them potential buyers of a product.

Defining Markets

A market for healthcare goods or services can be delineated in a number of different ways. The definition used depends on the purpose of the analysis, product involved, competitive considerations, and even the type of organization cultivating the market. Furthermore, the nature of the market depends on the orientation of the organization involved in marketing. For example, the market for cardiac care may be identified as a five-county referral area regardless of which providers offer cardiac care. In other words, everyone in that geographic area who potentially needs cardiac care is identified as the market. On the other hand, the term may refer to the market served by a particular healthcare organization—that is, Hospital X controls a five-county market area regardless of the services it offers. Several different ways of conceptualizing a market are discussed below.

actual or desired

The term *market area* as used here is comparable to service area for all practical purposes. Historically, the term *service area* has been used to identify the area served by not-for-profit organizations or areas officially defined as the territory for a particular organization. For example, a health clinic that has been assigned a specific service area by a regulatory authority or a territory based on a health plan contract can be thought to have an identified service area. For-profit healthcare organizations, pharmaceutical companies, and distributors of consumer-health products, on the other hand, are more likely to think in terms of market areas. Over time, as the healthcare industry has become more competitive overall and marketing has come to be more accepted as a healthcare function, an increasing number of healthcare organizations have begun thinking in terms of market areas.

Geographically Based Markets

The most common method of defining a market is on the basis of geography. A *geographically based market* is delineated in terms of specified geographic units. Most market research, in fact, focuses on a census tract, ZIP code, or county (or a group of any of these units) as the basis for analysis. This type of market area is typically delineated in terms of the boundaries of the geographic units chosen for analysis. Geographically based markets are popular because of the familiarity of both analysts and decision makers with established geographic boundaries, the correspondence between the formal operating spheres of many organizations and specified geographic boundaries, and the fact that necessary data are typically collected or reported for established geographic units. (An understanding of the various units of geography used by marketers is important, and Box 6.1 describes the most common units.)

In actuality, few markets (for healthcare or anything else) neatly follow political, statistical, or administrative boundaries. In fact, markets virtually always change faster than their formal boundaries, and some slippage between a geographically defined market area and the actual market area will inevitably occur. Furthermore, market areas are often "gerrymandered" to conform to geographic boundaries that represent a reasonable approximation of the service area under study. The primary reason for this, of course, is the fact that the available data are usually organized on the basis of these geographic units. In addition, it is difficult to visualize a market unless one can think in terms of concrete, recognized boundaries.

Population Segments

A market may also be defined in terms of a *population segment* or some component of the population. Marketers often report that the "market for

Box 6.1: Units of Geography for Healthcare Marketing

Virtually all health planning activities are linked to a particular geographic area. Public health agencies and community-based organizations typically have authority over or are designated to serve specific geographic areas. Private-sector healthcare organizations typically plan for markets delineated based on geography. Even when the target audience is a population segment rather than a geographic unit, this audience will ultimately be linked in one way or another to geography.

For our purposes the geographic units used by healthcare marketers can be divided into three major categories: political or administrative units, statistical units, and a residual category of units that do not fit into either of these categories.

Political or Administrative Units

Political or administrative divisions are the most commonly used geographic units in marketing. Many healthcare organizations' service areas coincide with political boundaries such as cities, counties, or states. Furthermore, it is convenient for private-sector organizations to use standard political or administrative units to establish their boundaries. Political units also are useful in spatial analysis, as many statistics are compiled on the basis of political boundaries. The following political and administrative units are frequently used in marketing.

Nation

The nation (in this case, the United States) is defined by national boundaries. Although a few national chains or consumer-health product companies may be interested in data at the national level, most healthcare organizations focus on lower levels of geography. However, national averages (e.g., mortality rates) are often important as a standard to which other levels of geography may be compared.

State

The major subnational political unit is the state, with data typically available for 50 states, the District of Columbia, and several U.S. territories. Because the individual states have responsibility for a broad range of administrative functions, many useful types of data are compiled at the state level. In fact, state agencies are a major source of health-related data. However, each state compiles data independent of other jurisdictions, resulting in uneven data reporting from state to state.

County

The county (or, in certain states, townships or parishes) represents the primary unit of local government. The nation is divided into more than 3,100 county units (including some cities politically designated as counties). The county is a critical unit for marketing because many healthcare organizations view their home county as their primary service area. States typically report most of their statistics at the county level, and the county health department is likely to be a major source of health data. Even healthcare organizations with regional markets are likely to consider the county as the building block for data collection.

City

Cities are officially incorporated urban areas delineated by boundaries that may or may not coincide with other political boundaries. Although cities typically are contained within a particular county, many city boundaries extend across county lines. Because cities are incorporated in keeping with the laws of the particular state, little standardization with regard to boundary delineation exists. For this reason cities do not make very useful units for market analyses. In many cases, however, city governments are involved in data-collection activities that may be useful to marketers.

Congressional District

Congressional districts are established locally and approved by the federal government. These districts are typically delineated by means of political compromise and do not correspond well with any other geographic units. Although the Census Bureau reports its data for congressional districts, limited data are collected at the congressional-district level. In addition, the boundaries tend to change over time, making these units not particularly suited for use in marketing.

State Legislative District

State legislative districts have similar characteristics to congressional districts. They are drawn up by the states based primarily on political compromise. Although the Census Bureau reports its data for state legislative districts, virtually no data are collected for such districts. Furthermore, their boundaries are subject to periodic change. For these reasons they are not very useful as units for purposes of healthcare marketing.

School District

School districts are established for the administration of the local educational system. Although theoretically reflecting the distribution of school-aged children within the population, other factors may play a role in determining the configuration of school districts within a community. While school districts may be sources of data useful in developing population projections, few statistics are generated for this unit of geography.

Statistical Units

Statistical areas are established to allow various agencies of government to collect and report data in a useful and consistent manner. The guidelines for establishing most statistical units are promulgated by the federal government. The most important statistical units for marketing purposes are discussed below.

Region

Regions are established for statistical purposes by the federal government by combining states into logical groupings. Four regions (northeast, south, midwest, and west) have been established by grouping states based on geographic proximity and economic and social homogeneity. Health statistics are sometimes reported at the regional level by federal health agencies. (The term *regional* is also used informally to refer to a group of counties or states delineated for some other purpose than data compilation.)

Division

For statistical purposes the federal government divides the nation's four regions into nine divisions. Each division includes several states, providing a finer breakdown of the nation's geography. Divisions are seldom used as a basis for health services marketing.

Metropolitan Statistical Area

Metropolitan statistical areas (MSAs) are delineated by the federal government as a means of standardizing the boundaries of cities and urbanized areas. Because each state has different criteria for the incorporation of cities, the MSA concept provides a mechanism for creating comparable statistical areas. An MSA includes a central city, central county, and any contiguous counties that could logically be included within the urbanized area. An increasing amount of data are available on MSAs, and this unit is often used to define a market area.

Urbanized Area

An urbanized area as defined by the Census Bureau includes the entire densely settled area in and around each large city, regardless of whether the area is within the corporate limits. Although limited amounts of data are available for urbanized areas, knowledge about urbanized areas is important in developing a full understanding of the population distribution within a metropolitan area.

Census Tract

Census tracts are small statistical subdivisions of a county established by the Census Bureau for data-collection purposes. In theory census tracts contain relatively homogeneous populations ranging in size from 1,500 to 8,000. For many purposes the census tract is the ideal unit for compiling market data. It is large enough to be a meaningful geographic unit and small enough to contribute to a fine-grained view of larger areas. The Census Bureau collects extensive data at the census-tract level, although this information is only available every ten years from the decennial census. In general, limited health data are available at the census-tract level, although some government agencies do collect and report data for this unit of geography.

Census Block Group

Census tracts are subdivided into census block groups that include approximately 1,000 residents. A tract is composed of a number of block groups, each containing several blocks. The block group provides an even finer picture of a community than the tract level, although fewer data elements are compiled at the block-group level. Little health data are available at the census-block-group level.

Census Block

Census block groups are subdivided into census blocks, the smallest unit of census geography. The term *block* comes from the fact that the typical block is bounded on four sides by streets, although some other visible feature (e.g., railroad track, stream) or nonvisible feature (e.g., city limits) may serve as a boundary. Census blocks tend to be the most homogeneous of any unit of census geography, with the average block housing approximately 30 persons. Only a limited amount of demographic data, and virtually no health data, are available for census blocks.

Block Numbering Area

Before the entire United States was divided into census tracts the Census Bureau divided untracted territory into block numbering areas (BNAs). In rural areas BNAs served the same purpose as census tracts. However, with the 2000 census, the two systems were combined and block numbering groups were phased out. BNAs remain useful when retrospective data collection is necessary.

ZIP Code Tabulation Area

ZIP code tabulation areas (ZCTAs) are a new statistical entity developed by the Census Bureau for tabulating summary statistics from the 2000 census. This new entity was developed to overcome the difficulties in precisely defining the land area covered by each ZIP code used by the U.S. Postal Service (see discussion below). ZCTAs are generalized area representations of U.S. Postal Service ZIP code service areas. They are created by aggregating the Census 2000 blocks whose addresses use a given ZIP code into a ZCTA with that ZIP code assigned as the ZCTA code. ZCTAs represent the majority of U.S. Postal Service's five-digit ZIP codes found in a given area. The Census Bureau's intent was to create ZIP code–like areas that would retain more stability from census to census.

Other Geographic Units

Certain other geographic units may be used by healthcare marketers. These units are often more suited to business-development activities than are political and statistical units.

ZIP Code

Unlike the geographic units previously discussed, ZIP codes do not constitute formal government entities. Their boundaries are set by the U.S. Postal Service and are subject to change as population shifts occur or as the needs of the Postal Service dictate. This lack of stability often means that ZIP codes have limited value for historical analyses or tracking phenomena over a long period. Furthermore, ZIP codes seldom coincide with census tracts or other political or statistical boundaries, making the synthesis of data for various geographies extremely difficult. ZIP codes tend to be much larger than census tracts, sometimes including tens of thousands of residents.

Nevertheless, the ZIP code is a useful unit for defining the market areas of smaller physician practices, smaller hospitals, and even specialty niches for larger health systems. Commercial data vendors compile a great deal of information at the ZIP-code level. Perhaps more important, healthcare organizations typically maintain ZIP codes for virtually every consumer with whom they come in contact, making this an accessible geographic identifier linked to every customer record.

Area of Dominant Influence

Taken from media advertising, the area of dominant influence refers to that geographic territory (typically a group of counties) over which a form of media (e.g., television, newspaper) maintains predominance. This concept is useful when healthcare marketers are interested in media promotions and want to determine the reach of a particular marketing campaign.

product x" is this or that market segment; in these cases they are typically not referring to a geographically defined market area but to a more nebulous market defined in terms of demographics, psychographics, or some other characteristic. Examples of markets defined in this manner are active seniors, women of childbearing age, or a psychographically defined segment such as "yuppies."

Markets conceptualized in terms of population segments can be exceedingly broad or quite narrow. If the senior population is defined as the market, this obviously cuts a broad swath through the U.S. population. On the other hand, if the senior population that requires nursing home care is depicted as the market, this is obviously a much narrower segment of the population. Similarly, the nature of the market could depend on whether one is speaking in terms of a broad range of services (e.g., comprehensive inpatient services) or a narrowly defined individual service (e.g., outpatient eating-disorder treatment).

Consumer Demand

A third way of delineating a market may be from the perspective of the service itself—that is, a market defined by *consumer demand*. For example, healthcare organizations may seek to identify geographic areas with large concentrations of potential patients for a particular service. In this instance markets are defined in terms of their healthcare needs. Examples of markets defined in this manner are the population in need of geriatric services or the one in need of behavioral health services. A hospital may consider virtually the entire population within its defined service area as part of its market for hospital services, whereas a home health agency may envision a narrowly defined subsegment of the population as its potential market. While markets defined in terms of consumer demand may sometimes coincide with established boundaries, they are just as likely to cross geographic boundaries.

Market Opportunities

A fourth way of looking at markets is in terms of the healthcare *opportunities* adjudged to exist in a given area. A certain geographic area may be viewed with interest because that area has a shortage of providers or a lack of facilities. An area characterized by a lack of competition obviously is attractive to an opportunistic organization. In other cases the number of providers may be adequate, but the fragmentation of providers may offer an opportunity for an organization that can appropriately package its services.

Additional opportunities may be offered by areas characterized by a high level of unmet healthcare needs. These may include areas (or populations) that appear to need a certain level or type of services but, for whatever reason, are not receiving the needed care. For example, a specified population, according to a demand model, should consume a certain number of mammograms per year based on its size and composition. If the number of mammograms being performed annually is significantly lower, this may indicate an unmet need. (Note that many unmet needs exist in populations with limited resources; depending on the type of organization performing the research, these populations may or may not be appropriate candidates for targeting.)

Similarly, opportunities may exist in areas in which a gap analysis indicates a shortfall in services or mismatch between needs and services. The number of physicians or hospital beds a given population should support can usually be determined using various computer models. If the number of physicians or hospital beds located in the area falls below the expected number, opportunities may exist in that market.

Market Without Walls

There is yet a fifth way to define a market—in this case the term *market without walls* may be appropriate. Increasingly, certain markets are no longer defined in terms of geographic units or population segments. For example, the markets for contact lenses, health-food supplements, and certain home-testing products have become less dependent on location as these products may be purchased by mail order, through television shopping services, or via the Internet. In addition, the advent of telemedicine allows a specialist in one location to receive electronically transmitted test results for a patient in a different location, thereby diminishing the importance of geographically defined markets.

Delineating Geographic Market Areas

The first step in developing an understanding of the market to be served involves the delineation of the current market area for the healthcare organization. A number of methods can be used to specify the market area, and the method will vary with the type of organization or service involved. In some cases it may be important to identify the primary, secondary, and even tertiary market areas.

Data Analysis

One method for delineating a geographic market area uses the internal data maintained by the organization on the characteristics of its patients. The point of origin of these existing customers is determined (e.g., in terms of county, ZIP code, or even address), with the subsequent plotting of all or a sample of the residences of active patients on a map. A growing number of healthcare providers are mechanizing this process, either purchasing basic mapping software or investing in desktop marketing systems that facilitate strategic marketing activities. The advantage of making market-boundary delineation routine is that it facilitates periodic assessment of boundary changes. Furthermore, data from patient satisfaction surveys, for example, can be linked to geographic information, thus enhancing the value of those data.

The geographic area (e.g., ZIP code, county) from which a pre-specified percentage of admissions are drawn may be designated as the provider's market area. As a rule of thumb it could be argued that the area from which 75 percent to 80 percent of the patients are drawn represents the core market area. (While it may be worthwhile in some cases to try to target the area covered by 100 percent of organization's patients, from a marketing perspective it may make more sense to focus one's efforts.)

It is not unusual to think in terms of market areas existing at different levels. For example, it may be useful to think in terms of primary, secondary, or even tertiary market areas. Thus, it may be determined that the area that accounts for 60 percent of patients will be considered the primary market area, while the area that accounts for the next 25 percent of patients may constitute the secondary service area. The area accounting for the remaining 15 percent of patients would be considered the tertiary market area. By taking this approach the healthcare organization is able to develop a more refined view of its overall market area; this information helps the marketer craft campaigns that address the respective needs of those in the primary, secondary, and tertiary markets.

Multiple market areas may exist for organizations that provide multiple services. The market area for the hospital's obstetrics service may differ significantly in size and configuration from its market area for trauma care or orthopedic surgery. The market area for general hospital services may be different, and much smaller, than that for more specialized offerings.

The delineation of market areas in this manner assumes that patients are originating at their residences when they seek care. While this is the case more often than not, the analysis should also account for patients who do not come from their residences but from other facilities (e.g., nursing homes) or from industrial or commercial sites (Pol and Thomas 2001).

Redefined Markets

In some situations the existing market may not be in keeping with the objectives of the organization. The composition of the identified market area may be changing, as reflected in the characteristics of resident consumers, or the organization's clientele may have moved away from the facility, as in the case of an inner-city hospital whose patients have moved to the suburbs but continue to patronize the facility. The question to ask becomes: Is this the appropriate market area to use as a framework for marketing?

In establishing the market area for a new service or new location, data on the patient origin for existing patients will not be available. One approach may be to determine the maximum distance or driving time that consumers are willing to travel for a given health service. Computer software is available to perform this task, although in rapidly changing areas driving times can be significantly altered over a relatively short period.

Untapped Markets

A third method focuses on establishing market-area boundaries for a service or services not yet offered. Delineating these boundaries is much more difficult and usually requires multiple techniques. One approach may be to determine the residential distribution of patients who use similar services. If another organization is offering the same or similar services, its market-area boundaries must also be estimated. Distance or driving-time data may be evaluated as well. However, a more subjective approach may be required because the service in question is new to the area. Data on the same service offered in a different market area may be available through professional networks. These data could help to establish time and distance parameters. Surveys of potential consumers of these services (e.g., physicians, patients) may also provide valuable time- and distance-sensitivity information.

Once delineated, market-area boundaries must be continuously monitored for change. Traffic patterns and driving times change and the entrance or exit of competition may occur, so market-area boundaries may be significantly altered over a short period. Changes in tastes and preferences for services either on the part of physicians (e.g., increased interest in home infusion therapy) or patients (e.g., increased demand for outpatient services) must also be monitored to determine their effect on market-area boundaries.

Nongeographic Boundaries

The identification of non–geographically based markets involves a potentially more complicated process. Most often these markets are defined in terms of size and composition, with the geographic area providing only the context. Thus, a national market would only consider the geographic boundaries of the United States as a framework within which to view submarkets. An example would be the population of women who have given birth in the last six months. With respect to a given service (e.g., mental health services for postpartum depression), the size of the effective market can be estimated.

When it comes to identifying market-area boundaries based on the location of non–geographically defined markets, the situation becomes more complicated. In an ideal world the mere presence or absence of a target population (e.g., active seniors, women of childbearing age, Hispanics, yuppies) would be adequate. However, situations are seldom this clear cut, and the non–geographically defined market is likely to be interspersed with populations with other characteristics. In other words, marketers seldom find an either/or situation but find that market concentrations are more a matter of degree. Thus, it becomes necessary to develop measures of the concentration of the target population within a geographic area.

Often the emphasis in data analysis is placed on identifying areas with high or low concentrations of persons susceptible to certain illnesses or areas with shortages or surpluses of healthcare providers. For example, if a healthcare provider is interested in geographic areas with high concentrations of older persons, several procedures can be used. Suppose the larger market is a particular state, and the substate markets of interest are counties within that state. The goal is to identify the counties with the highest concentrations of persons age 65 and older. The percentage of the population age 65 to 74 and 75 and older is used as the basis for index construction. The indicator chosen will depend on a number of factors, including the nature of the population, type of service, and marketing methodology employed. Ultimately, it may be appropriate to use a methodology that combines, for example, both number and percentage concentration.

When viewing markets from a nongeographic perspective, a different identification strategy is used. The point of reference is a larger population such as the United States or perhaps a region within the boundaries of the United States. The purpose of the exercise is to find concentrations of persons with certain characteristics within subgroups of the population. For example, if health insurance interests wanted to identify the segments of the population that had the highest rates of noninsurance, the composition of the nation's uninsured population could be examined.

One additional way of defining nongeographic markets may be in terms of consumer propensity to obtain a particular good or service. Market analysts in other industries have long identified population segments based on their willingness, ability, or interest in a particular product. While healthcare services cannot be viewed in exactly the same manner as these other products, there is increasing interest in identifying potential markets in terms of their propensity to be affected by a particular condition or to use a particular service. Often based on demographic or psychographic profiling, this approach attempts to identify those within the population who have a higher likelihood of needing or using a particular service. If, for example, 100 is used as the average for the use of a particular service, an index score of 200 for a specific segment of the population would suggest a propensity to use this service that is twice the average for the total population. On the other hand, a propensity score of 50 would indicate a use rate that is half the average.

Proxy Analyses

Because propensity data are unlikely to exist for the residents of a particular geographic area, inferences have to be made based on knowledge gained from the analysis of other populations. For example, if it has been found that the likelihood of HIV infection among Hispanics is a function of Puerto Rican ancestry, a specified level of education and income, and residence in a highly mobile urban area, it should be possible to develop a propensity score for the presence of HIV within various Hispanic populations. Thus, the propensity score for Hispanics in parts of New York City may be 250, whereas that for Hispanics in Miami may be only 45. In another example, it may be found that the propensity for obtaining laser eye surgery is related to certain psychographic, or lifestyle, segments. Thus, five lifestyle segments may be found to have a propensity score for laser eye surgery of 300 or more (or three times the average), whereas individuals in ten other lifestyle segments almost never obtain laser eye surgery. To the extent that the distribution of lifestyles can be specified for a target area it becomes possible to determine the potential market based on such an approach. (The variation in health services utilization from market to market cannot be overemphasized, and Box 6.2 presents evidence to support the existing disparities in the use of health services.)

Profiling Healthcare Markets

Once geographic boundaries for a market or the parameters for a non–geographically defined market have been established, key attributes of the pop-

---

Box 6.2: Geographic Variations in Health Services Utilization

Healthcare analysts long ago realized that significant variation exists in the utilization of health services from community to community in the United States. As early as the 1970s, research revealed that the rate of procedures performed even in adjacent states varied to a degree not explained by population differences. The rate of performance of procedures could range from 10 percent of the population in some markets to 50 percent in others. These studies suggest that the level of health services utilization is less a function of disease prevalence than a reflection of the characteristics of the medical community and the practice patterns of local physicians (Wennberg and McAndrew Cooper 1999).

Typical of the findings on this issue are the results of a study that compared the cities of Boston and New Haven in terms of their health services utilization patterns. While the two cities are similar in terms of the factors that *should* determine the use of health services, they differed dramatically on virtually every indicator of health services utilization. The hospital admission rate, for example, was nearly twice as high in Boston than in New Haven. Furthermore, residents of Boston were much more likely to be hospitalized for various acute and chronic conditions than residents of New Haven. The average annual per capita expenditure on healthcare in Boston was twice that of New Haven. However, the comparative utilization patterns were not always consistent. The rates of performance for certain procedures were much higher in Boston, but for others they were much higher in New Haven (Wennberg and McAndrew Cooper 1999).

It is now realized that a number of factors account for these seemingly inexplicable differences. A major factor is the variation in physician practice patterns from community to community. In some communities it is standard practice to treat a prob-

ulation within those boundaries may be quantified. This requires that markets be appropriately profiled in terms of relevant characteristics. A *profile* refers to the collection and analysis of detailed information about the market area(s) in question. Information on any and all characteristics relevant to service provision must be obtained from whatever primary and secondary sources are available.

Market Size

Markets can be distinguished along several dimensions. The first dimension is market size. *Size* here refers to the absolute number of potential consumers in a specific market area. The analyst often begins by determining the total population and refining this to determine the area's *effective market*. Thus, the first figure likely to be generated provides the universe of potential customers and must be pared down to reflect realistic market potential. For example, the analyst may determine within the total population the incidence of a certain phenomenon related to healthcare needs (e.g., births) relevant to the market analysis.

lem with surgery; in others the standard calls for less invasive treatment. In some communities conventional medical wisdom calls for hospitalization for certain diagnostic tests and procedures, whereas in others it is customary to handle such cases on an outpatient basis.

Other factors contributing to differential utilization rates include the relative supply of facilities and services. There is pressure, for example, to fill hospital beds if they are available and to use technology in which the organization has invested. In contrast to other industries, competition in healthcare often drives up both utilization levels and costs, thereby accounting for an additional degree of variation. Even the presence of a medical school may influence both the level of utilization and types of procedures performed. Increasingly, the level of managed care penetration is a significant factor influencing utilization rates.

Given these variations, how does the analyst know the appropriate level of utilization? Is the reported level of utilization high or low, or what should be realistically expected? Of course, one way to address this is to use some standard rate of utilization such as the health services utilization rates developed by the National Center for Health Statistics based on national surveys. These rates provide useful benchmarks, but because most analyses focus on local markets, how appropriate are these benchmarks for the market in question? There is no easy answer to this dilemma. The analyst must be able to gain enough knowledge about the local healthcare environment to make reasonable assessments about the level of utilization.

Source: Wennberg, V. E., and M. McAndrew Cooper (eds.). 1999. *The Dartmouth Atlas of Health Care.* Chicago: American Hospital Association.

The analyst can identify the largest markets for the widest range of health services simply by examining census data. For example, among the 50 states the largest market for total health services in 2000 was California. On the other hand, the largest market for services for persons age 85 and older was Florida. States can be ranked along other size dimensions, for example, using the number of persons enrolled in Medicare.

Market Composition

The second dimension is *composition,* or the makeup of the identified market. Composition is usually framed in terms of the number of persons in a given area with certain characteristics. These compositional characteristics typically include demographic, socioeconomic, and psychographic traits. This profile is also likely to include other attributes such as marital status and household structure, educational level, and income characteristics. More detailed data on economic characteristics (e.g., labor force traits, housing values) may also be considered. A basic profile includes data that would be useful for virtually any analysis. It almost always includes projections of future characteristics.

The demographic analysis is often accompanied by an assessment of the psychographic characteristics of the market-area population. Information on the lifestyle categories of the target audience can be used to determine the likely health priorities and behavior of a population subgroup, leading to a consideration of *consumer attitudes*. The attitudes displayed by consumers in a market area are likely to have considerable influence on the demand for almost all types of health services.

During the profiling process the situation with regard to insurance coverage is typically assessed. The emphasis on insurance coverage will vary depending on the nature of the organization. The *payer mix* of a market area (and of the organization being planned for) is perhaps more directly significant to specific healthcare providers whose financial viability is a function of their payer mix.

While many providers attempt to limit the number of self-pay patients they serve, a multibillion-dollar market exists for elective services not covered by insurance plans. The entire vanity market involving facelifts, tummy tucks, and other cosmetic procedures is strictly driven by patients paying out of pocket. Another example is the alternative therapy industry that has emerged to challenge mainstream medicine, built almost entirely on out-of-pocket payments.

The type of community is also a consideration when collecting baseline data on the market. Whether the dominant community type within the market area is urban, suburban, or rural will have important implications for both health status and health behavior. Consumer attitudes are also likely to be different for the various community types, and the existence of submarkets within the market area may be a complicating factor in the planning process.

The health status of the market-area population is part of the profile. *Fertility* characteristics refer to the attributes and processes related to reproduction and childbirth, and the importance of these characteristics varies depending on the type of organization and marketing emphasis. The number of births as well as the characteristics of those births, along with the attributes of the mothers and fathers of the children, form the basis for fertility analysis.

Historical patterns of fertility represent a major influence on current patterns of health services demand. A wide range of goods and services revolves around childbearing. Childbearing also triggers the need for such down-the-road services as pediatrics and contraception-related services. The demand for treatment of the male and female reproductive systems and the heightened interest in infertility treatment reflect services related to the reproductive process.

The level of *morbidity* within a population is a major concern for health services planners. Incidence and prevalence rates can both serve a useful planning purpose, and both may be employed as part of a planning analysis, depending on the nature of the project. This category includes disability indicators along with measures of morbidity in terms of disease prevalence. To the extent possible, planners need to project rates of incidence and prevalence into the future to plan for coming developments.

The study of *mortality* examines the relationship between death and the size, composition, and distribution of the population of the market area. Despite the fact that the current low death rate limits the usefulness of this indicator as a measure of health status, mortality data are always examined to determine what they can tell us about the health of the community.

Health Services Demand

The third market-distinguishing dimension involves the translation of needs and wants into the demand for health services. The needs of a market in terms of childhood immunizations can be translated into demand for a specified number of health department clinics and clinical personnel. The wants of a market in terms of facelifts and laser eye surgery can be translated into demand for a certain number of plastic surgeons and ophthalmic surgeons. In many cases, however, actual data on the market may not be available, and estimates of need will have to be calculated. Fortunately, a number of models have been developed for estimating and projecting the demand for a particular service. These modeling techniques require an understanding of the service area and the manner in which these models operate. Modeled data are never as good as actual data, but the estimates generated by methodologically sound models are adequate for most purposes. In any case, modeled data *must* be used if the level of need is being projected for some future time period.

Typically, the level of need will be expressed in terms of a percentage of the population or a rate of some type. For example, it may be found that 20 percent of the adult population is affected by a clinically identifiable emotional condition or that the crude birthrate is 15 per 1,000. The most common measures of need would be the prevalence and incidence rates used by epidemiologists and public health officials. These measures of the level of need provide the baseline data on which the rest of the analysis depend (Dever 1991).

Once the level of need has been identified for the delineated market area, it becomes possible to specify the actual number of potential cases. A high prevalence rate by itself does not ensure a meaningful market. Healthcare is a numbers game, and it takes a critical mass to support any service. The population projections carried out become important, and their accuracy becomes a critical issue. However, if the level of need has been determined and adequate population figures are available, estimating the potential cases is easy.

The extent to which the identified needs are being met is illustrated at least partially in the form of the health behavior of the market-area population. Health behavior includes both the formal utilization of health services and informal actions on the part of individuals that are designed to prevent health problems and maintain, enhance, or promote health. In terms of formal activities the potential indicators include hospital admissions, patient days, average lengths of stay, utilization of other facilities besides hospitals, physician office visits, visits to nonphysician practitioners, and drug utilization. Among the indicators that have become important more recently are the utilization of freestanding medical facilities and various types of alternative therapies.

Availability of Resources

The fourth dimension involves the availability of *health services resources*. Resources include healthcare personnel, facilities, and programs that offer the same services as the organization in question. The identification of resources will depend on the nature of the organization. A general hospital, for example, will want to identify the availability of other resources comparable to the ones it offers, whether they are offered by a competing hospital or by some other healthcare organization. A medical specialty group is likely to be interested in a much narrower range of resources because many of the resources in the community would not be relevant for that physician practice.

An important step in the examination of available resources is a determination of the nature of the competition. Certainly, the competitive environment in healthcare has become more complicated as a variety of new forms of healthcare organizations have emerged. In simpler times hospitals knew that other hospitals were their competition, cardiologists knew that other cardiologists were their competition, and so forth. Today the environment has changed, and competition can take a number of forms. In the case of hospitals many other types of organizations have begun competing with their services. These are not always outside interests, in fact, given that their own medical staffs may set up competing operations. The boundaries of specialty practice have become blurred as aggressive specialists seek to expand their range of services. The purveyors of alternative therapies have emerged to challenge mainstream physicians on many fronts.

In profiling the community the temporal component is important. Whether determining the needs of the target market or identifying competing services, three time horizons must be taken into consideration. Obviously, the current inventory of needs and resources is a starting point. However, it is also important to develop a sense of the historical trends affecting the community. Is the population growing or declining? Are the characteristics of the population different today than they were five years ago? Are the numbers of competitors increasing? The most important time frame, however, is the future—whether this means the next two, five, or ten years. The market-area profile should identify the future characteristics of the population, future health services needs of that population, and likely future developments with regard to competitive forces.

From Mass Market to Micromarket

When healthcare providers remained at the production stage of marketing the total population was considered the market for most of their services. Hospitals, for example, considered themselves to provide all things for all people. Thus, they sought to exploit an undifferentiated market using mass-marketing techniques. No attempt was made to distinguish between different segments of the population, and only the crudest distinction based on geography was made between markets.

Healthcare organizations operating in this mode typically emphasize a mass-marketing approach. This involves developing generic messages broadcast in shotgun fashion to the entire service area. No attempt is made to target specific audiences, identify likely best customers, or tailor the message to any particular subgroup. This approach involves the use of mass media (e.g., newspaper, radio, television) that blanket the market area. The message has to be general and tout the merits, rather than any specific services, of the organization.

As healthcare entered the marketing era, target-marketing techniques were incorporated. *Target marketing* involves the identification and subsequent cultivation of segments of the market-area population that have certain attributes. These may be segments of the population that reside in the particular geographic area or belong to demographic or psychographic subsegments of the population, or individuals falling into any number of other classifications.

The intent of target marketing is to deliver a particular message to a particular audience in an effort to attract members of this segment of the population as customers. Target marketing facilitates the communication of a message to the targeted audience in a manner that is efficient and cost effective. By eliminating segments of the population that are not being cultivated as customers, marketing effort and expense are minimized; target marketing thus offers the marketer more bang for the buck. While target marketing typically involves the use of traditional media, the media channels are carefully chosen to reach the target audience. Thus, wide-circulation newspapers and network television are eschewed in favor of special-interest publications, radio stations appealing to specific audiences, and cable channels with known viewer demographics.

In targeting audiences for specific goods and services certain established rules should be applied. Targeted markets must be amenable to being ranked and realistic in size, and targeted customers must be reachable and have some minimum level of response potential. Assuming the market is of adequate size, another consideration besides the potential number of cases is the actual geographic distribution of prospective customers within the service area. The importance of customer distribution varies with the type of service and characteristics of the population. Some services are supported by a local population and others by a more far-flung population. On the other hand, some populations are much more mobile than others or are otherwise more or less sensitive to travel times or distances.

In recent years many healthcare organizations have adopted a micro-marketing approach that involves identifying individuals or households for solicitation through a marketing campaign. This level of identification of prospective customers is usually not necessary to support healthcare marketing campaigns. However, in some situations it may be more efficient and cost effective to be able to identify the individuals or households that are the best prospect for a particular service. For example, if an ophthalmic surgeon has determined that individuals with certain demographic and psychographic traits are better candidates for laser eye surgery than those with other characteristics, the most effective approach may be to contact individuals with those attributes directly through direct mail or telemarketing rather than to use a more broad-based approach. Compared to the shotgun approach of mass marketing, this method represents a rifle approach to marketing; only those who have a high potential to respond are targeted.

The Effective Market

One of the peculiar aspects of healthcare is the fact that the potential market for a service may not correspond to the population that actually uses that service. Because the level of need within the target population may not correspond with the level of interest, it is important to determine the extent to which the population really *wants* the service. Although it may be possible to conduct a psychographic analysis of the market area and, from that, develop an idea of the level of interest in a particular service, many situations will require primary research. Ideally, no new program or service should be introduced without a consumer survey; the newer the service or the more unfamiliar the market being entered, the greater the need for such research. Many new programs have failed because the actual level of interest of the target population was much lower in reality than on paper (Thomas 1993).

Ascertaining the level of interest may be relatively straightforward. Market surveys often query consumers about their interest in the availability of such a service and their willingness to use it if available. Marketers in healthcare found out early on, however, that these responses have to be carefully qualified. Typically, respondents express an interest in any new service that appears to benefit them specifically or the community in general. However, when their use of the service is qualified by introducing locational factors or price considerations, their level of interest may change. For example, one survey found that a large portion of consumers in a target area would be interested in a hospital-sponsored fitness program. When the likely location was disclosed, interest waned somewhat. It waned even further when the proposed fee schedule was introduced. Obviously, the more elective the program(s) or procedure(s) under study, the more important these qualifiers become.

Payer Mix

A factor that has become increasingly important in developing a market profile is the consumer's ability to pay for health services. The analyst must determine the potential payer mix of the target population and estimate the level of reimbursement that may be expected for a particular service.

Given the fact that different payers (e.g., commercial insurance, Medicare) have different levels of reimbursement, the effective payer mix will ultimately determine the actual level of payment.

The two bases for determining the ability to pay on the part of the target population are its income level and the extent of insurance coverage. For major health problems (i.e., illnesses requiring hospitalization or intensive services) the level of insurance coverage is the more important consideration. Employer-sponsored commercial insurance generally affords the highest level of reimbursement. Other forms of private insurance (e.g., BlueCross) are also desirable. While payments under Medicare and Medicaid are essentially guaranteed, reimbursement rates under these government insurance programs have historically been lower than those of commercial insurance plans. For elective services the level of income is probably more important than the level of insurance coverage.

In some areas, underinsurance is an issue—one that has taken on increased significance during the economic downturn early in this decade. Certain segments of the population may technically have insurance coverage, but copayment provisions, restrictions on benefits, or limitations on reimbursement may reduce the value of such insurance.

The emergence of managed care as a force in the market has obviously changed the playing field. Unfortunately, the available information on managed care at the market level is limited, and an understanding of managed care penetration and the market shares of various managed health plans often requires primary research. Nevertheless, the impact of managed care on the healthcare environment requires the acquisition of any information that is available on the status of managed care plans in the target community.

Competition

Market potential must also be adjusted to take existing providers into account. Except in those rare cases in which the market is totally unserved, competitors for the potential customers will exist. These competitors may take a variety of forms; indeed, one of the characteristics of U.S. healthcare in the 1990s was the proliferation in the number and types of competitors involving a broad range of healthcare products. Some of these competitors may already be entrenched within the target area or population; others may be entering the market to challenge those that are already entrenched.

Regardless of the nature of the competition the available market must be adjusted to take its impact into consideration. A family practitioner opening an office in a community may face competition from other family practitioners, other primary care providers, public health clinics, urgent care centers, government-sponsored clinics, and even alternative therapists. A realistic assessment of the potential market requires that all of these factors be taken into consideration.

A related activity concerns measuring market shares for the organization and possibly its competitors. For these calculations, the numerator would be the number of "cases" recorded for the organization (or its competitors) and the denominator would be the total instances of that phenomenon for the market area from both a static and dynamic perspective. Internal records on procedures, discharges, or diagnoses may provide the numerators for market share calculations. Denominators may be derived from data made available as a result of reporting requirements. For example, hospital discharge data are often collected by state health departments and aggregated at geographic levels such as the county. A simple calculation divides the number of discharges from Hospital X in County Y by the total number of discharges in County Y.

In the absence of a clearinghouse for utilization data, denominators may be generated from estimates of the number of procedures and discharges using population and incidence information. The number of diabetes cases in a given market area can be estimated by multiplying national or regional incidence rates by population data specific to age or other enumerated factors known to differentiate the probability of being diagnosed with diabetes. Estimates can be used as proxies for the actual data when no market-specific count of procedures, discharges, or diagnoses exists to serve as the market share denominator. Case Study 6.1 describes the steps involved in determining the effective market for a particular service.

Evaluating Market Areas

Market identification and subsequent profiling provide the foundation for the eventual evaluation of market areas. Once data for potential target geographies or market segments have been gathered and analyzed, the analyst is in a position to evaluate the relative merits of the markets under study. The analyst must determine which markets appear to have more potential than others and which are probably not worth pursuing.

This evaluation includes an analysis of demographic trends (especially changes in population size and composition), socioeconomic trends, and psychographic characteristics. Relevant trends in terms of fertility, morbidity, and mortality should be identified. More to the point, the evaluation includes an analysis of trends in health services utilization and patterns of care. It is important to determine present and future demand for both inpatient and outpatient services. This should be specific to the service in question and at the lowest level of geography possible. Projecting trends into the future is important, as few health services can be introduced overnight. Many projects require a two- or three-year startup period, so the characteristics of the population today are not nearly as important as their characteristics tomorrow.

Depending on the service, the market evaluation involves an assessment of existing providers of the service in question. To the extent possible the characteristics of competitors, including their strengths and weaknesses, should be determined so that the organization can determine its market position and assess the extant level of competition. This becomes valuable later in making a realistic assessment of the capturable market.

The basic question to be addressed is how to differentially weigh the data that have been collected. While a high concentration of elderly people may be judged to be an essential characteristic of a prospective market, a high concentration may not be sufficient to declare this market viable. The high-concentration variable may provide the initial screening criterion, allowing other, less attractive market areas or populations to be eliminated from consideration.

Several mechanisms for evaluating the market are available. First, floor or ceiling values can be set for essential criteria, and any values that fall outside the specified range can result in the elimination of a market from consideration. Second, treat each variable as having equal importance (equal weight), and generate a composite index including all factors. Decisions on the elimination or further consideration of a market would be based on these index scores. Third, differential weights reflecting the assumed importance of various factors can be assigned and a weighted aggregate index produced. For example, in some cases the availability of insurance coverage may be given more weight than the presence or absence of competitors.

Even if the markets are not geography specific, similar approaches can be used. Indexes of actual or potential levels of demand on the part of different ages, racial groups, or other population segments can be examined. Those groups with the highest index scores are retained for further evaluation. Furthermore, combinations of factors such as age and race can specify markets, given that no one factor is likely to be accepted as a global measure of market differentiation.

Market evaluation also requires a return-to-basic business and marketing principles. Profit/loss statements, returns on investment, cash flow, mechanisms for service delivery, and options for marketing those services must all be addressed before decisions can be made. Given the information that has been developed, the next step is to calculate the likely costs and benefits involved in introducing the service. Information on market potential, possible pricing structure, vulnerability of the competition, and reimbursement potential must be taken into consideration in determining whether to initiate the service and, if initiated, at what level. Case Study 6.2 demonstrates assessment of the true utilization potential of a market.

The Changing Nature of Markets

The healthcare environment has historically been characterized by relative stability and predictability. However, this situation has given way over the past several years to an increasingly unstable and unpredictable environment. This development has had an inevitable impact on healthcare markets of all types and has introduced a dynamic that must be considered when markets are being analyzed. This dynamic has implications for the identification, profiling, and evaluation of healthcare markets.

Several factors contribute to the changing nature of healthcare markets. Many of these factors are inherent in the market areas themselves and are not directly health related. Market areas are constantly undergoing change in terms of demographic characteristics, with changes in population size, composition, and distribution being everyday occurrences. Changes in lifestyles have also become common in U.S. society.

The demand for services within a particular market or population segment may be influenced by a variety of factors, from changing consumer preferences to newly introduced technology. National or regional trends with respect to service usage, especially in the consumption of elective services, should be monitored. Finally, technological advances that make new procedures possible and old procedures better reshape both the constellation of services offered as well as the way (e.g., inpatient versus outpatient) services are delivered. Changing insurance arrangements could easily affect the level of demand for various services within a specific market.

Other factors that contribute to changing markets include the fluid competitive situation. Existing competitors may be changing locations, services, and marketing strategies. New competitors may be entering the market, and some competitors drop out. This situation has been complicated by the emergence of national chains that may enter a market and, essentially overnight, upset the competitive balance. National and state legislation that facilitates the creation of new partnerships (e.g., health alliances) or alters regulatory powers or procedures (e.g., for health maintenance organizations) reshape, and in some instances create, markets for services.

The smaller the market area, the more rapidly change can occur (Pol and Thomas 1997). For this reason measures of projected growth are required to capture the dynamic nature of these markets. Without an understanding and analysis of market change, marketing decision making cannot take place in a way truly useful to business marketers.

The ubiquity of change is one more reason to establish market research as an ongoing process rather than an ad hoc activity. The identification, profiling, and evaluation of markets is not a one-time activity that should only be returned to three, five, or ten years later. It should be seen as an ongoing process used to continually search for market opportunities and provide continuous evaluation of current strategy. Making these procedures routine, investing in the requisite hardware and software, and training personnel to perform these functions are sound investments for virtually all health services providers.

Summary

An understanding of the market to be served is a critical requirement for marketing professionals in any industry. To understand the intersection between healthcare and marketing, it is necessary to understand the societal framework in which both enterprises exist. The social, political, and economic characteristics of the target population must be thoroughly understood along with the lifestyles, attitudes, and other traits that characterize that group.

The market for healthcare goods or services can be delineated in a number of different ways. Markets can be conceptualized based on geographic coverage, population characteristics, level of demand, and market potential. With the emergence of the Internet, *markets without walls* have become common. Market or service areas for an organization can be delineated in a number of ways, and the approach used depends on the circumstances. The level of geography used in the analysis (e.g., ZIP code, county) depends on the characteristics of the organization and the type of services provided. Over time, healthcare marketers have moved from a mass-marketing approach to a target or even micromarketing approach in an effort to more effectively target consumers.

Once defined, a market must be profiled in terms of its salient characteristics, including demographic and socioeconomic traits, psychographic or lifestyle attributes, health status, and patterns of health behavior. The population's ability to pay for care is an increasingly important consideration. Market characteristics are constantly changing, and market areas must be examined in terms of past, present, and future traits.

A number of factors must be considered in the determination of the "effective" market for a healthcare organization. The total demand must be adjusted for such factors as ability to pay, consumer preferences, existing relationships, and the presence of competitors. A distinction must be made between consumer needs and wants when evaluating a potential market.

Discussion Questions

- How do we define "markets" in healthcare, and what determines how market delineation differs for various types of healthcare organizations?
- What are some of the bases on which markets may be delineated (e.g., geography, population segment, utilization), and what determines which approach should be used?
- For a startup organization with no history in a particular market area, how can the market area be delineated?
- What determines the level of geography (e.g., county, ZIP code, census tract) at which a market or service area should be delineated?
- Why is it sometimes difficult to delineate market or service areas using standard political boundaries?
- How can unmet needs that may indicate an untapped market be identified?
- To what extent has the Internet changed the manner in which markets are organized?
- How can patient volume and/or market share be used to delineate market or service areas?
- What are the most salient demographic characteristics for profiling a population, and how may these traits differ depending on the type of healthcare organization?
- Although lifestyle segmentation has been neglected in healthcare in the past, what arguments can be made for the use of psychographic analysis by healthcare marketers today?
- Why would some argue that the *payer mix* is the most important population attribute to be considered during a market assessment?
- What is the relationship between needs and wants when it comes to health services?
- What factors have contributed to the transition from a mass-marketing orientation to a target-marketing orientation in healthcare?

References

Dever, G. E. A. 1991. *Community Health Assessment*. Gaithersburg, MD: Aspen.

Pol, L. G., and R. K. Thomas. 1997. *Demography for Business Decision Making*. New York: Quorum.

———. 2001. *The Demography of Health and Healthcare, 2nd ed.* New York: Plenum.

Thomas, R. K. 1993. *Healthcare Consumers in the 1990s*. Ithaca, NY: American Demographics Books.

Additional Resources

Berkowitz, E. N. 1996. *Essentials of Healthcare Marketing*. Gaithersburg, MD: Aspen.

Harris, M. S. 2000. "Marketing Health Care to Minorities: Tapping an Emerging Market." *Marketing Health Services* 20 (4): 4–9.

DETERMINING THE EFFECTIVE MARKET

Southern Health Systems (SHS), a fictional organization, had established a satellite hospital in a growing suburban area ten years previously, and the hospital had become relatively successful. It had attracted adequate medical staff and maintained a fairly high occupancy rate. At the time of its construction SHS was not authorized to offer labor and delivery services. Now there appeared to be a significant market for maternity services, as the population had reached a critical mass and large numbers of young families had moved into the community.

SHS marketing staff were instructed to assess the situation and determine the potential for maternity services the market offered now and for the future. This assessment was not only necessary for rational decision making on the part of SHS; but also because a certificate-of-need must be filed with the state, the data would be required to make a case for the granting of a license for obstetrics beds. SHS market analysts were cognizant of the need to identify not only the gross potential for maternity services, but the *effective demand*.

As in any market research project the analysts began by delineating the service area likely to be served by the facility should it be approved. Once satisfied that a defensible service area had been specified, the analysts profiled the population within that service area. They determined the size and characteristics of the current population and developed projections for the future that reflected anticipated changes in its size and composition.

According to the most recent census data the population of the service area in 2000 was approximately 42,000 residents. Estimates for the service area purchased from a demographic-data vendor projected a population in 2010 of 50,000. It was felt that this represented the maximum population capacity of the area, as virtually all available residential land would be occupied by 2010. The demographic characteristics of the population in 2000 were determined and projected forward to 2010. While a wide range of demographic data were reviewed, the analysts focused on such relevant data as the age structure of the population (especially the proportion in the childbearing years), marital status of the population (unmarried suburban residents typically do not have babies), and racial and ethnic composition of the population. The last attribute was considered important given the disparities in birthrates among the various racial and ethnic groups. The psychographic (or lifestyle) characteristics of the service-area population were also analyzed on the grounds that individuals in different lifestyle clusters have different rates of childbearing.

The analysts also researched the situation with regard to insurance coverage. Because this information was not readily available, they had to carry out some primary research. A sample survey of the area's households revealed that 75 percent of the service-area population was covered by some form of commercial insurance. Small proportions were covered by Medicare, Medicaid, or some form of military coverage. A negligible proportion were uninsured. The high level of insurance coverage was a positive finding.

Satisfied that the number of childbearing-age women was adequate (i.e., 23 percent of the population, compared to 19 percent countywide) and that a significant proportion of the households were married couples with or without children (i.e., 55 percent, compared to 35 percent for the county), the analysts advanced the assessment. The next step involved a determination of current and anticipated levels of fertility for the service-area population. Because detailed data on the fertility patterns of the service-area population were not available, known figures for a similar population were applied.

The analysts first looked at the overall birthrate for the population (i.e., crude birthrate) and found that the rate estimated for this population—15 births/1,000 population—was well above the rate of 10/1,000 for the county overall. This was not surprising given the fact that the crude birthrate uses the total population as its denominator and this population was skewed toward childbearing-age women. To refine this figure the general fertility rate was examined for a comparable population to determine the fertility rate for women of childbearing age (i.e., those between age 15 and 44). The general fertility rate for this population was actually lower than that for the county overall (i.e., 58/1,000 women age 15 to 44, compared to 65/1,000). This provided a more realistic view of the likely level of fertility for this population because it adjusted for the size of the childbearing-age population.

Based on these figures it was estimated that the population would yield almost 700 births annually by 2010, with a 2003 estimate of 570 births. Thus, 700 births became the base figure for calculation of the effective market for obstetrics services. This figure had to be adjusted for the various factors likely to affect its conversion into demand for the hospital's maternity services. One demographic factor that needed to be considered was the projected growth in the proportion of the service-area population that was African American. Given the overall higher fertility rate of the African-American population, the anticipated number of 2010 births was adjusted to 750. However, psychographic data gathered on the service-area population indicated that its lifestyle orientation was not particularly child oriented. Thus, the anticipated number of births was adjusted back down to 725.

A major consideration was the drag on potential demand represented by competition from other resources. After all, this would be a new service and, with the exception of existing patients of SHS facilities who might transfer their business to the satellite facility, SHS would have to cultivate a new set of obstetrics customers. Realistically, many if not most of the women of childbearing age in the community are likely to have existing relationships with OB/GYNs. To capture these, the patients must be convinced to change to an OB/GYN affiliated with the new facility, or SHS would have to have the good luck of its existing OB/GYNs joining the staff of the new facility. Furthermore, many potential customers would be constrained in their use of facilities by the health plans that covered their obstetrics costs. One further consideration was the fact that some of these potential maternity customers had already delivered children at another facility (or had otherwise positive experiences with a competing hospital) and would not be inclined to change hospital loyalty without a good reason.

Based on their experiences elsewhere SHS analysts felt that the combined effect of these three factors (i.e., provider relationships, insurance steering, and previous experience) would reduce the potential market share to approximately 50 percent of the total in the short run, with SHS growing this to 60 percent by 2010. It was felt that a market share of 75 percent to 80 percent would be the best one could hope for; thus, a 60 percent share in 2010 was considered a reasonable estimate.

Based on adjustments for the effects of competition the analysts estimated that SHS could capture approximately 285 births during its first year of operation and approximately 420 births annually by 2010. Discounting a certain number of births captured because of the innovative nature of the facility (more early on, fewer later), these estimates were adjusted to an *effective* level of demand of 250 births in 2005 and 400 births in 2010. Given that a minimum of 200 births was felt to be required to justify the cost of establishing the facility, SHS analysts concluded that the effective demand was adequate to support going forward with the proposed maternity service.

6.2

IS THERE REALLY A MARKET FOR IT?

T he primary objective in analyzing any market is to determine the potential demand for some good or service being offered to that market. The market-analysis process typically determines the size and composition of the target market and profiles the identified area in terms of demographic and socioeconomic characteristics. The market is also typically profiled in terms of such health-related characteristics as disease incidence, utilization rates, and referral patterns.

The initial market analysis attempts to estimate the market potential on paper. The analyst would typically determine, for example, the age distribution, racial characteristics, and marital status of the target population along with such socioeconomic traits as income levels, workforce characteristics, occupational categories, and educational levels. Through this process the analyst compiles all of the information necessary to determine that market's potential for the goods or services being offered, or does he?

Years of experience with market analysis suggest that "paper" characteristics such as these need to be verified from as many perspectives as possible and be interpreted in light of any information on the community that may have a bearing on the issue. The analyst must be able to read between the lines and capture the essence of the market that may not be readily obvious from the raw data.

In some cases, especially when a new market is being entered, these secondary data may be all the analyst has access to. The analyst should verify this information by means of ground-level research using whatever means are available, even primary research. In fact, it may not be possible to determine the effective level of demand within a market without asking the residents.

A case in point involves a growing suburban area outside a medium-size southern city. The community had all the earmarks of an up-and-coming suburb. Its population was rapidly growing, with increasingly upscale housing units being constructed. Income levels were rising over time, and the socioeconomic status was steadily increasing for the resident population. An examination of the available data suggested a highly attractive market in terms of demographics. Psychographic data were examined to further specify the types of services likely to be in demand.

It was concluded that the market was composed of an upwardly mobile population with a high level of ambulatory care needs. The population appeared to be ripe for innovative programs (e.g., health maintenance organizations), progressive services (e.g., behavioral healthcare), and even trendy products like fitness centers. In short, the community appeared to be a marketer's dream in terms of offering new services. Even better, few healthcare providers had yet become established within the community.

Fortunately, the data-collection process included a survey of community residents. The survey was intended to confirm the conclusions drawn based on the secondary data. The first clue that things were not as they seemed came early in the interviewing process, when interviewers encountered high refusal rates and a generally hostile respondent population. When the survey data were eventually analyzed it was found that, contrary to the paper analysis, this population was anything but progressive. The residents of this suburb turned out to be very traditional in their approach to healthcare and resistant to any new or innovative services. Virtually no interest was expressed in such programs as women's services, fitness centers, or behavioral health programs, despite large numbers of residents who fit the profile for these services.

The attitudes of the respondents were further influenced by the high proportion of military personnel and retirees in the area. The situation for these residents was much different from that for typical suburbs in that their military affiliation and retirement health plans influenced their health services utilization patterns.

Ultimately, the community was offered a very basic package of primary care services. The gap between the residents' lifestyles and their socioeconomic status and the presence of a large military and retired population mitigated the development of the types of services typically offered to a growing, upscale suburban population. Luckily for the hospital planning the services the community survey provided the information necessary to prevent a serious strategic miscalculation based on the paper profile of the market area.

HEALTHCARE CONSUMERS AND CONSUMER BEHAVIOR

I n any industry the goods and services offered theoretically reflect the needs, desires, and preferences characterizing that industry's consumers. While this is true in healthcare to a certain extent, the industry defies this basic tenet in many ways. This chapter describes the different categories of customers in healthcare and the implications of their attributes for marketing. The unusual nature of consumer behavior in healthcare is described, along with the steps involved in the consumer decision-making process.

The Healthcare Consumer

Consumer, as the term is typically used in healthcare, refers to individuals with the potential to consume a particular good or service. As noted in Chapter 2, anyone who has a want or need for (and presumably the ability to pay for) a product could be thought of as a potential buyer. This being the case, the entire U.S. population represents a market for at least some type of healthcare good or service.

Healthcare organizations have generally failed to think of consumers this way. The notion that individuals are not true health consumers until they are sick has been a barrier to the development of healthcare marketing. Until recently, the generally accepted assumption was that none of the 285 million U.S. citizens were prospects for health services *until* they present themselves for care. Thus, healthcare providers made no attempt to develop relationships with nonpatients.

The approach taken by consumer-goods industries is drastically different in that they make the assumption that virtually everyone must have a need (or at least a want) that could be exploited. Their marketers do not wait to address the potential needs of the consumer population.

In healthcare, the thinking has advanced in recent years to include a much broader range of health services, including some that go beyond the traditional offerings. Thus, sick people are no longer the only target of healthcare marketers, and in some circumstances well individuals are more sought after than sick ones. Healthcare providers realize that the before-market and after-market around the patient episode holds many possibilities for product sales.

Today's market for fitness equipment, self-help books, health food, and a variety of other supportive goods and services is tremendous and increasingly exploited by healthcare organizations.

Ultimately, many healthcare purchases are in response to a health *want*. Today the demand for cosmetic surgery, laser eye surgery, skin care, and medically supervised weight-loss programs is growing. The conditions these procedures address are, in most cases, not life threatening or medically necessary.

Why Healthcare Consumers Are Different

Healthcare consumers differ from the consumers of other goods and services in a variety of ways. To a great extent, healthcare purchases are nondiscretionary. They are often ordered by a health professional for the good of the patient. The patient could, of course, refuse the treatment, but that does not happen often. In virtually no other situation in any industry is a good or service prescribed for the consumer and that consumer pressured to comply with the prescription.

Healthcare consumers are generally insulated from the price of the products they consume. Because of the manner in which health services are paid for and the buyer's lack of access to pricing information, healthcare users often do not know the price of the services they consume.

Healthcare consumers are hampered by other issues as well. They are uninformed concerning the operation of the healthcare system and seldom have direct experience with it. To evaluate the quality of services provided by health facilities and practitioners, consumers must assess the provider based on subjective criteria (e.g., friendliness of staff, quality of food) rather than objective considerations.

All healthcare encounters have an emotional component not present in other consumer transactions. Even stoic people are likely to be emotional in the face of potential health scare for a parent, child, or some other loved one. As stated in Chapter 2, whether this emotionally charged and personal aspect of the healthcare episode prevents the affected individual from seeking care, colors the choice of provider or therapy, or leads to additional symptoms, the choices made by the patient or other decision makers are likely to be affected. (Box 2.2 in Chapter 2 presents differences between healthcare consumers and other types of consumers.)

Why Healthcare Consumers Are Similar

While much has been made of the unique characteristics of healthcare consumers, they are perhaps more similar to consumers in other industries than the above discussion would suggest. While some healthcare episodes involve emergency or life-threatening conditions, the overwhelming majority do not.

Thus, a large proportion of the healthcare episodes that occur involve some discretion on the part of the end user or those involved in the decision-making process, and the consumption of many types of services is elective. Much like other consumers, healthcare consumers are likely to distinguish between needs and wants when it comes to the consumption of services. Clearly, most healthcare consumers would consider angioplasty to correct a heart condition—a need, whereas laser eye surgery would be considered a want; the latter might be considered a discretionary expenditure, whereas the former would be nondiscretionary.

Healthcare consumers are like other consumers in that their level of demand for goods and services is elastic. Years ago the conventional wisdom was that the demand for health services was essentially inelastic. It was assumed that those who were sick consumed services and those who were well did not. Not only does this assumption reflect a dated notion of health and illness, it also does not account for the vast amount of discretionary transactions that occur in healthcare. We now realize that the demand for health services is extremely elastic and that the level of demand can be influenced by a wide range of factors.

Furthermore, we now realize that the demand for health services can be manipulated. This book cites many cases in which consumers were made aware of a service that they previously did not know existed. Indeed, many consumers have been convinced that they have a condition they did not know they suffered from.

One final similarity relates to the ability to pay for services. A majority of patients pay for care through some type of insurance. Those without insurance must pay out of pocket or resort to a healthcare *safety net*. It has historically been felt that healthcare is such a necessity that individuals would find a way to pay for required services even if it meant going into debt. Furthermore, it could be argued that safety nets exist in various communities in the form of public health clinics, charity hospitals, and such facilities that would ensure that all health problems were taken care of in one way or another.

We now realize that the ability to pay for care is a major consideration affecting the demand for healthcare goods and services. Admittedly, for elective procedures and other products not considered medically necessary consumers may be unwilling to pay out of pocket and thus reduce the demand for services. Certainly, during periods of economic prosperity the volume of cosmetic surgery, laser eye surgery, and other vanity services increases; similarly, during periods of economic downturn the volume of such discretionary expenditures decreases.

Recent research, however, has unexpectedly revealed that the consumption of medically necessary services also reflects the ability to pay for care. Individuals without health insurance or other personal resources are less likely to obtain care even for conditions considered medically necessary. Thus, individuals facing this situation may be reluctant to seek care without the ability to pay for it. Indeed, their physician or hospital is likely to expect payment on the front end if they lack insurance. The inability to pay for healthcare is even more pronounced when prescription drugs are involved. A deathly ill patient can eventually be admitted to an emergency room, but he or she cannot obtain necessary drugs without payment. Ultimately, healthcare consumers must weigh the economic implications of consuming goods and services just as consumers in any other industry must.

The Variety of Healthcare Customers

One of the more important attributes of healthcare customers, which should be obvious by now, is their variety. As discussed below, we can think in terms of individuals as consumers of healthcare goods and services. Yet, health professionals and facilities are also major consumers of goods and services in the healthcare arena. While the needs may be different for organizations than for individuals, many of the same marketing issues remain.

Healthcare consumers fall into a variety of different categories, each with specific needs. We generally think of those requiring life-saving services as the typical patients. Although these are clearly rare occurrences, when they do occur they require dedicated personnel, equipment, and facilities so that they can be managed. Another, more common category of consumers is those that require routine health services. These include the typical person who presents himself or herself for treatment at a doctor's office, clinic, or therapy center. This category constitutes the bulk of episodes for those requiring formal healthcare. A third category includes consumers who desire elective health services, including goods and services considered elective or medically unnecessary.

Another major category of consumers is composed of those involved in self-care. Research has indicated that the amount of self-care is much greater than previously thought and that accessing the formal healthcare system typically occurs *after* other options have been exhausted. Thus, symptomatic individuals typically self-diagnose and self-medicate, employing the wide range of do-it-yourself healthcare products that have become available. Pharmacy shelves are stocked with a variety of products and devices for home testing and treatment, and the Internet has expanded the availability of such products.

For these and other reasons a number of different terms are applied today to the purchasers and end users of healthcare goods and services. At the practitioner level the term *patient* is giving way to other terms that more clearly reflect the contemporary healthcare environment. The major terms in use are described similarly in Chapter 4 and are reviewed below.

Individual Customers

Consumers

Consumer, as usually used in healthcare, refers to any individual or organization that is a potential purchaser of a healthcare product. Theoretically, everyone is a potential consumer of health services, and consumer research often targets the public at large. The healthcare consumer is often the end user of a good or service but may not necessarily be the purchaser. *Consumer behavior* refers to the utilization patterns and purchasing practices of the population of a market area.

Customers

The *customer* is typically thought of in healthcare as the actual purchaser of a good or service. While a patient may be a customer for certain goods and services, the end user (i.e., the patient) often may not be the customer. Someone else may make the purchase on behalf of the patient.

For this reason hospitals and other complex healthcare organizations are likely to serve a range of customers, including patients, staff physicians, health plans, employers, and a variety of other parties, who purchase goods or services from the organization. The customer-identification process in healthcare is therefore more complicated than in other industries.

Clients

A *client* is a type of customer who consumes services rather than goods. A client relationship implies personal (rather than impersonal) interaction and an ongoing relationship (rather than an episodic one). Professionals typically have clients, whereas retailers, for example, would have customers or purchasers. A client is likely to have a more symmetrical relationship with a service provider than a patient, who is typically dependent on and powerless relative to the service provider.

Patients

While the term *patient* is used rather loosely in informal discussion, a patient is technically someone who has been admitted into the formal system of healthcare. A prerequisite for this status is the individual being defined sick by a physician. Technically, a symptomatic individual does not become a patient until a physician officially designates the individual as such, even if he or she has consumed over-the-counter drugs or taken other measures for self-care. Under this scenario an individual remains a patient until he or she is discharged from medical care.

Enrollees

While health insurance plans have historically conceptualized their customers as enrollees, this concept has only recently become common among healthcare providers. However, with the ascendancy of managed care as a major force in healthcare, other healthcare organizations have begun to adopt this term. Thus, providers who contracted to provide services for members of a health plan began to think in terms of enrollees. This is a significant shift in nomenclature, as an enrollee has different attributes from a patient. The most important difference is the fact that a relationship is established with the individual *before* the onset of an illness episode, rather than once the person becomes ill. Furthermore, the relationship with the enrolled extends beyond the end of the illness episode. Enrollees may be variously referred to as *members, insureds,* or *covered lives.* (See Box 4.2 in Chapter 4 for a discussion of the significance of differing definitions of the healthcare customer for the operation of the system.)

End Users

The ultimate consumer of healthcare services, as in other industries, is referred to as the *end user,* and all of the terms above may be used variously to refer to the end user of health services. This term is typically not used by health professionals other than marketers. In healthcare the end user is typically the patient who is the direct recipient of a healthcare service or the eventual consumer of a consumer-health product or over-the-counter drug. The end user could also take the form of a health plan enrollee who eventually files claims for payment for medical care. The healthcare situation is unique in that the end user may not play an active role in the selection of the goods or services to be consumed and is often isolated from the cost of these goods and services.

Professional and Institutional Customers

Physicians

As noted above, the end user of healthcare goods and services represents only one of the customer categories found in healthcare. Much of the consumption of goods and services is carried out by health professionals and healthcare institutions. Although the physician is thought of as a provider rather than a consumer of services, physician practices actually represent a major customer for many goods and services. Hospitals solicit physicians to join their medical staffs (and service them once they join). Provider networks and health plans solicit the participation of physicians and other clinicians. Nursing homes, home health agencies, and hospices may depend on them for their referrals. Many physicians depend on referrals from other physicians.

Physicians also serve as customers for a variety of organizations providing support services, including billing and collection services, utilization review companies, medical supply distributors, biomedical equipment companies, and biohazard management companies. Physicians are also customers for information technology vendors who sell or service practice management systems, imaging systems, and electronic patient records. Physicians have traditionally been the primary customer for pharmaceutical companies. The lengths to which pharmaceutical companies will go to acquire physician loyalty to their drug lines are legendary.

Other Clinicians

Other clinicians are customers for many of the same goods and services as are physicians. Dentists, optometrists, podiatrists, chiropractors, mental health counselors, and other independent practitioners have many of the same needs as physicians and are cultivated by similar marketing entities. These providers require supplies, equipment, billing and collections, information technology, and other services just as physicians do.

Hospitals and Other Institutions

Hospitals and other healthcare institutional settings have a wide range of health-related requirements as well as the normal needs that any large organization must address. Like physicians, they require medical supplies and biomedical equipment. More so than physicians, they require durable medical equipment such as wheelchairs and hospital beds. They are customers for a wide range of support services, from billing and collections to physician recruitment to marketing. By virtue of providing food service, gift shops, and parking services, hospitals are customers for a wide variety of non-health-related goods and services. Hospitals and other healthcare facilities are heavy consumers of information technology and are major customers for information technology vendors and consultants.

Employers

Major employers represent customers for health plans, managed care plans, individual providers, and provider networks. Most health plans are employer based, and competing health plans seek to contract with employers for the management of their employees' health. Individual providers may seek to contract with employers that are self-insured or otherwise open to negotiated services. Employers are also customers for a variety of direct services from providers, including a wide range of occupational health services, employee assistance programs, fitness center programs, and various other services that providers may market directly to them.

Other Customers

Like organizations in other industries, healthcare organizations have various internal customers, and chief among them are their employees. Any organization must consider its workforce a customer; healthcare organizations have unfortunately not been in the forefront in this regard. It is important to continuously market the mission, goals, and objectives of the organization to these internal customers and regularly solicit their input.

Another internal customer would be the organization's board of directors. In most organizations the board of directors is charged with setting the direction of the organization and monitoring its progress. This body typically plays a critical role in the operation of the organization and should be considered an important customer by the staff of the organization.

Other, secondary customers should be considered as well. One of these is the general public. Most provider organizations and many other types of organizations in healthcare must maintain a positive public image. Not only is it important to create and sustain corporate goodwill, but it may be necessary to demonstrate at some point that the organization is a good community citizen and, in the case of not-for-profit organizations, deserves to retain its tax-exempt status.

Another customer for healthcare organizations is the media. The media requires cultivation to ensure that the organization's story is told and told in the right manner. Indeed, long before hospitals and other healthcare organizations had formal marketing functions they had public relations departments to deal with the media.

For many healthcare organizations one or more branches of government represent customers. Health facilities and health professions are regulated by government agencies and often maintain separate government- relations offices. If the organization is not for profit, its tax-exempt status depends on maintaining good relationships with the appropriate government agencies. In areas where certificate-of-need requirements exist healthcare organizations must maintain relationships with the appropriate agencies.

Characteristics of Healthcare Customers

The general characteristics of healthcare consumers have been described above and their unique attributes noted. Our understanding of the healthcare customer, however, is confounded by the variety of patterns that exist in the use of services. The types of attributes that influence the use of health services are discussed in more detail in Chapter 9; however, some of these bear discussion here because of their influence on the nature of healthcare customers and the implications of these characteristics for marketing planning.

Age

Age is considered by many to be the single best predictor of the utilization of health services. The amount and type of services used and the circumstances under which they are received will vary with the patient's age. Although it has become a truism in U.S. society that the consumption of health services increases with age, this idea primarily reflects the impact of hospital care. The rate of hospitalization for individuals under 45 is low, at 26.5 per 1,000 population, with the lowest admission rate in 2000 recorded for the 6 to 17 age cohort. The only exception to low rates at younger ages is for women during their childbearing years. After 45, however, admission rates begin increasing dramatically, with the rate more than doubling from the 15 to 44 age cohort to the 45 to 64 cohort (National Center for Health Statistics 2002, Table 90). In terms of emergency room utilization (for true emergencies), teens and those in their early 20s (particularly males) account for a disproportionate share because of injuries and accidents. Elderly people also comprise a large share of emergency room patrons.

Age differences exist in the utilization of physician services, although they are not as dramatic as those for hospital and nursing home care. With the exception of the youngest age cohorts, age has a direct relationship with the number of physician office visits. Overall, elderly persons visit physicians one and one-half times more than nonelderly persons do. Looked at differently, in 2000 those under 18 were nearly twice as likely to report no healthcare visit during the previous year as those 65 and older. This difference reflects the fact that a large proportion of visits for elderly people are for regular checkups and monitoring chronic conditions, not for acute problems (National Center for Health Statistics 2002, Table 72).

A significant difference exists in the utilization of specialists and the age of the patient. With increases in age, the utilization rate for primary care physicians decreases and that for specialists increases. For example, in

2000 more than half (53.5 percent) of elderly persons reported visiting a non–primary care specialist, compared to 20.3 percent of those under 18 (National Center for Health Statistics 2002, Table 85).

The relationship between nursing home utilization and age is predictable. Few nursing home residents are under 65. However, within the nursing home population itself significant differences in age distribution exist. Overall, fewer than 5 percent of those 65 and older resided in nursing homes in 1999, a figure that has changed little in two or more decades. However, of those 85 and older, 18.5 percent were institutionalized. Looked at another way, the age distribution of nursing home residents is around 13 percent of aged 65 to 74, nearly 35 percent of 75 to 84, and more than 50 percent of 85 or older (National Center for Health Statistics 2002, Table 97). Thus, as the U.S. population has aged, the average age of nursing home residents has actually increased. Similarly, those 65 and older account for 70.5 percent of home health patients, with clients for home health services concentrated in the 75 to 84 age group. A similar pattern exists with regard to the use of hospice services (National Center for Health Statistics 2002, Tables 88 and 89).

Age differences are also found in the use of other types of facilities. Among the older population, there is a preference for inpatient rather than outpatient care; the ingrained notion of better care and a more secure environment among older age cohorts tends to favor hospitalization. On the other hand, preferences for outpatient settings among the younger age cohorts have emerged. (This preference appears to be increasingly mitigated by the effect of changing reimbursement patterns and the influence of aging baby boomers.) The primary users of freestanding urgent care clinics, for example, are in the 25 to 40 age group. The under-45 population is also more likely to use other outpatient settings, such as freestanding diagnostic centers or surgicenters. These differences are partly a reflection of age-generated contrast in perceptions, but they also reflect the fact that younger age cohorts are more likely to be enrolled in some alternative delivery system.

Gender

In U.S. society women are more proactive than men with regard to healthcare and are consequently much heavier users of the healthcare system. They tend to visit physicians more often, take more prescription drugs, and use other facilities and personnel more often. Obviously only women will consume OB/GYN services, but they are also overrepresented in general practice settings because of their higher prevalence of chronic conditions. Driven by the use of obstetrical services, hospital utilization was significantly greater for females than males in 2000 (National Center for Health Statistics 2002, Table 90). In the case of tertiary care, however, males tend to predominate. Although males become sick less often than females, they are more likely to contract serious conditions. Males—particularly adolescents and young adults—are more likely to utilize hospital emergency rooms for true emergencies, primarily because of the large number of injuries and accidents occurring among this subpopulation.

Women comprise the majority of nursing home admissions, and the U.S. nursing home population is nearly 75 percent female. For the 85-and-older cohort the female proportion is more than 80 percent (National Center for Health Statistics 2002, Table 97). The higher mortality rate for males results in more female candidates for nursing home admission. Furthermore, men surviving into the older age cohorts are more likely to have a wife to care for them. Women account for nearly two-thirds of home health patients.

Race and Ethnicity

A correlation has been found between racial and ethnic characteristics and the utilization of certain types of health services. The clearest differences have been identified between the sickness behavior of African Americans and whites. Certain Asian populations and ethnic groups also display somewhat distinctive utilization patterns. To a limited extent, differences in utilization may be traced to differences in the types of health problems experienced. However, many of the differences in the use of healthcare resources reflect variations in lifestyle patterns and cultural preferences.

The hospital discharge rate for whites tends to be around 20 percent lower than that for African Americans, despite the older age structure of the white population. Discharge rates for Asians and Hispanics are much lower than those for whites, whereas those for Native Americans are between the white and African-American rates (National Center for Health Statistics 2002, Table 90).

Whites are overrepresented among the nursing home population. African Americans and other racial and ethnic groups tend to be underrepresented, although Hispanics increasingly report a pattern similar to that of non-Hispanic whites. This underrepresentation among African Americans is particularly telling in view of the heavy burden of chronic disease and disability affecting this population.

In general, whites tend to use physicians at a higher rate than do the rest of the population. In 1995 whites in the United States averaged 3.4 physician office visits, compared to 2.6 for African Americans. Thus, while African Americans constitute 12.6 percent of the U.S. population, they account for only 10.5 percent of the physician office visits, despite higher rates for many acute and chronic conditions (National Center for Health Statistics 1998). Looked at differently, 16.0 percent of whites reported no healthcare visits in 2000, compared to 17.3 percent of African Americans. Interestingly, larger proportions of Native Americans (21.2 percent), Asians (20.2 percent), and Hispanics (26.5 percent) reported no healthcare visits of any type (National Center for Health Statistics 2002, Table 72). Whites are overrepresented among the patients of specialists. While African Americans are overrepresented among the patients of obstetricians (primary care), they are underrepresented among the clients of ophthalmologists and orthopedic surgeons (specialty care).

African Americans are significantly more likely to use emergency room services than are whites. The rate of emergency room use for Hispanics is similar to that for whites, whereas Native Americans have the highest emergency room use rates of any group. Asians are the least likely to use emergency room services (National Center for Health Statistics 2002, Table 79).

Some ethnic group members (e.g., Hispanics) use alternative types of care in the form of traditional healers. Thus, their physician usage rate does not provide a full picture of their healthcare utilization. In fact, research into the use of alternative therapies by Americans suggests that the whole notion of the utilization of clinic services should be reviewed (Eisenberg et al. 1993).

Marital Status

Marital status is a surprisingly effective predictor of the utilization of health services. It is related not only to levels of service utilization but also to the type of services used and the circumstances under which they are received. (The categories of marital status for the discussion below are never married, married, divorced, and widowed.)

In general the married require fewer services because they are healthier. Yet, they use more of certain types of services because they are more aware of the need for preventive care; more likely to have insurance; and, it is argued, have a "significant other" to encourage them to use the healthcare system. This social support provided by marriage serves to forestall the need for intensive care by providing an environment that retards the progression of disorders and encourages individuals to use preventive care. The never married, divorced, and widowed, on the other hand, are more likely to be characterized by negative health behaviors.

The age-adjusted rate of hospitalization for married individuals is relatively low. Admission rates for the never married also tend to be relatively low, whereas those for the widowed and divorced are high by comparison. If rates of admission for various conditions are considered, the variation among marital statuses is even more pronounced.

Some differences related to marital status do exist in the utilization of physician services, although they are not as dramatic as those for hospital and nursing home services. Federal surveys have found that married women "see" a doctor (i.e., via visit or telephone) an average of seven times a year. The rate of contact for divorced and widowed women is slightly higher. The rate of physician contact for men is lower than that for women in every marital status category, although little difference exists from one marital status to another for men. Some differences, albeit small ones, exist in the utilization of specialists by marital status of the patient.

The patterns of utilization of dentists and other health professionals are similar to physician utilization patterns for the various marital statuses. While the married have fewer dental problems, they are more regular users of dentists than are those in the other marital status categories. No clear marital status differences are found for the use of podiatrists, chiropractors, and physical therapists.

The relationship between nursing home utilization and marital status is one of the clearest to be discussed in this section. Few nursing home residents are married. The bulk of nursing home residents are widowed, although small numbers are divorced or never married. Married individuals requiring nursing care are often maintained in the home and cared for by a spouse.

Income

Income is probably one of the better predictors of the utilization of health services. Income is related not only to levels of service utilization but also to the types of services used and the circumstances under which they are received. Hospitalization rates tend to decrease directly with income, and greater discrepancies exist among the various income groups than for any of the other social variables examined. The rate of hospitalization for the lowest-income group in the United States is the highest of any income group, reflecting the higher incidence of health problems (National Center for Health Statistics 2002, Table 90).

Lower-income groups are heavier users of hospital emergency room care, especially for nonemergency conditions. On the other hand, lower-income populations are less likely to utilize freestanding emergency clinics or urgent care clinics, presumably because of a lack of knowledge of their availability (such clinics are often located in suburban areas) and the fact that payment is typically demanded when care is rendered.

In the past significant differences have existed in the utilization of physicians in relation to income. Historically, the number of annual physician visits per capita has increased as income increases. The lowest-income groups tended to be infrequent users of physician services; in the past this reflected a lack of family physicians and the use of alternative sources of care such as public health clinics. This situation has changed since the 1960s because of the availability of government-sponsored insurance programs and programs that subsidize physician services in underserved communities. However, the lower-income groups continue to be underrepresented among the patients of private practice physicians and to be overrepresented among emergency department users (National Center for Health Statistics 2002, Table 79).

As income increases, the utilization rate for primary care physicians decreases and that of specialists increases (National Center for Health Statistics 2002, Table 85). A direct and inverse relationship also exists between income and dental care utilization. The more affluent view dental care as a preventive service, whereas the less affluent see it as an expensive service only to be used in emergencies.

Education

The relationship between education and the use of health services resembles that for income, and educational level is probably one of the better predictors of the utilization of health services. Education is related not only to levels of service utilization but also to the types of services used and the circumstances under which they are received.

The rate of hospitalization for the least educated segments of the U.S. population is low, despite the fact that the incidence of health problems is greater for the poorly educated than for any other group. The better educated, although less affected by health problems, have much higher rates of hospitalization. This is thought to be a function of a greater appreciation of the benefits of healthcare and more insurance coverage on the part of the better educated.

Physician utilization is considerably higher for the best educated than for the least. In general the number of annual physician visits per capita increases with education. The least-educated groups have the lowest rates of physician visits. As education increases, the utilization rate for primary care physicians decreases and that of specialists increases. This partly reflects the prestige dimension of medical specialists and the knowledge required to select a specialist. The presumed greater expertise of specialists makes them appealing to the well educated.

A direct and inverse relationship exists between education and dental care utilization. The better educated see dental care as a preventive service, whereas the least educated are less likely to appreciate its benefits.

The relationship between nursing home utilization and education is not clear. Educational differences are found, however, in the use of other types of facilities. Less-educated groups are heavier users of hospital emergency room care, especially for nonemergency conditions. On the other hand, better-educated populations are more likely to utilize urgent care centers. The better educated are also more likely to utilize other outpatient settings such as freestanding diagnostic centers or ambulatory surgery centers.

Occupational Status

Occupational status is related not only to levels of service utilization but also to the types of services used and the circumstances under which they are received. In general those in higher occupational categories (such as managerial and professional occupations) require fewer services because they are healthier. Yet, they utilize more of certain types of services because they are more aware of the need for preventive care and tend to have better insurance coverage.

Higher-status occupational groups have somewhat higher admission rates. The pattern identified for the various occupational statuses for patient days is comparable to that for admissions. The lower-status occupational categories make up for any differences in admissions with more patient days.

Some differences are found in the use of other types of facilities on the basis of occupational status. Income and educational levels no doubt play a role here, and the type of insurance coverage available (primarily a function of employment status) is important in the type of service used. Some differences related to occupational status do exist in the utilization of physician services.

Given the importance of these attributes in influencing the use of health services, it is worth reviewing the trends affecting the U.S. population in this regard (see Box 7.1).

Consumer Attitudes

Attitude refers to a position an individual has adopted in response to a theory, belief, object, event, or another person. It establishes a relatively consistent, acquired predisposition to behave in a certain way in response to a given object. Attitudes are typically thought to have three components:

Box 7.1: Trends in Healthcare Consumer Characteristics

Healthcare marketing is an evolving field, and marketing professionals continue to face challenges as they seek to establish legitimacy for marketing within healthcare. These challenges would be daunting enough if marketers were dealing with a stable pool of healthcare consumers. Unfortunately, this is not the case, and a major challenge lies in adapting marketing techniques to the changing nature of the U.S. population. Against the backdrop of a rapidly aging population, marketers are faced with high rates of immigration and internal migration, frequently changing lifestyles, and constantly changing family and marital status situations that contribute to the transformation of the American mosaic. The most important of these trends and their implications for healthcare marketing were discussed in Chapter 3 and are noted again below.

Changing Age Distribution

The implications of the aging of America for health services demand have been well documented, with age arguably the single most important predictor of the demand for health services. The emergence of elderly people as a consumer group in the U.S. population has not gone unnoticed by marketers.

Population growth within the older age cohorts (age 55 and older), particularly among the oldest old (age 85 and older), is faster than that for the younger cohorts, and significant differences have been identified between the young old, middle old, and oldest old. Even among those within the same age cohort, important differences have been found in other demographic characteristics, lifestyles, and health status and behavior.

The age-related development with the most implications for future healthcare demand is the movement of the huge baby boom cohort into middle age. This cohort grew up in affluence and comfort, and they are used to having things, including their health, in working order. When they have to contend with the onset of chronic disease and the natural deterioration that comes with aging, the healthcare system will be significantly affected.

Feminization

An automatic accompaniment to the aging of America has been the feminization of the U.S. population. The older the population, the greater the "excess" of females. Except for the very youngest ages, females outnumber males in every age cohort. Among older seniors females outnumber males two to one, and at the oldest ages there may be four times as many women as men. This results in an older age structure for women; in 2000 the median age for women was 38.0 years, compared to 36.5 years for men.

These trends have contributed to an increased role for women in the healthcare system. While women have no doubt historically directed much of the use of health services, only in recent years has the pivotal role of women in the healthcare system became clear to marketers. As the baby boomers age, an increasing proportion of healthcare consumers will be women, and it can be argued that baby boomers will drive the future direction of healthcare. It may be more accurate to assert that baby boom *women* will be the dominant force in healthcare for the foreseeable future.

Increasing Racial and Ethnic Diversity

Another demographic trend that characterizes U.S. society today is its increasing racial and ethnic diversity. The level of immigration is at an all-time high, and long-established ethnic and racial minorities are growing at faster rates than those of native-born whites. The cumulative effect of the trends of the past several years has been a diminishing of the relative size of the white population (especially the non-Hispanic white population) and the growing significance of the African-American, Asian, and Hispanic components of the U.S. population.

Given the fact that the U.S. healthcare system has historically been geared to the needs of the mainstream white population, the trend toward greater racial and ethnic diversity cannot help but have major implications for the future of the system. Any marketing activities must take into consideration the changing characteristics of the population and the demands these changes will make on the system.

Changing Household and Family Structure

Another demographic development characterizing U.S. society is its changing household and family structure. This trend is no surprise to demographers, although it has seldom been linked to health issues. For decades the family has been undergoing change; first it was high divorce rates, then fewer people marrying (those who did marry did so at a later age), then fewer people having children (those who did have children had fewer of them, at a later age). What is popularly considered the typical American family (two parents and x number of children) has become a rarity, and nontraditional households have become the norm.

As with marital status, the changing household structure has important implications for both health status and health behavior. The typical patient is less and less likely to be part of an intact nuclear family and more likely to live in a nontraditional family arrangement. The marketing approaches for two-parent families, single-parent families, and elderly people living alone are quite different.

(1) a *cognitive component* related to what the individual knows or believes about an object or act, (2) an *affective component* related to what the individual feels emotionally about an object or act, and (3) a *behavioral component* related to how the individual is disposed to behave toward an object or act.

When consumer attitudes are considered in healthcare, they typically refer to the attitudes that influence the preferences, expectations, and behaviors of the end user or purchaser of health services. Thus, attitudes held by consumers toward the healthcare system in general, physicians, particular facilities, certain treatments, and so forth are thought to color their consumer decision-making processes. Willingness to utilize urgent care centers rather than emergency rooms, health maintenance organizations rather than traditional health plans, and chiropractors rather than orthopedic surgeons may be a function of the attitudes held by consumers.

Attitudes are not restricted to the consumers of health services, and physicians and other health professionals also bring attitudes to the situation. The attitudes of physicians, for example, have been documented to have an effect on the likelihood of a malpractice suit being filed. Even organizations may be predisposed to certain attitudes, as in the case of healthcare organizations that are prejudiced against the use of consultants or tailor their service offerings to reflect the organization's religious underpinnings.

As stated in Chapter 3, today's consumer is much more knowledgeable about the healthcare system, open to innovative approaches, and intent on playing an active role in the diagnostic, therapeutic, and health maintenance processes. These new attitudes are concentrated among the under-50 population and among certain demographically distinct groups. These groups have also provided the impetus for the rise of alternative therapies as a competitor for mainstream allopathic medicine.

The baby boom population is more patient centered and more likely to emphasize the nonmedical aspects of healthcare. Baby boomers are less trusting of professionals and institutions and are more self-reliant than previous generations of patients. They pride themselves on getting results and extracting value for their money. They are increasingly in positions of power, which allow them to influence the reshaping of the healthcare landscape.

Such new attitudes toward healthcare reflect the rise of consumerism. *Customers* (as opposed to *patients*) expect to receive adequate information, demand to participate in healthcare decisions that directly affect them, and expect the healthcare they receive to be of the highest possible quality. They want convenience, service, and value when it comes to healthcare.

Segmenting the Market for Healthcare Products

Once healthcare moved away from mass marketing as a means of cultivating consumers, it began to adopt a more targeted marketing approach. Of particular importance in this approach is the market-segmentation process. Market segmentation, long used in other industries, is used to identify specific segments of the population that are subsequently singled out for cultivation.

Not every subgroup within a population qualifies as a target market, and certain rules of thumb help marketers identify a meaningful market segment. A viable market segment should be *measurable* in that accurate and complete information on customer characteristics can be acquired in a cost-effective manner. It should be *accessible* in that it is possible to communicate effectively with the chosen segment using standard marketing methods. It should be *substantial* enough to be considered for separate marketing activity. A segment should also be *meaningful* in that it includes consumers who have attributes relevant to the aims of the marketer. In examining market segmentation as applied to healthcare, Berkowitz (1996) adds that a viable market segment should also evidence a desire for the product and have the ability to pay for it. Market segmentation can take a number of different forms; some of the more common are described below.

Demographic Segmentation

Market segmentation on the basis of demographics is the best known of the approaches to identifying target markets. The links between demographic characteristics and health status, health-related attitudes, and health behavior have been well established. For this reason demographic segmentation is always an early task in any marketing planning process, and demographically distinct subgroups are typically defined relative to various goods and services.

Geographic Segmentation

An understanding of the spatial distribution of the target market has become increasingly important as healthcare has become more consumer driven. One implication of this trend has been the increased emphasis on the appropriate location of health facilities. The market-driven approach to health services has demanded that healthcare organizations take their services to the population, and the major purchasers of health services are insisting on convenient locations for their enrollees. Knowledge of the manner in which the population is distributed within the service area and the link between geographic segmentation and other forms of segmentation is critical for the development of a marketing plan.

Psychographic Segmentation

For many types of goods and services an understanding of the psychographic, or lifestyle, characteristics of the target population is essential. The lifestyle clusters that can be identified for a population often transcend (or at least complement) its demographic characteristics. Most important, psychographic traits can be linked to the attitudes, perceptions, and expectations of the target population as well as to the propensity to purchase various services and products. While psychographic analysis in healthcare has lagged behind its use in other industries, health professionals are finding increasing numbers of applications for this approach, and growing amounts of healthcare data are being incorporated into psychographic segmentation systems.

Usage Segmentation

A common form of segmentation long used by marketers is now being applied to healthcare. The market-area population can be divided into categories based on the extent of use of a particular service. In the case of urgent care clinic usage, for example, the population can be divided into heavy users, moderate users, occasional users, and nonusers. This approach can be applied to a wide range of services but may have its most important applications when elective goods and services are under consideration. This information provides a basis for subsequent marketing planning that can be tailored differently, for example, for existing loyal customers and non-customers. The willingness of individuals to use certain services, especially elective procedures, often reflects the extent to which they fall into the category of adopters (see Box 7.2).

Payer Segmentation

A form of market segmentation unique to healthcare involves targeting population groups on the basis of their payer categories. The existence of insurance coverage and the type of coverage available are major considerations in the marketing of most health services. Furthermore, health plans cover some services and not others, and this becomes an important consideration in marketing. For elective services paid out of pocket, a targeted marketing approach is typically required. The payer mix of the market-area population has come to be one of the first considerations in profiling target populations.

Benefit Segmentation

Different people buy the same or similar products for different reasons. Benefit segmentation is based on the idea that consumers can be grouped according to the principal benefit sought. The benefits consumers consider

Despite its emphasis on research and innovation, the healthcare institution is relatively conservative. It only adopts new techniques or treatment modalities after extensive testing; even then, practitioners are often reluctant to forsake tried-and-true procedures. Similarly, most healthcare consumers tend to be conservative in their approach to care, preferring to stick with proven treatments rather than opt for more experimental approaches.

This approach, however, is not true across the board, and segments within the population eagerly seek out innovations, even in healthcare. Indeed, the openness of the baby boom generation to innovative approaches has led to the introduction of a wide range of novel health services, from urgent care centers to freestanding diagnostic centers to progressive birthing centers. Clearly, some segments of society have a greater predilection for innovation than others.

Marketers have studied the process through which individuals come to adopt a new procedure or therapeutic modality. This analysis focuses on the mental processes through which an individual passes from first hearing about the innovation to final adoption. Based on a review of previous research, the population can be subdivided into five categories:

1. *Innovators* typically represent the first to adopt a new service and account for about 2.5 percent of the population. They are eager to try new ideas and products, almost to the point of obsession. They have higher incomes, are better educated, and are more active outside their communities than noninnovators. They are less reliant on group norms, more self-confident, and more likely to obtain their information from scientific sources and experts.

2. *Early adopters* represent on average the next 13.5 percent to adopt the product, adopting early in the product's life cycle. They are much more reliant on group norms and values and are much more oriented to the local community than innovators, who have a more cosmopolitan outlook. Early adopters are more likely to be opinion leaders because of their closer affiliation to groups. Because of their personal influence on others, they are regarded as the most important segment for determining whether a new product will be successful.

3. The *early majority* represent the next 34 percent to adopt. They will deliberate more carefully before adopting a new product, collecting more information and evaluating more options than will the early adopters; therefore, the process of adoption takes longer. They are an important link in the diffusion process, as they are positioned between the earlier and later adopters.

4. The *late majority* represent the next 34 percent to adopt. They are described as skeptical, and they adopt because most of their friends have already done so. Because they rely on group norms, adoption is the result of the pressure to con-

form. They tend to be older, have below-average income and education, and rely primarily on word-of-mouth communication rather than the mass media.

5. *Laggards* represent the final 16 percent to adopt. They are similar to innovators in not relying on the norms of the group. They are independent because they are tradition bound, making decisions in terms of the past. By the time they adopt an innovation, the innovation has probably been superseded by something else. Laggards have the lowest socioeconomic status.

Healthcare marketers can improve their effectiveness by determining the point at which their goods and services are in the product life-cycle process and using this information to target the components of the consumer population most likely to adopt the product. Efforts directed toward those unlikely to adopt a new good or service will be wasted.

Source: Assael, H. 1992. *Consumer Behavior and Marketing Action.* Mason, OH: South-Western.

when making a purchase decision related to a given good or service include such product attributes as quality, convenience, value, and ease of access. Healthcare marketers should be able to differentiate consumer segments based on their particular "hot buttons."

Consumer Behavior

Consumer behavior refers to the patterns of consumption of goods and services that characterize healthcare consumers, along with the factors that contribute to this behavior and processes that lead up to a purchase decision. Because marketing is driven by consumer needs, an appreciation of the behavioral dimension of any target population is essential. The marketing plan ultimately seeks to influence this behavior. (Note that this discussion focuses on individual consumers, not the behavior of professionals or organizations in their role as consumers; these other consumer categories should be considered separately.)

Decisions with regard to the use of health services are influenced by many factors that do not play a role in other consumption decisions. These decisions are likely to involve an emotional component, and healthcare consumers may be facing life-threatening situations that affect them or their loved ones. The fact that many consumers cannot bring themselves to even say the word cancer supports this view. Emotions like fear, pride, and vanity come into play. For example, who would have thought 20 years ago that men would overtake women in the use of cosmetic surgery?

Despite the differences between healthcare consumers and other consumers, the decision criteria for healthcare consumers can be classified in the same manner as in other industries. The categories of factors that influence purchase decisions include technical, economic, social, and personal criteria. Technical criteria include quality of care, clinical outcomes, environment, and the amenities that influence the decisions of healthcare consumers. Economic factors, perhaps the least relevant in healthcare, include the price of goods and services, mechanism for payment (e.g., insurance), and perceived value of the service rendered. Social criteria include such factors as the status associated with the professional, facility, or procedure performed; influence of the social group; and other factors related to the social environment. Personal criteria include factors related to the emotional aspects of the service, self-image issues, and even moral and ethical considerations.

It is traditional to think in terms of a hierarchy of needs in setting the context for the analysis of consumer decision making. Most refer to Maslow's theory of motivation in addressing this issue. Maslow (1970) contends that the first order of need for human beings involved physiological needs for food, water, air, shelter, sex, and so on. Once these basic needs are met, society members can begin to think in terms of their safety and security needs, including freedom from various threats and the establishment of security, order, and predictability in their lives. At this stage health begins to emerge as a value in its own right.

With this foundation, society members can begin to think in terms of social or companionship needs—the next level in the hierarchy. These needs include friendship, affection, and a sense of belonging. To these needs would eventually be added esteem or ego needs, including the need for self-respect, self-confidence, competence, achievement, independence, and prestige. Finally, at the top of the needs hierarchy individuals have a need for self-actualization. This includes the fulfillment of personal potential through education, career development, and general personal fulfillment. Few societies in the history of the world have achieved this level of need fulfillment for any significant portion of their population.

This model is important to marketers for a couple of reasons. First, the level of the hierarchy at which an individual or population functions says a lot about the healthcare needs it faces. At the lower levels of the model, survival needs dominate the healthcare arena. Society members face threats from pathological agents and a hostile environment. At the higher levels of the model the threats common at the lowest levels have been moderated; rather than attempting to preserve life and limb, society members can focus on health maintenance and enhancement. Their needs shift from life-saving procedures and public health considerations to self-actualization needs such as weight control, fitness programs, and cosmetic surgery.

From a marketing perspective individuals at the survival level are only likely to be responsive to marketing initiatives that address their immediate needs. They do not respond to promotions for services that enhance their quality of life or require out-of-pocket expenditures. (This helps explain the difficulty involved in convincing individuals with precarious financial situations that they ought to invest in healthy lifestyles.) As individuals progress up the hierarchy they are more open to discretionary services and appreciate the importance of maintaining and enhancing their health status. Indeed, body imaging may become a means of raising status and self-concept.

Ultimately, the types of healthcare goods and services to which consumers respond, the method for reaching individuals at different levels in the needs hierarchy, and the message that is appropriate will reflect one's position in this model. Marketers are faced with the challenge of matching the product, medium, and message to the status of the target audience vis-à-vis the needs hierarchy.

Consumer Decision Making

In virtually every other industry the end user is responsible for the purchase decision, and the decision maker actually consumes the good or service. This is often not the case in healthcare, in which the end user of the service (i.e., the patient) does not make the decision to purchase the service. Thus, a physician is likely to determine the what, where, when, and how much of the service is provided. Alternatively, the decision maker may be a health plan representative, employer, or family member, not the party who eventually consumes the service. The marketer is faced with the challenge of determining where to place the promotional emphasis under these circumstances.

Another unique characteristic of healthcare that has implications for the marketing plan is the fact that the end user of a service may not be the ultimate target of a marketing initiative. In fact, healthcare marketers have identified a number of other categories of target audiences that may be more important than the end user. For example, various categories of *influencers* have been identified. These could be family members, counselors, or other health professionals that encourage consumers to use a particular good or service. The role of various *gatekeepers* might also be considered. These could include primary care physicians, insurance plan personnel, discharge planners, and others who have responsibility for channeling consumers into certain services. Another category involves the *decision makers* who make choices for the consumer. These could be family members, primary care physicians, or caregivers who act on behalf of consumers for various reasons. Finally, the category of *buyers* of healthcare services includes employers, business coalitions, and other groups that may indirectly control the behavior of consumers by determining which services they can and cannot utilize.

One of the most important findings from recent research relates to the importance of women in the healthcare decision-making process. It has already been established that women use a disproportionate share of healthcare resources. By virtue of being inordinately heavy users of health services for themselves, women effectively make the majority of purchase decisions on the consumer side. Furthermore, women generally make most of the decisions for their children and often their husbands as well. They are also likely to be involved as healthcare decision makers for their parents or other dependent family members. While women consume at least half of the personal health services in the United States, they could conceivably account for 80 percent or more of the decisions to purchase goods or use services.

A basic understanding of the process consumers go through in the purchase decision-making process is important for marketing planning purposes. The following steps in the consumer purchase model should be taken into consideration in the development of a marketing plan (Berkowitz and Hillestad 1991). The point at which the target market is located in the consumer behavior progression will determine the focus of the plan. The steps listed below in the decision-making process represent an amalgam of various approaches to this process overlaid with a healthcare perspective.

- *Problem recognition.* The first step in the purchase decision process occurs when the consumer recognizes a problem or need. The task for the marketer is to identify the circumstances or stimuli that trigger a particular need and use this knowledge to develop marketing strategies that trigger consumer interest.
- *Information search.* At this stage of the decision process the consumer is aroused to search for more information. The consumer may evidence heightened attention to the condition or initiate an active information search. (See Box 7.3 for a discussion of healthcare consumers' similarities and differences with other types of consumers in the approach to information searches.)

- *Initial awareness.* Awareness refers to the initial exposure of the target population to the good or service being marketed. Thus, during the information search the healthcare consumer becomes exposed to the various options that exist for addressing the problem at hand.
- *Knowledge emergence.* Knowledge concerning the options crystallizes as the healthcare consumer begins to understand the nature of the good or service and appreciate its potential for addressing the problem at hand.
- *Alternative evaluation.* At this stage the consumer is in a position to use the accumulated information to evaluate the available options and make a rational purchase decision. Various options may be ruled out and others maintained in the pool at this point.
- *Contract assessment.* Contract assessment is a step unique to healthcare in that many goods and services will not be considered for purchase if the provisions of the consumer's insurance plan do not cover them or the available provider does not accept the type of insurance carried (Berkowitz 1996).
- *Preference assignment.* Preferences develop at the point at which the consumer expresses a tendency for one good or service (e.g., a podiatrist rather than an orthopedic surgeon) or decides between different providers of the same service (e.g., Podiatrist A rather than Podiatrist B).
- *Purchase decision.* At this point the healthcare consumer makes a decision (or has it made for him or her) with regard to the good to be purchased or the service to be used. Healthcare is different from other consumer contexts in that a variety of players may be involved in the purchase decision at this point.
- *Product usage.* At this point the healthcare consumer actually buys the product in question or utilizes the service. This could be as simple as buying Band Aids at the neighborhood pharmacy or as complex as undergoing a heart transplant.
- *Postpurchase behavior.* This is the stage in the purchase decision process at which consumers take further action after purchase. It involves some type of assessment of the outcomes of the consumption episode and may involve input from family and other parties. Postpurchase behavior involves some assessment of satisfaction with regard to the experience, and the consumer subsequently becomes an advocate for the product or service (or a detractor if dissatisfied).

| **Box 7.3: Information Seeking by Healthcare Consumers** | The information search process for healthcare consumers tends to differ considerably from the process followed by consumers in other industries. The healthcare industry is unique in many ways and does not offer the same sources of information typically available to other consumers. This situation, of course, differs with the goods and services being offered. Personal health items like Band Aids, over-the-counter pharmaceuticals, and nutriceuticals are marketed in much the same |

manner as other consumer products. The primary difference arises, however, in the marketing of healthcare services.

The healthcare delivery system involves a complicated structure, and it is difficult for even career health professionals to fully understand it. For healthcare consumers faced with a choice with regard to a practitioner, facility, or program, the necessary information is seldom available. The most important difference is the lack of accurate and detailed information on the service providers in healthcare. Despite the growth of advertising in healthcare, it is just not possible to convey issues of quality, value, and outcomes as they relate to physicians, hospitals, and other providers in the same manner in which promotional material can describe other services.

In the face of this lack of information, where does the healthcare consumer turn? Traditionally, healthcare consumers have access to two primary sources of information on healthcare—one informal and one formal. The primary source of health information historically has been friends, relatives, neighbors, and work associates—individuals who can be informally accessed for information. Based on experience and information they have gathered, these associates can offer information seekers insights into various providers. The formal source, which may be somewhat less common but more authoritative, is physicians and other health personnel. By virtue of their position within the system and their presumed knowledge doctors in particular have been a major source of information for the consumer.

These two major sources have been supplemented by information gleaned from the media. This has historically included news obtained from print media (e.g., magazines, newspapers) and electronic media (e.g., radio, television). Newsletters geared to the needs of healthcare consumers have become common, and there is no end to the number and variety of self-help books published for healthcare consumers.

These sources of knowledge continue to be important to healthcare consumers today, but they have begun sharing space with others. With the introduction of Medicare and Medicaid in the 1960s and the emergence of managed care in the 1980s, healthcare consumers have been increasingly turning to their health plans in search of information on healthcare providers. This development reflects to a great extent the restrictions on the use of practitioners, facilities, and programs imposed by the health plans, but it also indicates the growing importance of health plans as a valuable source of information on the system. Managed care plans have been particularly aggressive in establishing call centers and encouraging their enrollees to seek information prior to making any health-related decisions.

The other source of healthcare information that came to the fore in the 1990s was the World Wide Web. The Internet has become a major source of health-related information, and a majority of "wired" healthcare consumers have accessed the Internet for information on a health issue they or someone else faced. Consumers are increasingly armed with Internet-generated information when they present themselves at the doctor's office. While the quality of the available data and the impact of better informed patients on the practice of medicine certainly merit discussion, the Internet is clearly replacing most traditional sources as the first resort in healthcare consumers' information searches.

Virtually every step in the consumer decision-making process has to be modified to allow for the special case of healthcare. While the framework for healthcare decision making is comparable to that for other types of consumers, numerous quirks in healthcare serve to create a unique situation. Familiarity with this process is important for the marketer, and the approach to the consumer will vary depending on the point in the process at which the consumer is located.

Summary

Although the consumer is the primary concern of virtually every industry, it is only in recent years that healthcare has come to think in terms of consumers. Most healthcare providers in the past thought of consumers until they entered the system as a patient. The prepatient and postpatient phases were neglected, and well people were not considered candidates for health services.

As healthcare has become more market driven, the importance of the consumer has been increasingly recognized. Healthcare organizations have begun to redefine patients as customers and appreciate the variety of customers that most healthcare organizations serve. Today, healthcare constituents take the form of consumers, customers, clients, patients, and enrollees, each of whom has unique characteristics. Other customers may include employees, board members, government agencies, the press, and the general public.

Healthcare consumers are different from consumers in under industries in a number of ways. These differences primarily reflect the unique characteristics of the healthcare industry. At the same time, healthcare consumers have a number of characteristics in common with consumers of other goods and services.

A number of demographic factors influence the behavior of health-care consumers. These include age, sex, race/ethnicity, marital status, income, and education. The attitudes held by consumers also plan an important role in the formal and informal health behavior of various groups within the population. Marketers can segment consumers along a number of dimensions, including geographic distribution, demographics, psychographics, usage, and desired benefits.

The decision-making process for healthcare consumers is generally the same as it is for other consumers. The same steps are followed, beginning with recognition of a need and ending with postpurchase behavior. However, the process for healthcare consumers is influenced by the unique characteristics of healthcare, and these consumers face some issues not experienced by consumers of other products.

Discussion Questions

- Why can it be argued that everyone in society (although perhaps involuntarily) is considered a potential consumer of health services?
- Why has the healthcare industry not historically thought of its customers as "consumers" in the sense that other industries have?
- In what ways are healthcare consumers different from the consumers of other goods and services?
- In what ways are healthcare consumers similar to the consumers of other goods and services?
- How can we distinguish between the different "varieties" of healthcare consumers (e.g., patients, clients, end users, enrollees)?
- What are some examples of *institutional* customers that must be considered by healthcare marketers?
- Explain the contention that healthcare organizations typically have a much broader range of customers than do organizations in most other industries.
- What are some of the demographic traits that are likely to influence the behavior of healthcare consumers?
- In what ways do psychographics (or lifestyles) influence the behavior of healthcare consumers?
- What role do attitudes play in influencing the behavior of healthcare consumers?
- What major shifts in attitudes have characterized healthcare consumers over the past few years?
- What are some of the bases for market segmentation that healthcare marketers may consider?

• What are the major steps in the decision-making process for health-care consumers, and how do these steps differ from those in other industries?

References

Berkowitz, E. N. 1996. *Essentials of Healthcare Marketing*. Gaithersburg, MD: Aspen.

Berkowitz, E. N., and S. G. Hillestad. 1991. *Healthcare Marketing Plans: From Strategy to Action*. Boston: Jones and Bartlett.

Eisenberg, D. M., R. C. Kessler, C. Foster, F. E. Norlock, D. R. Calkins, and T. L. Delbanco. 1993. "Unconventional Medicine in the U.S.—Prevalence, Costs and Patterns of Use." *New England Journal of Medicine* 328: 246–52.

Maslow, A. 1970. *Motivation and Personality, 2nd ed*. New York: Harper & Row.

National Center for Health Statistics. 1998. *Health United States, 1998*. Washington, DC: U.S. Government Printing Office.

———. 2002. *Health United States, 2002*. Washington, DC: U.S. Government Printing Office.

Additional Resource

Muschis, G. P., D. N. Bellenger, and C. Folkman Curasi. 2003. "What Influences the Mature Consumer?" *Marketing Health Services* 23 (4): 16–21.

HEALTHCARE PRODUCTS AND SERVICES

The first task for any marketer is to develop an understanding of the products being marketed. Although many healthcare sales involve goods, most deal with services, and the nature of the product depends on who the customer is. This chapter addresses the issues involved in determining what the product to be marketed is and explores the challenges faced in making this determination in healthcare. The implications of defining the product in various ways are reviewed, and the emerging retail aspect of healthcare sales is discussed.

Defining the Product

As stated in Chapter 4, the definition of marketing refers to the promotion of ideas, goods, or services as in any industry. Goods and services are considered types of products for our purposes, although the term *product* is often used interchangeably with healthcare *service*. In contrast to other industries, it is often difficult to precisely specify the product to be marketed, and marketers expend a great deal of effort in determining exactly what they are marketing.

In most industries, an organization's "product" would be obvious. Indeed, it would be its raison d'etre. The situation is not this simple in healthcare, and health professionals are not used to thinking in terms of products. The initial response to the question above is likely to be something like "quality care," "improved health," or "treatment and cure." While it is hoped that healthcare organizations provide these types of benefits to their customers, these answers are not very helpful to the marketer.

Product Mix

Many healthcare organizations offer a variety of products to their customers. An organization's *product mix* refers to the combination of goods, services, and even ideas it offers. Certainly, the hospital is an example of an organization that offers a wide range of goods and services. Indeed, a major hospital will offer hundreds, if not thousands, of different procedures. In addition, hospitals offer a variety of goods (in the form of drug doses, supplies, and equipment) that are charged to the customer.

Healthcare organizations mostly promote ideas—intangible concepts that are intended to convey a perception to the consumer. Image is an idea likely to be conveyed through marketing activities. The organization may want to promote the perception of quality care, professionalism, value, or some other subjective trait. Establishing a brand, for example, involves the marketing of an idea. The assumption that familiarity will breed utilization is the basis here.

Again, when advertising was first incorporated by healthcare organizations in the 1980s most of the attention was on promoting ideas. In particular, early marketers promoted the organization's image and establish it as the preferred provider in its market. While the trend has been away from image advertising toward service advertising, many healthcare organizations continue to market ideas to their target audiences. While the intangible benefits of healthcare may be among the most important, they are often difficult to conceptualize and effectively market.

Goods Versus Services

The primary distinction between goods and services is their degree of tangibility, or the extent to which they can be examined, touched, or experienced prior to purchase. Services tend to be consumed at the time they are provided (e.g., an immunization), whereas many goods tend to endure for an indefinite period (e.g., a home blood pressure cuff). These variations clearly determine the types of marketing strategy developed for each category.

A *good* refers to a tangible product typically purchased in an impersonal setting. The purchase of goods tends to be a one-shot episode, while obtaining *services* may be an ongoing process. While we generally think of healthcare as a service, the sale of goods is ubiquitous in the industry. Consumer-health products, such as toothpaste and soap, are household articles, and virtually everyone buys pharmaceuticals—whether prescription or over the counter. Home-testing kits and therapeutic equipment are acquired by consumers, and the sale and rental of durable medical equipment are common.

Consumer Products Versus Industrial Products

Goods can be classified by the types of users who buy them. *Consumer goods* are goods purchased by the ultimate consumer. *Industrial goods* are products purchased for use in the manufacture of other products that will at some point be purchased by the ultimate consumer. Both consumer and industrial goods have several variations. While we are mostly concerned with consumer products, we will make a distinction between personal consumer goods and goods purchased for professional or institutional use.

Consumer products may be classified in terms of the amount of effort and type of search the consumer uses in selecting the product. Thus, consumer goods in most industries fall into three categories: (1) convenience goods, (2) shopping goods, and (3) specialty goods. *Convenience goods* are products consumers purchase frequently with little deliberation or search before purchase; cold remedies, analgesics, and dietary supplements are examples. Because the consumer engages in little deliberation, name recognition and product distribution are critical concerns for the marketer. The makers of over-the-counter drugs, for example, expend considerable effort in establishing brand identity and ensuring prominent display in retail outlets.

A second type of consumer good is the shopping good. *Shopping goods* are products for which the consumer engages in a significant amount of search to compare competing brands on selected attributes such as price, style, or features; fitness equipment, computers, and cameras are common examples. Marketers of shopping goods must differentiate their brand from their competitors' on the attributes that are important to their customers. Salespeople often play a major role in helping the consumer learn about alternative brands (Berkowitz 1996).

The third category of consumer goods includes specialty items. *Specialty products* are those the consumer specifically seeks out. Often the consumer is loyal to a particular brand and will go to great lengths to find the particular item; common examples include exclusive brands of jewelry, perfume, and electronic equipment. Few goods in healthcare fall into the specialty category.

Industrial products have two broad levels of classification. *Production goods* are used to become part of a final product. Raw materials fit into this category and are of limited interest here. A second type of industrial goods is known as *support goods,* items used to assist in the production of other goods and services. Examples include a CT scanner, examination table, or the printer used to generate patient bills.

Nondurable Goods Versus Durable Goods

Goods can also be divided into two groups: nondurable goods and durable goods. A *nondurable good* is an item that can be consumed in some defined period; examples include food products, drugs, and bandages. A *durable good* is a product that lasts over an extended period. Items such as hospital beds, wheelchairs, and computers would be classified as durable goods.

The differences between goods and services and between nondurable and durable goods reflect important considerations for any marketing initiative. Nondurable products are often heavily advertised because consumers frequently purchase such products. Many pharmaceuticals are heavily advertised directly to the consumer. Retail store displays play a major role in direct marketing to the consumer; for durable products, personal sales often play a major role. Durable products usually cost more than nondurable products and are often far more complicated to use. For these products personal sales are essential to help answer customer questions and explain the intricacies of the product (Berkowitz 1996).

Quantifying Goods and Services

As mentioned in Chapter 4, services are difficult to conceptualize. Services are intangible in that they do not take on the concrete form of goods. They are more difficult to quantify, and consumers evaluate them differently. Because services are often more personal than goods (especially in the case of healthcare), they are likely to be assessed in subjective rather than objective terms. Services are variable; they cannot be subjected to the quality controls placed on goods but rather reflect the variations that characterize the human beings who provide them. Services are inseparable from the producer because they are dispensed on the spot, without any separation from the provider. Because services are perishable, they cannot be stored and once provided have no residual value. Because provision of services does not involve transfer of tangible property, ownership of services is also viewed differently from that of goods.

Healthcare providers are generally more concerned with the promotion of services than goods. Services are defined as intangible activities or processes offered to customers to solve problems, for which the organization is typically reimbursed. A physical examination, a flu shot, and open-heart surgery are examples of healthcare consumer services. While most people would recognize these activities as health services, the nature of services in healthcare is often difficult to describe. While a physician may break services down by procedure code, few services truly stand alone. The group of services that constitutes a particular surgical procedure, for example, may be *bundled* together. While clinicians (and their billing clerks) may see them as discrete services, the patient perceives them as a complex of services related to heart care, diabetes management, or cancer treatment.

Healthcare is different from other industries in that various parties are likely to have differing perceptions of the services offered. In the case of childbirth, for example, the mother is likely to see this as a natural experience, the physician as a medical episode, and the hospital administrator as an accounting event. Looked at differently, the mother is likely to see it as a unitary episode, the physician as a series of discrete activities, and the accounting department as a grouping of billable and non-billable services.

The healthcare marketer may see such an event in a different light from any of these other stakeholders. The marketer's task is to conceptualize the product and package it in an appropriate way for marketing purposes. Ultimately, however, the marketer has to conceive of the service in a manner to which the consumer can relate.

Product or Service Lines

In the 1980s, following the lead of other industries, healthcare organizations began to develop *product* or *service lines*. Other industries typically think in terms of product lines, but in healthcare service lines seem to be more appropriate. The establishment of service lines involved organizing the programs of the hospital into vertical groupings centered around clinical areas. These most typically included women's services, cancer services, cardiology, orthopedics, and pediatrics. Each service line was considered semi-autonomous and was charged with managing the vertical integration of its services. Thus, the service line administrator had broad control over the range of activities (including marketing) that supported the service line.

Some observers contend that services lines represented little more than the packaging of services for marketing purposes. While cases in which the service line was more in the packaging than in the substance certainly exist, in most cases a certain level of reorganization occurred around the specific clinical area. The use of the service line approach in healthcare remains controversial, and its merits are still being discussed today (see Box 8.1).

Ways to Conceptualize Products

A marketer may conceptualize the products offered by healthcare organizations in a number of ways, and an in-depth understanding of these distinctions is important. The nature and complexity of the product must be established, as the marketing approach will be a reflection of the manner in which the product is conceptualized.

Level of Care

Products may be categorized in terms of the level of care they represent. *Primary care* refers to the provision of the most basic health services. These generally involve the care of minor, routine problems, along with the pro-

Box 8.1: Healthcare Service Lines and Marketing	Over the past few years service line management has become the business design of choice for hundreds of hospitals nationwide. Service line management has evolved over the past 20 years as hospitals have looked for ways to become more agile, move closer to their customers, strengthen relationships with physicians, become more profitable, and go beyond cost cutting and reengineering to develop more innovative and effective ways to serve their patients.

A service line is a tightly integrated, overlapping network of semiautonomous clinical services and a business enterprise that bundles needed resources to provide specialized, focused care and value to a patient population. The most common service lines include cardiovascular services, orthopedics, rehabilitation, women's services, children's services, and oncology services. Service lines can be "virtual," in that all components are not usually under one roof; some services are horizontal and cross departments and disciplines. Indeed, the focus is not on the facility but on the services. A service line may be created around a business that is already well established, or the concept can be used to focus on a new service or niche.

The product line idea was developed by pacesetters in other industries—most notably Procter & Gamble, General Electric, and General Motors—as a way to decentralize decision making and strategic planning to make them more effective; improve cost management and productivity; enhance communication and collaboration; and, most important, get product line management teams closer to understanding the needs of their customers.

The product line management concept emerged in the healthcare industry in the 1980s as an organizational effort to deal with prospective reimbursement, a tight economic environment, declining revenues, and intense competition that drove the need for improving the way hospitals did business. However, accountability was limited, and product line management responsibility was heavily focused on marketing and public relations. In healthcare this concept has probably been carried furthest by pharmaceutical companies, which organize their business enterprises by product lines.

Many of the gains from product line management were erased with the advent of a new wave of change that began in the late 1980s. Hospitals became overwhelmed with the rise of managed care and integrated healthcare systems that spawned mergers, total quality management, restructuring (again), and redesign (or reengineering).

vision of general examinations and preventive services. For the patient primary care usually involves some self-care, perhaps followed by the seeking of care from a nonphysician health professional such as a pharmacist. For certain ethnic groups this may involve the use of a folk healer.

Formal primary care services are generally provided by physicians with training in general or family practice, general internal medicine, obstet-

The need to contain and reduce costs became critical, as did the need to build volume and profits.

As hospitals began to renew their patient focus in the 1990s the service line concept reemerged. This revitalized service line management model defines a hospital's clinical services and allocates organizational resources—human, financial, and strategic—to these service lines and clearly assigns accountability for performance to a service line leader.

This new service line platform integrates clinical and support services on a matrix management grid to create a horizontal integration of clinical services along a traditional continuum of care and a vertical integration of support services. Also built into this platform are education and wellness programs, retail models, business development (attracting and winning business directly), and physician relationship development, all with an increased emphasis on creating enhanced quality and value for patients.

Because the service line is closer to its costs and operational dynamics, its customer, and its competition, hospitals and health systems are decentralizing the accountability for strategic, operational, and financial performance from the corporate or executive office to the clinical service line. This shift in accountability to the service line maximizes hospital capacity by focusing on the best use of space and resources and provides more flexibility, or agility, in managing growth.

Whether the service line concept is an effective approach to healthcare strategy development is still open to debate, and little hard evidence documents the merits of this approach. This approach does facilitate the marketing of services in many ways, and the close relationship that can develop between operations and marketing represents an advantage. The focusing of marketing resources in this manner does have its benefits.

There is some question about the significance of service lines to customers. Ideally, service lines are designed to address consumer needs. However, it could be argued that most consumers do not think about healthcare in terms of vertical silos of care but as a continuum of services that extend across clinical lines. As service lines become more entrenched in healthcare a better understanding of their meaning for consumers should be established.

Source: Ireland, R. C. 2003. "Service Line Management Primer." *Service Line Leader* Newsletter. [Online article; retrieved 10/15/03.] http://www.snowinst.com/articles/sll-primer.htm.

rics/gynecology, or pediatrics. These practitioners are typically community based rather than hospital based, rely on direct first contact with patients rather than referrals from other physicians, and provide continuous rather than episodic care. Physician extenders like nurse practitioners and physician assistants are taking on a growing responsibility for primary care. In the mental health system, psychologists and other types of counselors constitute the primary level of care. Medical specialists may also provide a certain amount of primary care.

Primary care is generally delivered at the physician's office or some type of clinic. Hospital outpatient departments, urgent care centers, neighborhood clinics, and other ambulatory care facilities also provide primary care services. For certain segments of the population the hospital emergency room serves as a source of primary care. The home has increasingly become a site for the provision of primary care. This trend has been driven by the financial pressures on inpatient care, changing consumer preferences, and improved home care technology.

In terms of hospital services, primary care refers to those services that can be provided at a general hospital. These typically involve routine medical and surgical procedures, diagnostic tests, and obstetrics services. Primary care also includes emergency care (although not major trauma) and many outpatient services. Primary hospital care tends to be unspecialized and requires a relatively low level of technological sophistication.

Secondary care reflects a higher degree of specialization and technological sophistication than primary care, in keeping with the increased severity of the health problems. Physician care is provided by more highly trained practitioners such as specialized surgeons (e.g., urologists, ophthalmologists) and specialized internists (e.g., cardiologists, oncologists). Problems requiring more specialized skills and more sophisticated biomedical equipment fall into this category. Although much of the care is still provided in the physician office or clinic, these specialists tend to spend a larger share of their time in the hospital setting. Secondary hospitals are capable of providing more complex technological backup, physician specialist support, and ancillary services than primary care hospitals. These facilities are capable of handling moderately complex surgical and medical cases and serve as referral centers for primary care facilities.

Tertiary care addresses the most complex of surgical and medical conditions. The practitioners tend to be subspecialists housed in highly complex and technologically advanced facilities. Complex procedures such as open-heart surgery and reconstructive surgery are performed at these facilities, which provide extensive support services in terms of both personnel and technology. Tertiary care cases are usually handled by a team of medical or surgical specialists who are supported by the hospital's radiology, pathology, and anesthesiology physician staff. Tertiary care is generally provided at a few centers that serve large geographic areas. Frequently, a single hospital is not sufficient for the provision of tertiary care; a medical center may be required. These centers typically support functions not directly related to patient care, such as teaching and research.

Some procedures often performed at tertiary facilities may be considered as *quaternary care*. Organ transplantation—especially involving vital organs like heart, lungs, and pancreas—are included. Complicated trauma care is another example. This level of care is restricted to major medical centers, often in medical school settings. These procedures require the most sophisticated equipment and are often performed in association with research activities.

The level of care plays an important role in the type of marketing carried out. Consumers often have more discretion when it comes to primary care than for more specialized forms of care. Consumers can typically choose their primary care physician (although their insurance plan may impose limitations), and they can obtain primary care through urgent care centers or emergency rooms in the case of urgent or emergent situations. It is more difficult, however, to access specialists, especially those involved in tertiary or quaternary care. Typically, specialists require a referral from another physician or health professional, a situation that may be reinforced by the reluctance of insurance plans to reimburse for the services of a specialist who was not accessed in the proper manner.

For the marketer this means that the consumer is more of a target for primary care services than for more specialized services. Marketing tertiary or quaternary care to the general public is not likely to be very effective because in the typical case someone other than the patient will make the treatment decision. This does not mean that a hospital, for example, should not advertise the services of its specialists to the general public. Consumers need to be made aware of all of the available services, even if they cannot access them directly.

Level of Urgency

Another consideration is the level of urgency of the condition; health problems are generally thought to be routine, urgent, or emergent. Routine health problems comprise the bulk of primary care episodes; many, if not most, urgent care episodes involve routine care provided during off hours. True emergent care typically involves at least secondary care, if not tertiary or quaternary care.

While marketing can influence the use of all three categories of care, some are more amenable to marketing than others. Routine care, like primary care, represents more discretion on the part of consumers, and emergency care represents the least. Therefore, it makes sense to market primary care services directly to consumers. In some ways potential urgent care patients may be more amenable to marketing than even routine care patients. Often, users of urgent care centers do not have a regular source of care and are likely to be swayed by marketing when the need for care arises. The challenge here lies in the unpredictable nature of urgent care, and many segments of the population resist the use of such services.

Emergency services are perhaps the most difficult to market effectively to the general population. Emergency room use is a rare event, and many within the population do not have preconceived notions about emergency care. In situations in which the affected individual chooses the hospital emergency room, his or her doctor's affiliations or health plan restrictions are likely to be considerations. Someone other than the patient is likely to make the choice with regard to emergency department when the need arises. Thus, the marketing of emergency services may be more appropriately directed to ambulance companies, emergency medical technicians, police dispatchers, and other decision makers rather than the general public.

Inpatient Versus Outpatient Services

Health services may also be classified as inpatient or outpatient. Inpatient services require at least an overnight stay and are typically provided in hospitals. Outpatient (or ambulatory) services include care that involves less than a 24-hour stay within a health facility. As above, outpatient services are likely to be characterized by more consumer discretion than inpatient services. For many outpatient services consumers may present themselves for care without any prior relationship or even an appointment. The use of inpatient services requires at a minimum a referral or admission by a physician and possibly authorization by the patient's health insurance plan. While targeting the general public for outpatient services makes sense, the marketing approach for inpatient services should focus on the establishment and cultivation of a loyal medical staff and astutely negotiated contracts with health plans.

Medical Versus Surgical Services

A distinction is made for some purposes between medical services and surgical services. While we often speak of "med-surg" wards where both medical and surgical procedures are performed, the distinction between the therapeutic modalities needs to be noted. Medical procedures involve treatments based primarily on drug therapy, whereas surgical procedures refer to therapies that primarily involve surgery of some type. Of course, when any surgery is performed some drugs are administered, and when drug therapy is administered some surgical procedures, however minor, may be required.

These two approaches to care are obviously quite different and are implemented by different specialists. Medical therapy is typically carried out by internists and internal medical specialists (e.g., nephrologists, gastroenterologists), whereas surgery is performed by either general surgeons or, more frequently, surgical specialists (e.g., ophthalmic surgeons, orthopedic surgeons). While both types of therapies carry risks, the general public is more likely to attribute risks to surgical procedures. In either case the marketer must emphasize the benefits and minimize the risks of the procedures involved.

Diagnosis Versus Treatment

Differentiation between diagnosis and treatment is also common. Diagnostic procedures are used to diagnose conditions and test for the presence of a pathological condition. Treatments (or therapeutic procedures) are used to treat the condition once it has been diagnosed. Many diagnostic procedures are routine and administered at regular intervals to asymptomatic individuals; these may be referred to as screening tests. Tests administered in response to symptoms may be referred to as diagnostic tests. Hence, we have screening mammograms and diagnostic mammograms. This distinction is significant in that the same test may be marketed in a different manner depending on its use. Clearly, the approach to marketing differs depending on whether the product is a diagnosis or treatment. The emphasis with the former will be on prevention and early detection, with the intent of maintaining health. The emphasis with the latter is on treatment and cure, and the intent is to restore health.

Clinical Versus Nonclinical Services

Marketers may also distinguish between clinical and nonclinical services. Clinical services involve the administration of some formal medical procedure; these are what come to mind when we think about health services. Clinical services include an examination, diagnostic test, or therapeutic procedure, with administration by a clinical practitioner of some type.

Healthcare providers have added a number of nonclinical services to their practices. Hospitals provide numerous examples of this with their parking services, television services, and chaplain programs. Many practitioners offer social support services that complement their clinical services (e.g., support groups for patients of an oncology practice). Others may offer child care or transportation.

Obviously, one would market nonclinical services differently from clinical services. While clinical services may appear to be by far the most important—indeed, they generate the most revenue—it should be noted that consumers are more likely to evaluate their experiences based on nonclinical services. Thus, nonclinical services need to receive adequate attention from marketers.

Elective Versus Nonelective Procedures

Finally, a distinction may be made between elective procedures and non-elective procedures. Nonelective procedures are considered medically necessary; elective procedures are those that patients voluntarily choose to obtain. Nonelective procedures include those we think of as life-saving measures, although medically necessary services do not always deal with life-threatening conditions. Elective procedures include nontherapeutic abortions, laser eye surgery, facelifts, and hair transplants. Some joint surgery (e.g., for tennis elbow) may not be considered medically necessary and thus are classified as elective.

While elective and nonelective procedures may be marketed in much the same manner, significant differences should be noted. First, the decision maker is likely to be different. Nonelective surgery is generally prescribed by a medical practitioner and, being medically necessary, is covered by health insurance plans. The decision to undergo an elective procedure is generally made by the patient, perhaps with the advice of a medical practitioner. Because of their elective nature, these procedures are typically not covered by insurance. For this reason the appeal to the consumer is likely to be quite different. For nonelective procedures the demand cannot be influenced by marketing. Thus, the emphasis must be on influencing the choice of provider when a condition arises. In fact, a hospital seeking patients for nonelective procedures may focus its marketing on admitting and referring physicians to channel these procedures into its system.

Marketing elective procedures has a lot in common with the marketing of nonmedical services. Providers of these services are much more prone to advertise their services and often compete on the same basis as providers of other types of services. Thus, eye surgeons and plastic surgeons advertise their low prices, convenient locations, and efficient customer service. In addition, it may actually be possible to *create* demand for these services. Most balding men were probably happy to suffer in silence with their hair loss until they saw promotions for hair restoration. By introducing this new service a market was essentially created where one did not exist before.

One other way to categorize products is in terms of their point in the product life cycle (see Box 8.2).

Common Healthcare Products

While we have described the nature of healthcare products in a variety of ways, we have not described these products in detail or noted the types of healthcare organizations that provide them. This information is critical

✗ Read

| Box 8.2: The Product Life Cycle | Healthcare products, like other products, experience a natural life cycle that includes four distinct stages: introduction, growth, maturity, and decline. For marketers an understanding of the stage of the product life cycle is critical. If the organization is primarily involved in providing inpatient services, an appreciation of the point in the product life |

cycle where inpatient services can be placed is required. If a marketing plan is being developed for a specific procedure, the point in the life cycle where this product resides must be determined.

Introduction or Market Development

The first stage in the life cycle of a product is the introduction or market development stage. At this point a new product is launched. Because the product is likely to be innovative, most of the marketing effort is directed toward creating awareness and cultivating early adopters in the market. At this stage there are relatively few competitors, and goods and services are not standardized. Entry into the market is relatively easy because there are few established players; the introduction of desktop computers in the 1980s is an example of this stage.

Growth

The second stage is the growth phase. At this point the industry has become established, and the good or service has been accepted by the market. Expansion is rapid as new customers are attracted and additional competitors enter the arena. Products or services become increasingly standardized, although enhancements may continue to contribute to product evolution. Marketing planning at this stage emphasizes differentiation of the organization, product, or service. The rapid growth of home health care during the 1980s provides an example of this type of expansion.

Maturity

During the third stage the product achieves maturity. At this point most of the potential customers have been captured and growth begins to trail off. Because few new customers are available, competition for existing customers increases. Product features and pricing are highly standardized, and little differentiation remains between competitors. The number of competitors decreases as consolidation occurs among the various players in the market, and it becomes increasingly difficult for new players to enter the market. Marketing activities emphasize retaining existing customers or capturing competitors' customers. Traditional hospital inpatient services are an example of a product that has reached the maturity stage.

When a product reaches maturity it must adapt to its new state to remain viable. At this point there are three strategies for stretching the life of the product: (1) product modification, (2) market modification, and (3) product repositioning. Hospitals have attempted to employ all of these strategies in the face of product maturity. Hospitals have attempted to add goods or services to ensure that utilization does not continue to decline.

Hospitals have changed, or attempted to change, their image from one of inpatient services to a community resource offering a wide range of goods and services.

Decline

At the final stage the product experiences a period of decline. The number of customers decreases as consumers substitute new products or services. A "shakeout" typically occurs among industry players as the dominant competitors squeeze out the less entrenched, and other competitors adopt a different strategic direction. Competition among the remaining players for existing customers becomes even more heated. Because no innovations are being introduced and the customer base cannot be expanded, the remaining competitors increasingly emphasize reducing costs to maintain profitability.

Marketing's Role

The role of marketing will differ depending on the product's stage in the life cycle, which is likely to influence the packaging of goods and services, promotional techniques, approaches to competitors, and relationships with other organizations. During the introductory stage, when the product represents an innovation, the marketer's primary task is to educate consumers concerning the product and facilitate a first-to-market approach. During the growth stage the marketing emphasis is on differentiating the product from that of the competitors, capitalizing on its attributes, and penetrating new markets.

During the maturity stage the role of marketing shifts dramatically. Few new customers for the product exist, so the emphasis must be on retaining current customers and capturing customers from competitors. This is likely to be a period of market consolidation, and the marketer may be involved in perpetuating the organization's image during a period of turmoil. During the decline stage of the life cycle the marketer must focus on maintaining current customers and presenting the product in creative new ways to help expand its life span.

from the marketer's perspective in that the marketing team will generally focus on a specific service for its marketing campaign rather than the more generalized marketing of the organization. The marketing of ideas was discussed earlier and receives no further attention here.

Categories of Goods

While healthcare is considered a service industry, a significant amount of goods are sold by healthcare organizations, including healthcare providers. Hospitals provide a wide range of goods to their patients, including bandages, supplies, medication, food, and other nondurable goods. They also sell durable goods in the form of crutches, braces, and prosthetic devices. Hospitals may provide home monitoring or treatment equipment. They may even sell high-end durable goods such as hospital beds and wheel-chairs. They may also sell other goods through a gift shop, resource library, or other retail-type enterprises.

Some of the service line extensions of hospitals may also be involved in the sale of goods on a retail basis. For example, the fitness center might sell nutritional supplements, athletic attire, and fitness equipment. The cardiac rehabilitation program may sell videos, books, and other resources used in the rehabilitation process. (Box 8.3 describes the emergence of retail medicine.)

Other institutions for inpatient care may provide similar goods, although none is likely to offer the range of a hospital. Nursing homes, residential treatment centers, and assisted-living centers are likely to provide supplies, medication, food, and other nondurable goods to their patients or residents. Some of these goods are considered part of the room charge or surgical fee, and others are itemized on the patient's bill.

Physicians perform many of the same procedures on their patients that are carried out with hospital patients, so they provide many of the same goods, including wound dressings, casts, disposable supplies, and medications. These are typically not itemized separately for the patient but are included in the overall cost of the professional services. Some physicians have become increasingly involved in the retail aspect of healthcare, offering their patients a range of related goods. For example, a cardiologist may sell videos, audiotapes, and cookbooks describing ways to maintain heart health. A dermatologist may offer a range of skin-care products that address various conditions, some of which may not be clinically significant. A number of types of physicians may offer nutritional supplements and vitamins. While these retail activities are not always encouraged by the American Medical Association, it appears that they are becoming entrenched in physician practices in a number of specialties.

Among other practitioners, some sell numerous goods, whereas others sell relatively few. A major part of an optometrist's business (and, to a lesser extent, an ophthalmologist's) is the dispensing of eyeglasses and contact lenses. While dentists primarily provide a service, for many a considerable portion of revenues are derived from the sale of dentures, braces, and other orthodontic devices. Other practitioners, such as chiropractors and podiatrists, provide little in the way of goods for sale. Similarly, the array of psychological therapists and counselors who practice independently seldom offer goods to their clients.

Categories of Services

The primary function of healthcare providers is to offer services aimed at addressing a particular healthcare need. It would be impractical to itemize

<table>
<tr><td>

**Box 8.3:
The
Emergence
of Retail
Medicine**

</td><td>

The concept of *retail medicine,* or healthcare available to the masses outside a traditional institutional setting, is coming to occupy a new niche in the elective outpatient medicine marketplace. According to surgicenteronline.com the $5 billion retail esthetic medicine market encompasses everything from preventive medicine to cosmetic surgery. While there is no definitive estimate of the number of retail medicine centers in the United States, established outpatient facili-

</td></tr>
</table>

ties are cashing in on the trend and diversifying their existing menus of diagnostic and surgical services.

Preventive imaging centers are growing in number, and the variety of procedures is increasing. Many new centers are promoting general body imaging, heart scanning, lung screening, and virtual colonoscopy. The setting for screening and imaging varies from outpatient radiology clinics to hospital campuses to wellness centers. Radiology practices are also expanding the use of expensive diagnostic equipment to the large group of individuals who are currently without symptoms but are concerned about prevention. The United States has an estimated 100 privately owned or institution-affiliated screening centers, and the number is growing rapidly.

The retail medicine trend is also introducing new buzzwords within the healthcare community, including *medical entrepreneurs* who market their services to the *worried well* and *worried wealthy.* Early on, typical consumers were wealthier, proactive by nature, and independent thinkers not relying solely on physician advice. The interest level has broadened as more middle-class individuals have friends, colleagues, or family members who have succumbed to diseases discovered at a late stage. In addition, thousands of scanned individuals talk about their experiences, and advertising and media stories are pervasive.

all of the services offered by a large healthcare organization, but the major categories are noted here.

The hospital is the focal point of the U.S. healthcare system and the venue for a wide variety of services. The fee schedule for a hospital would include thousands of individual services, creating quite a challenge for those trying to understand the system. These services are categorized in a variety of ways to bring some order to the process.

One way of looking at these services is in terms of clinical areas. Thus, services may be classified as obstetric, pediatric, cardiac, oncology, orthopedic, and so forth. The variety of services provided to obstetric patients, for example, are grouped together, as are those for the other clinical categories. The prospective payment system introduced by Medicare recognized these categories and made them the industry standard. Various clinical support services, such as radiology and laboratory services, are generally established separately and serve patients in all clinical categories.

Aging baby boomers—the majority of the individuals who consume retail medicine—are more concerned about their health than any previous generation, and they drive much of the interest in retail marketing. One of the most sought-after components of the retail medicine trend is the full-body scan, which medical entrepreneurs say will reveal abnormalities in the body that can be addressed before they have a chance to become life threatening. CT scans promise to detect latent signs of conditions ranging from tumors to gallstones, clogged arteries to cancer.

Retail medicine often emphasizes prevention, an aspect of care largely ignored by hospitals and physician practices. Proactive citizens frequently will pay out of pocket for more sophisticated or attentive medical services. The owners of screening centers are giving the public what they inherently understand—prevention is better than a cure, and early detection is the key to successful preventive strategies. Also included as examples of retail medicine are the variety of fitness and wellness programs that healthcare organizations offer to the general public.

There has also been a trend toward the retailing of various goods through physicians' offices. Cardiologists may offer resources like books, videos, and audiotapes on heart health and rehabilitation for purchase by their patients. Obstetricians and pediatricians may sell resource materials on childbirth and parenting. Dermatologists may offer a range of products for skin care, sun protection, and hair growth. A variety of practitioners vend nutritional supplements and vitamins as a sideline to their practices.

Source: Pyrek, K. M. 2003. [Online information; retrieved 10/29/03.] http://www.surgicenteronline.com/articles/2c1feat2.html.

Another way of classifying the services provided by hospitals (and certain other facilities) is into facility-based services and professional services. Services associated with the hospital stay include room charges, nursing fees, and supplies as well as some overhead costs. Many of these services are bundled in the per diem room fee, but services that involve variable costs (e.g., breathing treatments) may be charged separately by the hospital as part of the facility fee. Professional fees are typically charged separately by attending and consulting physicians because they are not employed by the hospital but rather provide services (and bill) independently. Hospital-based physicians (e.g., radiologists, anesthesiologists, hospitalists) also submit separate bills that may be combined with the facility fee.

The services provided by a hospital may also be divided into diagnostic and therapeutic categories; in fact, different coding systems may be used for them. Routine diagnostic procedures (e.g., x-rays, blood tests, urinalyses) as well as specialized diagnostic tests (e.g., mammograms, CT scans, bone density tests) are offered in the hospital setting. Hospitals typically provide the widest array of diagnostic capabilities of any healthcare organization, and few diagnostic tests offered by other clinicians are not available within the hospital.

Therapeutic procedures cover the wide range of treatments provided within the hospital. These may range from simple procedures such as administration of medication and intravenous fluids to complex procedures such as open-heart surgery and organ transplantation. As noted above, these are typically grouped into clinical categories and supervised by administrators dedicated to that clinical sphere. (At least a basic understanding of the coding systems used in healthcare is necessary, and Box 8.4 provides an overview.)

One other distinct category of services provided by the hospital is emergency care. The emergency department is designed to handle cases that are urgent enough that they cannot be processed through the normal admission procedures. Theoretically, these departments handle serious injuries and health conditions that require immediate attention. They are staffed with physicians and nurses trained in emergency medicine and backed up with an array of hospital personnel. Emergency departments maintain or have access to the diagnostic equipment for expeditiously determining the condition of the patient. Services provided in the emergency department are charged separately from those for inpatients. Like inpatients, emergency patients are charged both facility and professional fees.

Hospitals are also likely to offer spin-off services related to their inpatient activities. For example, many hospitals have established occupational health programs and sports medicine programs to serve their patients and the community. Some hospitals offer home health, rehabilitation, and hospice programs as "follow along" services for their core activities. While these extension programs may contain a few unique services, for the most part they represent the repackaging of existing services into these focused programs. For example, a fitness program targeting the hospital's employees and community residents may combine existing services such as physical examinations, stress testing, cardiac rehabilitation services, and recreational therapy with services typically provided by nonmedical fitness centers such as personal trainers and aerobics instruction.

Other categories of services likely to be offered by hospitals include prevention, education, and community outreach programs. Patient educators may teach prevention to hospitalized patients or provide educational programs outside the hospital to patients or the general public. Nurses may provide educational services to postsurgery and obstetrics patients, while nutritionists may offer guidance to a wide range of patient types. Some of these prevention and education services are built into the facility fee; others are charged separately to the patient. Community outreach programs

> **Box 8.4:
> Coding
> Systems in
> Healthcare**

The healthcare marketer is likely to be overwhelmed by the variety of coding schemes used in the U.S. healthcare system. A number of different systems are in use, and it is impossible to understand healthcare without a working knowledge of the manner in which conditions and procedures are classified and recorded. The classification systems briefly described below are commonly used; however, more information than can be provided here will ultimately be required to gain an understanding of these various systems.

International Classification of Diseases

The most widely recognized and used disease classification system is the *International Classification of Diseases* (ICD) developed by the World Health Organization. The ICD system is designed for the classification of morbidity and mortality information and for indexing diseases and procedures that occur within hospitals and certain other healthcare settings. The present classification system includes two components: diagnoses and procedures. Two sets of codes are assigned to the respective components, and the codes are detailed enough that fine distinctions can be made among different diagnoses and procedures. (A different system is used for recording procedures in physicians' offices and other outpatient settings.)

The disease classification component is composed of 17 disease and injury categories, along with two supplementary classifications. Within each of these major categories specific conditions are listed in detail. A three-digit number is assigned to the various major subdivisions within each of the 17 categories. These three-digit numbers are extended another digit to indicate a subcategory within the larger category (to add clinical detail or isolate terms for clinical accuracy). A fifth digit is sometimes added to specify any factors further associated with that particular diagnosis. For example, with the ICD-9 version Hodgkin's disease, a form of malignant neoplasm or cancer, is coded 201. A particular type of Hodgkin's disease, Hodgkin's sarcoma, is coded 201.2. If the Hodgkin's sarcoma affects the lymph nodes of the neck, it is coded 201.21.

The supplementary classifications are a concession to the fact that many nonmedical factors are involved in the onset of disease, responses to disease, and use of services. These additional categories attempt to identify causes of disease or injury states external to the biophysical system.

Procedure categories were introduced for the first time with the ICD-9 version. The procedure component is divided into 16 categories. Of these, 15 are keyed to specific body systems (e.g., nervous system, digestive system), and one involves diagnostic procedures and residual therapeutic procedures. A two-digit scheme is used, with a code being carried out to two decimal places when necessary to provide more detail. The system was designed to accommodate use in both hospital and ambulatory care settings.

Current Procedural Terminology

While the ICD classification system focuses on procedures performed under the auspices of a hospital or clinic, the *Current Procedural Terminology* (CPT) system relates exclusively to procedures and services performed by physicians. Physician-provided procedures and services are divided into five categories: medicine, anesthesiology, surgery, radiology and pathology, and laboratory services. In its fourth edition (CPT-4) this system identifies each procedure and service with a five-digit code number. This method attempts to facilitate accurate, specific, and uniform coding for physician offices.

Examples of coded procedures include surgical operations, office visits, and x-ray readings. The most accurate descriptor is determined from the CPT guidebook by the provider, and that code is assigned. In addition to the identifying code, the five-digit number allows for modifiers to be appended. Modifiers may indicate situations in which an adjunctive service was performed. The manual also contains some useful information on accepted definitions for levels of care and extensiveness of consultation. Some 7,000 variations of procedures and services are cataloged.

Another set of codes has been developed to supplement the CPT codes. The Healthcare Common Procedure Coding System (HCPCS) is administered by the Centers for Medicare and Medicaid Services (CMS). HCPCS involves a listing of services provided by physicians and other providers that are not covered under the CPT coding scheme. These include certain physician services, along with nonphysician services such as ambulance, physical therapy, and durable medical equipment.

Diagnosis Related Groups

In response to the financial demands placed on the Medicare program, the Medicaid program, and other federally supported healthcare initiatives, the federal government introduced the prospective payment system (PPS) as the basis for reimbursement for health services rendered under Medicare. PPS limits the amount of reimbursement for services provided to each category of patient based on rates determined by CMS.

The basis for prospective payment is the *diagnosis related group* (DRG). Using the patient's primary diagnosis as the starting point CMS has developed a mechanism for grouping all hospital patients into more than 500 DRGs. The idea is to link payment to the consumption of resources, with the assumption that a patient's diagnosis should be the best predictor of resource utilization. The primary diagnosis is modified by factors such as coexisting diagnoses, presence of complications, patient age, and usual length of hospital stay to derive the diagnostic categories.

involve information and referral, health education, and wellness training generally geared to the general public. They could also include home visits by hospital staff to monitor health problems.

No other institutional setting provides the range of services of a general hospital, although some specialty hospitals may provide some services that are unique to that specialty. Specialty hospitals may be dedicated to a

For many purposes (e.g., general reporting, statistical analysis, planning), DRGs represent too fine a distinction among conditions. For these purposes DRGs have been grouped into 23 major diagnostic categories based primarily on the different body systems.

DRGs are categorized as either medical DRGs or surgical DRGs. In the calculation of reimbursement for services each DRG is given a weight, which is the major factor in a complicated formula for determining the rate of reimbursement for each hospital participating in the Medicare program.

Although introduced for use in federal healthcare programs, the DRG system was quickly adopted by other health plans as a basis for reimbursement. This system has become the standard classification system for hospitalized patients in the United States and has been adopted by other countries around the world.

Ambulatory Payment Classification

In view of rising outpatient costs CMS developed a system similar to DRGs for the outpatient environment. This system is referred to as *Ambulatory Payment Classification* (APC). As with DRGs, APCs focus on the facility component of healthcare costs, not on physician charges. The basis for the fee is the patient visit, rather than the entire episode as in the case of DRGs. An APC-specific diagnosis code has been developed, and CPT codes continue to be used to classify procedures and ancillary services. Introduced in August 2000, APC codes are now widely used in outpatient facilities.

Diagnostic and Statistical Manual

The definitive reference on the classification of mental disorders is the *Diagnostic and Statistical Manual* (fourth edition), commonly referred to as DSM-IV. Published by the American Psychiatric Association, the DSM remains the last word in mental disease classification, despite long-standing criticism of the classification scheme. Its 17 major categories of mental illness and more than 450 identified mental conditions are considered exhaustive.

The DSM classification system is derived in part from the ICD system. It is essentially structured in the same manner, using a five-digit code. The fourth digit indicates the variety of the particular disorder under discussion, and the fifth digit refers to any special consideration related to the case. The nature of the fifth-digit modifier varies depending on the disorder under consideration. Unlike the other classification systems discussed, the DSM system contains rather detailed descriptions of the disorders categorized therein and serves as a useful reference in this regard.

particular population (e.g., women, children) or specific condition (e.g., substance abuse, mental illness). In the case of the former, similar services as in a general hospital are likely to be performed, although the emphasis is on specialized services for women and children, respectively. Some unique services may be provided for children (and to a lesser extent women) in such hospitals. With regard to the latter, specialized services for the treatment of substance abuse and mental illness will likely be used in these institutions. Many general hospitals are not staffed or equipped to manage these types of conditions, so specialized facilities develop certain unique services.

Hospitals also provide a wide range of support services of which the patient is seldom aware; these are bundled into per diem or overhead charges. Some of these may be more obvious than others, such as janitorial services, landscaping, and parking services. Others, such as medical records management, information systems operation, research services, and marketing services, are not so obvious.

Other facilities that house patients on an inpatient basis include nursing homes and residential treatment centers. Assisted-living facilities in their various forms may occasionally provide health services, but not typically. The term *nursing home* is something of a misnomer in that a limited amount of actual medical care is provided. Most services provided in a nursing home are custodial and involve the personal care of patients. To the extent that nursing home residents require medication administration, chronic disease monitoring, and other forms of routine care, these services are carried out by some category of nursing personnel. Physicians are on call but not typically in residence. Unlike for a hospital patient, most services provided to nursing home patients are covered under their monthly fees. Nonroutine health services are typically covered by a third-party payer such as private insurance, Medicare, or Medicaid.

Residential treatment facilities provide a narrower range of services than hospitals but typically cover a broader range than nursing homes. Unlike nursing homes, residential treatment facilities are involved in the active treatment of most of their residents. Facilities for the treatment of addictions or mental disorders, for example, typically provide a range of appropriate services, usually folded into the per diem charges of the treatment center.

Physicians are the most common type of practitioner with whom the public comes in contact in seeking health services. The range of services the physician provides varies with the specialty involved, although most specialists provide a core group of procedures. Most physicians perform routine medical examinations (although the emphasis may vary with the specialty) and diagnostic tests such as x-rays, blood tests, and urinalyses. Specialists may not perform a full examination but rather focus on their particular area. An ophthalmologist, for example, is not likely to be concerned with other body systems beyond the eyes unless complications affect vision (e.g., with diabetes). Many patients of specialists have been referred to them by their primary care physicians, and the basic examination is presumed to have already occurred. The circumstances dictate the extent to which a specialist will reexamine the referred patient.

The range of diagnostic and treatment procedures offered by physicians (including osteopaths) is understandably more narrow than that provided by a hospital. Most specialties list hundreds of procedures on their fee schedules, but it could be argued that the 80/20 rule applies—that is, 20 percent of the procedures account for 80 percent or more of the patients. Physicians do not charge separate facility fees, and overhead charges are built into the office visit fee. Patients are charged separately for nonroutine diagnostic tests (e.g., x-rays) and any treatments provided (e.g., injections).

Most physicians provide primarily nonelective or medically necessary services, and more or less standard fee schedules cover these diagnostic and treatment services. In fact, the allowable fees established by third-party payers generally set the parameters for physician fee schedules. However, some physicians provide a mix of elective and nonelective procedures (e.g., orthopedic surgeons), and some provide exclusively elective procedures (e.g., many cosmetic surgeons). With elective procedures there are fewer guidelines and more latitude in terms of the fees that can be charged. For this reason physicians seldom compete on price for nonelective procedures but often attempt to provide a price advantage on their elective procedures. Thus, an ophthalmic surgeon may be essentially limited in terms of charges for Medicare-reimbursed cataract surgery but has considerable discretion in terms of fees for elective laser eye surgery.

The services offered by other practitioners vary depending on the profession. Optometrists offer examination services and provide a limited range of therapy. Chiropractors perform examinations and typically provide a narrow range of procedures aimed at spinal manipulation. Podiatrists perform examinations and offer a range of medical and surgical procedures for the treatment of foot problems. These procedures generally fall into the standard coding classifications used by physicians and hospitals.

Various mental health providers also offer a range of services geared to the treatment of mental disorders. The diagnostic categories used are likely to be unique to the mental health field, whereas the procedures performed typically fall into the standard coding classifications. While the range of diagnosis is extremely broad, mental health services typically fall under about a dozen major procedures.

Alternative therapy providers offer a wide range of services reflecting the diversity of therapeutic approaches that exist. Chiropractors were noted above, but practitioners of acupuncture, massage therapy, homeopathy, naturopathy, and other alternative therapies provide a variety of services that may not be specifically listed in the standard classification systems. As these procedures become more common, they will likely be added to the standard fee schedules.

One other category of service providers that should be considered in this context is social service organizations. While most social service organizations are not in the business of providing medical care, many do perform services that are considered health-related and often reimbursable by third-party payers. For example, agencies addressing HIV/AIDS issues may provide diagnostic tests for HIV, and a family planning agency may provide physical examinations and perform clinical procedures. As our definition of health expands, the boundaries between healthcare providers and social service agencies can be expected to blur.

Summary

The first task for any marketer is to develop an understanding of the products being marketed. The healthcare industry, however, is not used to thinking in terms of products, and marketers often have to help health professionals define the goods and services they are offering the consumer. Many healthcare organizations offer a variety of products to their customers, and the prevalence of services in healthcare makes marketing more of a challenge than it is in some industries. Because of the nature of healthcare, healthcare organizations frequently market ideas, concepts, or images rather than discrete goods or services.

Healthcare marketers must be able to distinguish between different types of goods and services and appreciate the differences in marketing approaches required. Healthcare is complicated by the fact that products may reflect differing levels of complexity, urgency, or means of distribution. Service line management has been adopted by some healthcare organizations in an effort to bring more organization to the management and marketing of various types of care.

Discussion Questions

- Why have healthcare organizations not historically been concerned about carefully defining their products?
- What is it about healthcare products that makes clearly defining them difficult?
- What are the important distinctions between goods and services, and what are the implications of these distinctions for marketing?
- What are some of the different goods that healthcare organizations may offer?

- Why is the service configuration for healthcare organizations often more complicated than that for other industries, and why is this complexity a concern for marketers?
- What is *service line management,* and what are the pros and cons of using a service line management approach in healthcare?

Reference

Berkowitz, E. N. 1996. *Essentials of Health Care Marketing.* Gaithersburg, MD: Aspen.

Additional Resources

Following are some examples of commercially available market research reports:

Freedonia Group. 2003. *Disposable Medical Supplies.* Cleveland, OH: Freedonia Group.

Kalorama Information. 2002. *The U.S. Market for Home Care Products.* New York: Kalorama Information.

Theta Reports. 1999. *Disability and Rehabilitation Product Markets.* New York: Theta Reports.

FACTORS IN HEALTH SERVICES UTILIZATION

Marketing is all about identifying and responding to the demand for goods and services, and in healthcare the demand for health services ultimately drives all healthcare marketing activities. The determination of demand in healthcare is particularly complex and requires an understanding of the many factors that influence the ultimate utilization of health services.

Most decisions about whether to offer a service will be predicated on presumed levels of demand. Once a service is offered, virtually all decisions related to the continued provision of that service will be a function of the level of demand. For this reason health marketers spend a great deal of their time and effort trying to determine current and future levels of demand for total health services or the specific services offered by the organization involved in the marketing process.

The factors influencing the level of demand for health services have become increasingly complex, and past utilization patterns are seldom predictive of future utilization. The significant demographic, socioeconomic, and psychographic transformation the U.S. population has been undergoing has served to modify the level of demand. At the same time, managed care arrangements and other developments in healthcare influence the level of demand for health services. Indeed, a frequent function of marketing is the creation of demand (see Box 9.1). These developments have made the task of projecting demand for health services increasingly challenging at a time when the ability to do so is critical to the survival of most organizations.

Defining Demand

Demand is an imprecise concept as applied to health services, and the term is often used interchangeably with other terms. In fact, no one definition of

[handwritten marginalia: "need want desire of a product"]

demand is in common use. The concept is sufficiently vague and used in so many different ways that it is difficult to provide an operational definition.

Part of the confusion in defining (and measuring) health services demand stems from a lack of agreement as to *who* the customer for health services is. This is seldom an issue in other industries, but it is of paramount importance in healthcare. Typically, the services demanded by the end user—usually the patient—are the primary consideration. However, other customer groups, such as physicians, health plans, and employers, may play a part in determining demand. For health plans the customer may actually be the benefits manager for an employer-sponsored plan. For medical supply or equipment companies the customers may be retail distributors.

An important aspect of consumer demand in healthcare is the fact that demand may not be generated directly by the end user but by some

---

Box 9.1: Creating Demand for a Healthcare Product

The introduction of healthcare products to a market generally represents a response to the demand for healthcare demonstrated by the market. In the typical case providers of healthcare goods and services develop their products in response to an established health condition or other felt need. It is not unusual today, however, for purveyors of goods or services to proactively identify new conditions that can benefit from an existing product. In this manner healthcare organizations *create* demand for a product in response to an identified health problem that did not previously exist.

Pharmaceutical companies have been particularly aggressive in their attempts to define new health conditions that could benefit from one of their products and subsequently promote that product to both consumers and those writing prescriptions. To create demand, however, the healthcare organization must demonstrate to the public and the medical community that (1) an identifiable health problem exists and (2) the company has a product for treating that problem.

Marketers may create demand for a healthcare product in several ways, including classifying ordinary processes or ailments of life as medical problems, portraying mild symptoms as portents of a serious disease, defining personal or social problems as medical ones, conceptualizing risks as diseases, and maximizing disease-prevalence estimates to enhance the perceived size of a medical problem.

Examples of campaigns to create demand for a particular product are unlimited. Conditions for which case studies may be presented include hair loss, irritable bowel syndrome (IBS), social phobias, osteoporosis, and erectile dysfunction. Each of these conditions has been subjected to demand-generation techniques in one way or another.

IBS may be considered as an example. Based on research conducted in Australia, analysts identified a concerted effort on the part of a pharmaceutical company to create demand for products developed to treat this condition. IBS has long been considered a common functional disorder, yet it is currently experiencing something of a global

intermediary. Thus, physicians may determine patient demand for hospital care and pharmaceuticals, insurance companies may influence the demand for services by virtue of the treatments they cover, and so forth.

Perhaps the best way to approach the demand concept in the case of healthcare consumers is by examining its component parts. From a marketing perspective demand can be conceptualized as the ultimate result of the combined effect of (1) healthcare needs, (2) healthcare wants, (3) recommended standards for healthcare, and (4) actual utilization patterns (Berkowitz, Pol, and Thomas 1997).

Healthcare Needs

Healthcare needs can be defined in terms of the overall health status of a population, or more specifically in terms of the number of conditions within

makeover. Without question, many people with the condition are affected by their symptoms, but the arrival of new drugs has seen manufacturers seeking to change the way the world thinks about IBS.

In this case a medical communications company was engaged to formulate a medical education program to promote the perception of IBS as a "credible, common, and concrete disease." The educational program was part of the marketing strategy of the manufacturer of a leading drug for the treatment of IBS. The key aim of the educational program was to establish IBS in the minds of doctors as a significant and discrete disease state. Furthermore, the campaign sought to convince patients that IBS is a common and recognized medical disorder for which a new, clinically proven therapy exists.

This process for generating demand involved the establishment of an advisory board to provide advice to corporate sponsors on current opinion in gastroenterology and on opportunities for shaping perceptions. Further work included the development of best practice guidelines for diagnosing and managing IBS. This effort was supported by the production of a newsletter in the prelaunch period to establish the market and convince the medical specialists that the condition is a serious and credible disease. This was accompanied by a series of "advertorials" directed at general practitioners. Other groups to be targeted with promotional material included pharmacists, nurses, and patients.

Although portrayed by the pharmaceutical company as a medical education plan, the intent was clearly to change public perceptions about IBS, establishing it in the public domain as a clinically identifiable condition and thereby creating a demand for a drug for treating this condition. While pharmaceutical companies may be particularly aggressive in attempting to create demand for a good or service, such activities are widespread among healthcare organizations of various types.

Source: Moynihan, R., I. Heath, and D. Henry. 2002. "Selling Sickness: The Pharmaceutical Industry and Disease Mongering." *British Medical Journal* 324 (April 13): 886–91.

that population that require medical treatment. The health conditions included here are those an objective evaluation (e.g., a physical examination) would uncover within the population. These may be thought of as the *absolute* needs that exist in nature, without the influence of any other factors. All things being equal, the absolute level of need should not vary much from population to population. These epidemiologically based needs that a team of health professionals would identify in a sweep through a community could be considered to represent the true prevalence of illness within the population.

A population with certain characteristics can be expected to experience a specified level of certain health conditions based on these characteristics. However, these absolute needs, at least in contemporary societies, do not translate directly into demand. In fact, the mismatch between these baseline needs and the ultimate utilization of services is substantial. Many conditions go untreated (indeed, even undiagnosed) for various reasons. Treatment is obtained for many other conditions that would not be identified among the absolute needs of the population. For example, no team of epidemiologists assessing the healthcare needs of a community is likely to identify sagging facial skin as a health problem, yet tens of thousands of facelifts are performed in the United States every year by medical doctors. The existence of a clinically confirmed need is not a prerequisite for the presence of demand for a service.

Healthcare Wants

Healthcare wants can be conceptualized as the wishes or desires for health services on the part of a population. Arguably, healthcare consumers are likely to obtain care for basic needs without a lot of promotion from marketers. Even so, any number of social marketing initiatives are currently underway to encourage consumers to obtain care for these basic needs. On the other hand, the level of wants is likely to be elastic and amenable to influence by marketers. Unlike needs, wants would not necessarily be uncovered by a sweep of public health investigators through the community. Wants are shaped less by the absolute needs of the population than by the variety of factors that influence the consumption of goods and services besides healthcare. In fact, many of the health services consumed are considered medically unnecessary or elective and reflect the operation of wants rather than needs. Examples of these services include tummy tucks and laser eye surgery for nearsightedness. The U.S. healthcare system has adapted to the existence of wants as well as needs, and important components of the system cater to those desiring elective services.

At the organizational level the type of organization and the services it offers will dictate whether needs or wants are the main consideration.

Certainly, an AIDS clinic deals with basic needs, and few elective procedures are relevant to the treatment of patients with AIDS. On the other hand, a plastic surgeon specializing in body sculpting is likely to focus on the want-driven demand generated by those motivated by vanity (see Box 9.2 for a discussion of marketing approaches for an elective procedure). At the same time, if this plastic surgeon also maintains a reconstructive surgery practice for trauma victims, both wants and needs may be a consideration.

Recommended Standards for Healthcare

The third dimension of the demand for healthcare services involves recommended standards for the provision of healthcare. As healthcare professionals have become more attuned to prevention and health maintenance the number of recommended procedures has increased. This component involves primarily diagnostic procedures or disease management procedures recommended for patients with certain symptoms or those at risk for certain health problems.

The medical community has developed standards that call for diagnostic tests at a certain frequency, performance of certain medical procedures at specified times, and implementation of various treatment plans for certain patients. A wide range of diagnostic procedures are now indicated for certain age groups and other population segments at risk for various health conditions. For example, an annual mammogram is recommended for all women over 50 and regular prostate exams are recommended for all men over 40.

As Americans have become increasingly health conscious a growing number of standards have been put into place. For example, a few years ago cholesterol tests were limited to patients actively under medical management. Today, cholesterol tests, along with a growing number of other diagnostic and screening procedures, are recommended for everyone at specific intervals. Many of these standards are considered important for public health purposes and as such may be subjected to social marketing efforts by various organizations.

Health Services Utilization

The fourth dimension of demand involves the actual utilization of health services. The utilization level is frequently used as a proxy measure for demand in that usage rates can be calculated for virtually any type of healthcare good or service. More data related to health services utilization are available than for the other dimensions of demand, primarily because utilization data are routinely collected for administrative purposes whenever a health service is provided. Utilization rates indicate the true level of activity within the healthcare system as opposed to theoretical demand.

**Box 9.2:
Marketing an
Elective
Procedure:
The Case of
LASIK**

Customer profiling is a common practice in most industries but has attracted limited attention in healthcare. The lack of interest in customer profiling reflects the same factors that have discouraged direct-to-consumer marketing and other targeted approaches to reaching healthcare consumers. Historically, the end user was not the one to make the decision with regard to choice of health service. Why spend resources, the argument went, on patients when their physicians or health plans would ultimately determine which health services they used?

This argument, of course, makes less and less sense in today's environment. With the resurgence of consumerism driven by the baby boom generation, the search for alternative therapies, and the emerging interest in defined contributions, the consumer may actually become king in healthcare for the first time in decades. The growing interest in direct-to-consumer marketing has been spearheaded by pharmaceutical companies, but numerous other opportunities for the application of this approach exist in healthcare today.

One area ripe for the application of such direct marketing methods is elective surgery. Elective procedures (i.e., those not considered medically necessary and thus not reimbursable under insurance) constitute a significant proportion of the procedures performed in healthcare and include everything from elective knee surgery to laser eye correction (LASIK) to facelifts. Not only are these procedures truly elective—usually the consumer, not the physician or health plan, makes the choice—but patients for many types of elective surgeries are characterized by a particular profile; thus, individuals obtaining facelifts or tummy tucks do not represent a cross-section of the population.

Many companies in varied industries have used profiling to determine the characteristics of their best customers. *Best customers* are typically defined as those who use the company's services often, spend above-average amounts, do not default on payments, and so forth. In the healthcare context a best customer for an elective medical procedure would be, for instance, someone who responded to a direct-mail solicitation, such as an invitation to a seminar, and then went through with the surgery or treatment. Private-pay customers can be considered best customers for many healthcare services for which negotiated rates are low and payment may be delayed. Identifying a profile of healthcare consumers who are most likely to fall into these desirable categories therefore has clear implications for the profitability of a private healthcare practice.

The most effective approach to customer profiling involves obtaining actual patient data that will allow for the development of a reasonably accurate profile of the best prospects for that particular service. Aggregate data on the patients obtaining facelifts or elective knee surgery would provide the basis for developing a methodology for identifying look-alikes within the population. Even better, however, are actual patient names and addresses. This information can be used to link the patients to a variety of consumer databases to develop a more in-depth profile of the typical candidate for a procedure. Thus, patients for a particular service can be profiled in terms of their demographic characteristics, lifestyle clusters, and consumer behavior, among other characteristics.

Furthermore, these detailed data can be subjected to sophisticated statistical analyses to empirically validate the profile.

LASIK represents a useful case study in healthcare customer profiling. LASIK has grown in popularity as new techniques have been perfected and outcomes improved. In many ways LASIK is the poster child for this type of study: it is almost always an elective procedure requiring out-of-pocket expenditure on the part of the patient, it is relatively expensive, and it appeals disproportionately to certain segments of the population. Interest in LASIK is particularly high today, with the burgeoning potential represented by near-sighted baby boomers and the drying up of other types of surgical opportunities for oph-thalmic surgeons.

For this particular analysis patient data were obtained from a successful laser sur-gery clinic. Although information could have been obtained on the characteristics of the patients, only patient names and addresses were requested for this analysis. The clinic provided the names and addresses of three groups of patients: (1) those on whom they had performed surgery; (2) those who had presented themselves for surgery but turned out to be clinically ineligible; and (3) those who had indicated an interest in LASIK at some point but, as far as was known, had never obtained the procedure. The analysis involved approximately 700 LASIK patients (and medically ineligible prospective patients) and more than 1,200 prospective patients who did not have the surgery after an initial inquiry. In addition, a random sample of 1,000 consumers was drawn from the ZIP codes predominant among the patients and prospects.

The Experian consumer database provides three types of "enhancement" data for each consumer:

- Individual-level data, such as age, marital status, and gender
- Household-level data, such as home ownership, estimated household income, and presence of children
- Geographic-area data, such as the median household income of the census block group in which the consumer lives; racial and ethnic profile of the block group; median home value; and a lifestyle cluster code (the Experian Mosaic cluster), which classifies the ZIP+4 into one of 62 demographic and lifestyle cluster

To ensure that the patient and random samples represented the same underlying population, any consumers whose ZIP codes fell outside the primary area served by the LASIK clinic were removed from the research database.

When the characteristics of the patients, prospects, and matched general popula-tion were compared, significant differences were found in the demographics and house-hold characteristics of the three groups. Differences were found in terms of age, gender, race, marital status, income levels, and rate of home ownership. Little distinction was found, however, between the patients and the other groups in terms of educational sta-tuses or occupational characteristics.

When the groups were compared in terms of Mosaic lifestyle clusters, four of these clusters were determined to be negatively associated with a propensity for LASIK. These clusters generally typified lower socioeconomic-status neighborhoods. Based on these comparative data a logistic regression model was derived to predict the probability that a given consumer would fit the profile of previous LASIK patients. Prospects who failed to obtain LASIK surgery were eliminated from the analysis; the contrast groups were patients (including medically ineligible persons) and random consumers.

The model ultimately settled on demonstrated reasonable predictive validity. Overall, 63 percent of the sample was correctly classified as either a patient or nonpatient based on the consumer data readily available from the Experian database. While a logistic regression model will yield both false positives and false negatives, this overall result—with 60 percent of the positives correctly classified and 66 percent of the negatives correctly classified—indicated that this model could be employed to significantly increase the probability of identifying prospects for LASIK in the market served by the ophthalmic surgery practice.

In the final analysis the characteristics that had the most predictive power (in no particular order) were race, age category, gender, marital status, and income. While these factors all contributed to the likelihood of obtaining LASIK, certain occupational statuses and lifestyle categories reduced the likelihood of becoming a patient.

The ability to predict classification of an individual as a patient versus a nonpatient was improved dramatically using this approach. Using this model as a basis for identifying targets for direct mail would increase the hit rate significantly, and careful use of the model (i.e., targeting those who fall into the top three deciles in terms of propensity) should increase marketing effectiveness by 300 percent. This can have tremendous bottom-line impact for an ophthalmic surgery practice.

Source: Barber, F., R. K. Thomas, and M. C. Huang. 2001. "Developing a Profile of LASIK Surgery Customers." *Marketing Health Services* 21 (2): 32–35.

Because of the perceived relationship between demand and utilization, analysts may sometimes work backward from utilization levels and use them as a proxy for demand. However, utilization does not equal demand, and, depending on the circumstances, the level of demand may exceed actual utilization; conversely, utilization levels may exceed reasonable demand for services. For example, less utilization than expected may occur because of limited access to health services. On the other hand, some services may be overutilized for various reasons (e.g., insurance coverage, physician practice patterns) unrelated to the level of demand.

While all of these factors influence the demand for health services, they do not directly translate into utilization. Ultimately, the marketer is concerned with who uses what services. Motives and underlying causes are important, but what consumers actually *do* is more important and more concrete. (See Pol and Thomas 2001 for a detailed review of the relationship between demographic characteristics and both health status and health behavior.)

Factors Influencing Demand

The factors that influence the level of health services demand are multiple, and their interactions are complex. However, the correlation between the morbidity profile of a population and its healthcare utilization is not very direct. While biological characteristics may predispose the individual to various health problems, other factors may eventually determine the type and amount of health services used. Biological factors are comparable to the healthcare needs described earlier and may or may not translate into utilization.

Knowledge of the cultural background, lifestyle patterns, and financing arrangements of a population may be a better predictor of the type and level of services that will be used than knowledge of the actual level of morbidity characterizing a population. The following section describes some of the factors influencing the level of demand.

Population Characteristics

A variety of population characteristics influence the demand for health services. These can be categorized in terms of their effect on both health status and health behavior.

Psychological Factors

The psychological factors correlated with health services demand include personality types and attitudinal traits as well as the emotional responses evoked by health problems. Clearly, fear, vanity, and pride come into play in the use of health services. The relationship between these factors and health behavior can become exceedingly complex, as can be seen in the case of the hypochondriac or in cases where fear pushes one person to seek treatment but prevents another from visiting the physician. In the contemporary U.S. healthcare environment fear, vanity, and pride play a large role in the demand for many elective procedures (e.g., cosmetic surgery, stomach resection).

In other industries marketers pay more attention to psychological motivations, and personal individualized traits are frequently important in driving consumer behavior. Because of the individualized nature of psychological traits, they are difficult to directly correlate with health services utilization. In any case limited useful data on psychological characteristics are available to marketers.

Demographic Factors

As mentioned in Chapter 7, demographic characteristics influence utilization. Age is probably the best predictor of health services use. It is related to the type of services used and the circumstances under which they are received. This is true whether the indicator is for inpatient care, tests and procedures performed, or virtually any other measure of utilization. Different conditions are associated with each age cohort, resulting in demands for differing types of services.

The gender of the consumer is another factor influencing utilization rates. In the United States women are more involved in the healthcare system than men and are heavier users of health services in general. They tend to visit physicians more often, take more prescription drugs, and use other facilities and personnel more often. Women are also more aware of the health services that are available and quicker to turn to health professionals when symptoms occur.

Racial and ethnic characteristics influence the demand for health services, with the clearest differences identified between African Americans and non-Hispanic whites. Certain Asian populations and many ethnic groups also display distinctive utilization patterns. While differences in utilization may be traced to differences in the types of health problems experienced by these populations, many of the differences reflect variations in lifestyle patterns and cultural preferences. Different perceptions of and expectations for the healthcare system are also likely to exist among various racial and ethnic populations.

Marital status is related not only to levels of demand but also to the type of services used and the circumstances under which they are received. Different levels of morbidity are associated with each marital status category, resulting in demands for differing levels and types of services. The lifestyles associated with various marital statuses probably have more effect on utilization than do actual differentials in morbidity.

The income level of a population is probably one of the best predicators of the utilization of health services. A correlation exists between income level and the amount of health services used as well as between the types of services utilized and the circumstances under which they are received. This is true whether the indicator is for inpatient care, outpatient care, tests and procedures performed, or virtually any other measure of utilization.

The relationship between educational level and utilization resembles that for income. The distribution of health problems within the population is to a certain extent associated with educational status, and the educational level of the population is probably one of the better predictors of the demand for health services. Education is related to both the type and level of health services utilization.

A relatively direct and positive relationship exists between occupational and industrial characteristics of a population and health services utilization. The type of occupation, as well as occupational status, has been correlated with use of health services. Different levels of morbidity are associated with each occupational status category, resulting in demand for different levels and types of services.

Associations between religious affiliation and degree of religiosity and health behavior are probably the most idiosyncratic of any of the demographically related associations. These relationships have been exposed to limited research, so clear patterns are difficult to discern. Furthermore, in the United States, religious affiliation and participation tend to be associated with so many other variables that isolating the influence of these variables per se is difficult. Nevertheless, there is evidence that health status, and the subsequent use of services, is correlated with measures of religiosity.

Lifestyle and Psychographic Factors

Lifestyle and psychographic factors have important implications for healthcare wants, needs, and behavior. The propensity to utilize health services may be more highly correlated with lifestyle characteristics than with other variables. A specific constellation of health behaviors can be associated with each lifestyle category, making lifestyle an important predictor of health behavior. To a certain extent lifestyles override, or at least refine, differences based on demographic traits. (See Box 9.3 for a discussion of lifestyle segmentation systems.)

Other Factors

The healthcare technology available to a society has a significant influence on the consumption of health services. Other factors that influence the utilization of health services should be noted; however, these are of less importance to the marketer as they are generally outside the control of marketers or even healthcare administrators. These factors include technological developments and structural factors such as reimbursement arrangements, availability of facilities and services, and extant practice patterns of healthcare providers.

Advances in technology usually lead to higher levels of utilization of the services supported by the new technology. Indeed, some operations, like laser eye surgery, could never have been performed without certain technological advances. Thus, the availability of certain types of technology to providers is a controlling factor with regard to the services that can be performed. Technological advances have contributed to the shift from inpatient to outpatient care and facilitated the emergence of home health care

Box 9.3: Lifestyle Segmentation Systems

Lifestyle segmentation systems have been used for decades in other industries but never received wide acceptance in healthcare. For the most part healthcare provider organizations depended on physicians or health plans to channels patients to them; they had little interest in the characteristics of their patients.

Certain organizations, however, did have an interest in the characteristics of their patients, especially if they were involved in elective procedures or consumer-oriented products. They needed to target certain categories of patients who were not particularly bound to referring physicians or health plans or were buying health-related products directly. Unfortunately, such companies could obtain little guidance in the past because the existing lifestyle segmentation systems had not been adapted for use in healthcare. It was possible to access profiles (and develop a targeted mailing list) for financial services customers, packaged-goods consumers, or automobile purchasers, but not healthcare consumers.

The new healthcare environment demands increased attention to customer segmentation. The market has become much more consumer driven, and individuals are taking a much more active role in healthcare decision making. The pharmaceutical companies have led the way with a heavy investment in direct-to-consumer marketing. Healthcare providers such as plastic surgeons, orthopedic surgeons, and eye surgeons, who often perform elective procedures, are demonstrating increased need for segmentation capabilities. With the emergence of defined contributions as an option for employee benefits, growing numbers of health plans, health services providers, and other organizations are expressing an interest in customer segmentation and target marketing.

The first lifestyle segmentation systems, also referred to as psychographic segmentation, were developed in the 1970s. This initial approach to segmenting the population was developed in response to perceived deficiencies in demographic profiling. Marketers had come to realize that people in the same demographic category may fall into different groupings based on lifestyle despite being similar on paper. A case in point is senior citizens, who were once all grouped into the over-65 category. Lifestyle research discovered that within this demographic category were various lifestyle categories that had a greater effect on consumer behavior than age.

as a major component of the industry. The effect of technology has been particularly felt in the area of diagnostic testing in recent years. The variety of tests that can be performed has increased dramatically and includes the expanded use of home-testing procedures.

An important indicator of reimbursement potential is the type and extent of health insurance coverage for individuals and families characterizing the market. Indeed, the availability of insurance has been identified as one of the best predictors of the demand for services. When insurers

The best-known early lifestyle segmentation system—the values and lifestyle system (VALS)—was developed by Stanford Research International in the 1970s and inspired a variety of subsequent systems. The VALS system never benefited from widespread use, but three subsequent systems are widely used today: Claritas's PRIZM, Experian's Mosaic, and CACI Marketing Systems's "A Classification of Residential Neighborhoods" (ACORN). While the various systems are built using similar methodologies, they do differ in terms of the specific procedures used to create the categories.

The concept behind all segmentation systems is the use of geodemographic data in conjunction with data on consumer behavior, attitudes, and preferences to establish distinct lifestyle clusters that cover the entire population. This allows marketers and researchers to classify customers and potential customers into distinct categories, each with particular characteristics. Once the lifestyle segments have been identified for a population, a broad range of characteristics may be attached to the respective categories.

PRIZM may be the best-known system, primarily because of the clever names it gives its lifestyle categories. Individuals may be classified as, for example, "Patios and Pools," "Shotguns and Pickups," or "Executive Suites" among the 62 clusters. The PRIZM system is the only one that has been used extensively to link health characteristics to the lifestyle clusters. This information, however, is proprietary and can only be obtained by becoming a client of Inforum, the data vendor that developed the health-care links to the various clusters.

U.S. Mosaic is the latest version of the Experian lifestyle classification system. This system also includes 62 lifestyle clusters, grouped into 12 major categories. The naming scheme is somewhat more straightforward than for the PRIZM, with the "upscale singles" category, including such clusters as "high-income urban singles in apartments" and "urban, upper-mid-income seniors in apartments."

A number of multivariate statistical methods were applied to create the ACORN system. The most pertinent consumer characteristics were identified from a wealth of data using principal components analysis and graphical methods. CACI carefully analyzed and sorted the country's 226,000 neighborhoods by 61 unique lifestyle characteristics such as income, age, household type, home value, occupation, education, and other key deter-

introduce copayments or higher deductibles into their insurance plans, the use of health services often declines in response. When reimbursement for a service is improved, the use of those services tends to increase.

Frequently changing reimbursement arrangements also exert an influence on practice patterns. Hospitals face restrictions imposed by health plans on the services they can provide as the plans try to control claims. Changing reimbursement patterns and regulatory pressures are forcing physicians to change their practice patterns as well.

minants of consumer behavior. Next, the market segments were created by a combination of cluster analytic techniques. The techniques were selected to produce statistically reliable solutions and handle an immense amount of information. This process results in the assignment of more than 220,000 neighborhoods to 43 lifestyle segments.

Each developer of lifestyle segmentation systems makes a wide range of data available by cluster. All will perform lifestyle analyses for clients, and in some cases lifestyle data can be linked directly to household databases. CACI makes software available that clients can use to perform their own analyses.

The emergence of managed care as a dominant organizational structure within healthcare has also had an effect on utilization patterns. In fact, the goal of managed care is to control their enrollees' utilization of services. For this reason, health plans encourage their enrolees to obtain certain services while discouraging them from obtaining others.

The availability of health services in the form of facilities and personnel has an understandable effect on the level of utilization. In some situations the demand for services is not being met because of a lack of facilities or personnel. In others an oversupply of facilities or personnel may result in the overutilization of health services.

Research over the past two decades has revealed a surprising variation in the patterns of practice of physicians and, to a lesser extent, hospitals. Far from being an exact science, medicine involves frequent value judgments on the part of physicians and other practitioners. While individual differences exist among physicians within the same market area in terms of the volume and types of services provided to similar patients, even more striking variations exist from market to market (Center for Evaluative Clinical Sciences 1999). Local practice patterns significantly influence the level of service utilization, creating differences of several magnitudes between market areas in some instances.

The Elasticity of Health Services Demand

The recorded level of health services utilization reflects a combination of the needs, wants, and recommended standards of the population as well as the effect of the structural factors noted earlier. While each category of demand represents a different challenge for health services marketers, the real challenge is to be able to determine what combination of these factors is relevant for a particular situation. The determination of demand is clearly a multifaceted process that involves a number of different dimensions. While it may be appropriate, depending on the situation, to use need, want, recommended standards, or utilization as a proxy for demand, ultimately some type of blended concept must be developed to more precisely specify the level of demand.

Measuring Health Services Utilization

Health services researchers have developed a number of indicators for measuring service utilization. The indicators commonly used to measure health services utilization are discussed in the sections that follow.

Facility Indicators

Hospital admissions is one of the most frequently used indicators of health services use, as the hospital represents the focal point for treatment in the system. The terms *admissions* and *discharges* are used to refer to episodes of inpatient hospital utilization. The hospital admission rate serves as a proxy for a variety of other indicators because hospital admissions are correlated with tests conducted, surgeries performed, and allocation of other resources. Because hospital care is both labor and capital intensive, one admission carries a great deal of weight in terms of significance in overall healthcare expenditures. Admissions may be measured for the entire community or particular facility or be decomposed into components of utilization. This could involve the calculation of admission rates by clinical specialty, demographic attribute, geographic origin, payer category, and so on.

Patient days refers to the number of hospital days generated by a particular population and is calculated in terms of the number of patient days generated per 1,000 residents. This indicator refines hospital admissions as an indicator by reflecting the total utilization of resources, as measuring patient days serves to adjust for variations in length of stay for various conditions. Like admission rates, patient days may be calculated by diagnosis, type of hospital, patient origin, or payer category. Changes in reimbursement procedures have made the patient day more of a standard unit for the measurement of resource utilization than the actual hospital admission.

Another indicator used to measure hospitalization is the *average length of stay,* typically reported in terms of the average number of days patients remain in the facility during a specified time period. This indicator provides a good measure of resource utilization as well. In fact, Medicare and many health plans reimburse hospitals on a per diem rate.

Several other facility indicators may also be mentioned. While not all carry the significance of hospital admissions, each is important in its own way. Utilization rates may be calculated for nursing homes; hospital emergency rooms or outpatient departments; or freestanding emergency centers, minor medical centers, surgery centers, and diagnostic centers.

Personnel Indicators

Perhaps one of the most useful indicators of health services utilization is the volume of physician encounters. This is typically measured in terms of *physician office visits,* although telephone contact and physician visits to hospitalized patients are sometimes considered. The physician is the gatekeeper for most types of health services, and physician utilization is a more direct measure of utilization levels than hospital admissions because virtually everyone uses a physician's services at some time. Physician utilization rates are often broken down by specialty, as the utilization of different specialties varies dramatically.

Utilization rates may be calculated for other types of personnel. Most, like physicians and dentists, are independent practitioners who practice without the supervision of other medical personnel. Examples include optometrists, podiatrists, chiropractors, nurse practitioners, and physician's assistants as well as various mental health counselors and therapists. Other healthcare personnel who generally cannot operate independently but for whom utilization rates may be calculated include home health nurses and various technical personnel. Physical therapists and speech therapists are other categories of healthcare personnel for whom utilization rates may be developed if, for example, the analyst was involved in marketing for rehabilitation services.

Other Indicators

As the importance of home health care has grown in recent years, the volume of *home health care visits* has taken on more importance. The range of services provided has been expanded, and a much broader segment of the patient population is considered appropriate for home care. Home care utilization is typically measured in terms of visits by various types of personnel. Thus, a population may be considered to have a certain number of home nurse visits or home physical therapist visits as indicators of utilization. Alternatively, the number of residences (i.e., the rate per 1,000) receiving home care may be calculated.

Another indicator of the use of health services is the level of *drug utilization.* Although patient care providers typically have limited use for information on drug utilization, analysts representing other entities such as pharmaceutical companies do have a need for such data. These analyses typically focus on the consumption of prescription drugs because these (rather than over-the-counter medicines) are thought to more closely reflect actual utilization of the formal healthcare system. While the level of drug prescribing can be determined from physician and pharmacist records, rates of consumption for nonprescription drugs must be determined more indirectly.

Rates of prescription-drug utilization are typically calculated in terms of the number of prescriptions within a given year per 1,000 population. Alternatively, the average number of prescriptions written annually per person may be calculated. Occasionally, the level of drug consumption may be estimated based on the quantities of pharmaceuticals prescribed.

Predicting the Demand for Health Services

Knowledge about the current level of demand for health services, however measured, is important for the marketing process. Even more important, however, is the anticipated future level of demand characterizing the population under study. A variety of techniques have been developed for projecting future demand; three are discussed below.

Traditional Utilization Projections

The simplest and most straightforward approach to projecting the utilization of health services involves straight-line projections that extend historical trends. For example, it was common in the past to review several years' experience with hospital admissions and extrapolate this trend into the future. This approach was intuitive in that, if the trend had been upward, it continued to rise. On the other hand, if a downward trend had been recorded, the assumption was that historical patterns would persist in the future.

Few market analysts would use this approach in today's healthcare environment. Developments external to the healthcare arena have such an effect on the demand for services and ultimate patterns of utilization that extrapolating from the past is not practical. The past is no longer a guide to the future when it comes to the utilization of health services. This situation has forced a much more sophisticated approach to the projection of utilization.

Population-Based Models

The most powerful factor in terms of predicting health services utilization is the size of the population. A change in the number of people served tends to have the greatest effect on utilization expected in the future. Because of the importance of population size and because population projections are likely to be both readily available and fairly reliable, population-based projections have become the most common predictive technique used to forecast health services utilization.

The simplest approach is to multiply the projected population by known utilization rates. Thus, population-based models involve two components: (1) appropriate population estimates and projections and (2) accurate utilization rates. Population estimates and projections are available from a variety of sources and for various levels of geography.

While some benefit can be derived from basing the demand estimates on the total population, the analysis typically examines utilization in terms of age and gender. Changes in age distribution occur frequently and can have a major effect on utilization. Utilization patterns for males and females vary significantly and must be taken into consideration. The easiest way to express the effect of age is to employ sex- and age-specific use rates. As more data become available the population may also be examined in terms of race and income. In some cases it may be possible to decompose the population in terms of payer category.

Thus, utilization rates may be expressed in terms of hospital admissions or physician visits per 1,000 residents per year, patient days per 1,000 residents per year, live births per 1,000 females age 15 to 44 per year, and so forth. These rates can be adjusted to account for regional differences when appropriate. The utilization rates of interest can be applied to different age or gender categories and adjusted for other attributes to the extent they are available.

While population-based demand-projection models in all of their permutations offer an intuitively appealing approach, their usefulness has limitations. On the one hand, the mobility of the U.S. population introduces an element of uncertainty into the projection process. Furthermore, the cohort affect plays a role in determining differential utilization patterns, and analysts cannot contend, for example, that the utilization patterns of 65 year olds today will be the same as those of 65 year olds 20 years ago. Thus, applying an age-specific rate to today's elderly population based on past experience may be risky.

Utilization rates themselves are given to change. All things being equal in terms of population characteristics, numerous factors influence utilization rates. Many of these have already been discussed and include availability of services, financing arrangements, and level of managed care penetration. Who could have predicted, for example, the decline in hospital admissions that resulted from the introduction of the Medicare prospective payment system and the emergence of managed care? Developments like these make the prediction of future levels of utilization a challenge.

Econometric Models

Econometric models include a variety of techniques for projecting future phenomena in complex situations. In their simplest form econometric models represent a type of time series analysis. In effect, they attempt to statistically improve on the projection model that extrapolates past trends into the future.

Econometric models use equations that project utilization as a function of the interplay of various independent variables. With a complex phenomenon like the utilization of health services, it makes sense to consider forecasting based on multiple factors rather than a single one. The more factors recognized in predicting future utilization, the greater the probability of incorporating significant changes. Econometric prediction addresses such factors in a series of mathematical expressions. The equation ultimately used is the one that best fits the curve in terms of historical demand. However, for this complex form of econometrics to work, projections are needed for numerous independent variables in the equation. Many analysts have attempted to apply econometric models to the prediction of health services demand. Today, however, econometric models have limited utility because of the unpredictability and instability in the healthcare environment.

One emerging approach to predicting consumer demand that has been used in other industries and is only now being incorporated into healthcare involves lifestyle segmentation. As discussed earlier in this chapter, the identification of the lifestyle clusters characterizing a population can serve as a useful tool for predicting the types and levels of health services to be used by a target population (see Case Study 9.1).

Summary

The determination of demand in healthcare is particularly complex and requires an understanding of the many factors that influence the ultimate utilization of health services. From a marketing perspective, demand can be conceptualized as the ultimate result of the combined effect of (1) healthcare needs, (2) healthcare wants, (3) recommended standards for healthcare, and (4) actual utilization patterns.

The demand for health services is surprisingly elastic, and a number of factors influence the level of demand. These include population characteristics such as demographics, psychographics, and social group affiliation. They also include structural factors such as availability of and access to personnel and facilities, financial arrangements (especially the availability of insurance), technological resources, and community practice patterns.

A variety of indicators are available to measure utilization rates. These include admissions, patient days, and length of stay for hospital utilization and office visits, procedures performed, and drugs prescribed in the outpatient setting. The utilization indicator(s) chosen will depend on the type of organization and the product being marketed.

There are many circumstances in which actual utilization data are not available, and some methodology must be used to generate estimates and projections of the level of demand for various services. These techniques include projection into the future based on historical trends, population-based estimates and projections, and econometric forecasts. Currently, lifestyle-based demand estimates are being introduced into healthcare.

Discussion Questions

- Why is *demand* in healthcare a complicated issue, and what are some of the components that may contribute to the level of demand?
- Why is the correlation between health services demand and health services utilization imperfect?
- What are some of the demographic factors that influence the demand for health services?
- What role do psychographic or lifestyle factors play in influencing the demand for health services?
- How can we explain the fact that the mere presence of health services may increase the demand for healthcare?
- Is it possible to create demand for a service like healthcare?
- What is the role of health insurance in determining the demand for health services?
- How can we explain the fact that the patterns of health services utilization vary widely from community to community, although the characteristics of the population differ little?

References

Berkowitz, E. N., L. G. Pol, and R. K. Thomas. 1997. *Healthcare Market Research*. Burr Ridge, IL: Irwin Professional Publishing.

Center for Evaluative Clinical Sciences. 1999. *The Dartmouth Atlas of Health Care*. Hanover, NH: Center for Evaluative Clinical Sciences.

Pol, L. G., and R. K. Thomas. 2001. *The Demography of Health and Health Care, 2nd ed*. New York: Plenum Press.

USING LIFESTYLE ANALYSIS TO PREDICT THE USE OF BEHAVIORAL HEALTH SERVICES

During the last quarter of the twentieth century *behavioral health services* emerged as an important sector within the U.S. healthcare system. This umbrella term covers a wide range of conditions, including psychiatric problems, emotional disturbances, substance abuse, hyperactivity in children, and other conditions thought amenable to treatment by mental health professionals. Behavioral health services were considered a different category from services for the treatment of physical illness, and a separate industry developed for the management of behavioral health problems. Many health plans "carved out" behavioral health services, and eventually national managed care plans that specialized in the provision of such services emerged.

By the late 1990s the primary purchasers of behavioral health services (i.e., major employers) were facing increasing financial pressure as a result of increasing healthcare costs. Behavioral health services were particularly problematic because of the open-ended nature of many behavioral health conditions. At the same time, however, regulations that mandated parity between provisions for physical and behavioral health coverage were put into place. Employers who wanted to offer behavioral health coverage to their employees were faced with a major cost-containment challenge.

ABC Health Services was a major player in the behavioral health arena, reporting an enrollment of more than three million employees in its managed care plans. ABC was faced with the same issues as other behavioral health plans: customers who could not distinguish between plans and were shopping for the lowest price. As a result ABC was losing clients to other, sometimes less capable, plans that quoted lower prices.

In response to this situation ABC developed an innovative approach to the market using lifestyle segmentation analysis. Based on the records maintained on enrollees who participated in its behavioral health plans,

ABC believed that the likelihood of using behavioral health services could be linked to different lifestyle categories among employees. Furthermore, it was felt that for those who used services the type and intensity of the services could be correlated with lifestyle cluster.

ABC subsequently profiled existing clients in terms of their Mosaic lifestyle clusters (see Box 9.3). They found approximately a dozen Mosaic lifestyle clusters (a total of 62) associated with a high propensity to use behavioral health services. Another ten lifestyle clusters were virtually never associated with the use of such services. For example, the cluster containing middle-class suburban families tended to be characterized by high utilization levels, whereas the cluster involving low-income rural families was characterized by low utilization levels. The remaining cluster did not display a correlation with use or nonuse.

It was further found, for example, that the older affluent suburban household cluster had a high propensity for use of alcohol abuse services but not drug abuse services. On the other hand, the single, affluent urban high-rise cluster had a high propensity to use drug abuse services but not alcohol treatment services. Some clusters were characterized by episodic use of services (e.g., in response to some stressful event), whereas members of other clusters were characterized by recurrent use of services, indicating more deep-seated problems.

ABC Health Services was able to use this information in marketing its behavioral health plan to existing customers as well as prospective clients. ABC representatives offered to profile the employees of existing customers, for example, to determine the extent to which the package of services offered was meeting the needs of the employees. This not only allowed ABC to more efficiently serve the existing client population but also facilitated the prediction of future use of behavioral health services. The service mix could subsequently be adjusted to more efficiently and cost effectively serve the existing enrollees.

In the case of a prospective client, ABC was able to distinguish itself from other behavioral health plans through its ability to determine the configuration of needs characterizing the target group of employees. By serving in a consultative role in this manner ABC could demonstrate greater expertise in the management of behavioral health clients than its competitors. Furthermore, ABC could offer a package of services tailored to the specific needs of that employer population rather than the one-size-fits-all plan offered by other firms. By developing an in-depth knowledge of the target population using lifestyle segmentation analysis ABC was able to provide more effective services at competitive prices while raising the satisfaction level of both employers and employees.

III

HEALTHCARE MARKETING TECHNIQUES

Marketing is used in its broadest sense in this book and encompasses perhaps a wider range of activities in healthcare than in other industries. This section reviews the various healthcare marketing techniques, their advantages and disadvantages, and their relative effectiveness. The applicability of marketing techniques from other industries is considered.

Chapter 10 focuses on the topic of marketing strategy, describing the manner in which the options among various strategies are assessed and the need to interface marketing strategy with the organization's overall strategic plan. It emphasizes the importance of an integrated strategy in the development of effective marketing initiatives.

Chapter 11 provides an overview of the traditional promotional techniques, including advertising, personal sales, public relations, and sales promotion in which the healthcare marketer is likely to be involved. It also includes a discussion of the application of direct marketing techniques to healthcare. The modifications of traditional marketing approaches necessary for healthcare are addressed.

Chapter 12 presents an overview of new and emerging marketing techniques that are either unique to healthcare or adopted from other industries. Two categories of techniques are discussed—those that emphasize organization changes and those that capitalize on contemporary technology. Numerous applications of innovative marketing techniques are provided and their compatibility with healthcare considered.

MARKETING STRATEGIES

I n today's environment few healthcare organizations can successfully compete without a well-thought-out marketing strategy. Strategies serve
numerous purposes for the organization, and a number of different
strategies may be employed. In this chapter, the factors to be considered
in strategy development are reviewed and the steps involved in formalizing
marketing strategies are outlined.

Strategy Defined

The term *strategy* is used in a variety of ways by different students of marketing. For our purposes it refers to the generalized approach to be taken
in meeting the challenges of the market. Strategies set the tone for marketing activities (tactics) and in effect establish the parameters within which
the marketer must operate. The strategy chosen will influence the nature
of the marketing plan that is ultimately developed and will guide any subsequent marketing initiatives.

Marketers often think in terms of different levels at which strategies
may be developed. These could include a corporate strategy that deals with
the overall development of an organization's business activities, a business
strategy that indicates how to approach a particular product or market, or
a marketing strategy focusing on one or more aspects of the marketing mix.
The marketing strategy is the most relevant for our purposes and may be
thought of as the marketing logic by which an organization hopes to achieve
its marketing objectives. The organization's marketing strategy is reflected
in the specific strategies established for target markets, marketing mix
selected, and level of marketing expenditures.

Ideally, strategies are carefully thought out and deliberately formulated as a result of strategic planning, and much of this chapter deals with
the process of developing strategies. The absence of an articulated strategy,
however, does not mean that no strategy exists. Acts of commission or omis-
sion ultimately serve to create a strategy, and the lack of a formal strategy

could actually be considered a strategic approach in a technical sense. Indeed, many healthcare organizations end up with de facto strategies that were not deliberately formulated.

Unplanned strategies are referred to as *emergent strategies,* derived from a pattern of behavior not consciously imposed by senior management. They are the outcome of activities and behaviors that develop unconsciously but nevertheless fall into a consistent pattern. Although many healthcare administrators would concede that they do not have a strategy in place, some strategies, albeit unstated, almost invariably exist.

Before discussing various types of strategies it may be worth reviewing the reasons for developing strategies. Any strategy developed should

- *Provide direction for the organization or program.* The strategy should constitute the "how to" aspect of organizational development.
- *Focus the effort on one of many possible options.* Because there will always be numerous strategic options from which to choose, focusing on a particular strategy prevents confusion of purpose and diffusion of effort.
- *Unify the organization's actions.* The chosen strategy should provide the purpose and direction for the organization necessary to get everyone on the same page and unify the actions of organization members.
- *Differentiate the organization.* The strategy chosen should serve to solidify the organization's identity and distinguish it from competitors.
- *Customize the organization's promotions.* The strategy should provide guidance in the development of promotional material, with all materials presenting an image that is both distinct and consistent.
- *Marshall the organization's resources.* The strategy should provide guidance in the allocation of resources, allowing the focusing of resources on one approach rather than many.
- *Support decision making within the organization.* The strategy should provide a basis for making decisions, implicitly establishing criteria that can be used to frame issues that require a decision.
- *Provide a competitive edge for the organization.* Ultimately, strategy development is about positioning the organization vis-à-vis the market. The approach should capitalize on the organization's strategic assets and provide an advantage over competitors.

The Strategic Planning Context *Call Jo Action*

Strategic planning is a well-established activity in most industries and to many has become synonymous with corporate planning. The strategic plan should serve as the primary mechanism for adapting to an ever-changing environment. The emphasis it places on positioning underscores its central role in organizational development. Strategic planning allows the organization to adapt to the moving target the healthcare arena has become. Ultimately, a strategically oriented organization is one whose actions are aligned with the realities of the environment. The strategic mind-set adopted by the organization should ultimately spawn a marketing mind-set.

The strategic plan should be the basis for marketing resource allocation, particularly when scarce resources are being dispensed. The strategic plan should also provide the basis for relationship development in an environment increasingly driven by provider networks, integrated delivery systems, and referral relationships. The planning process should address the appropriateness of existing linkages and identify potential additional relationships.

Most important, the strategic plan should be a call to action. Indeed, many healthcare organizations have spun their wheels for years waiting for a clear direction to present itself. The strategic plan should not only embody the organization's strategy, but it should convey the vision of the organization and lay out the scenario for what it will be when it "grows up." This vision should generate the range of marketing activities necessary to support the organization's strategic initiatives.

Healthcare administrators sometimes have a tendency to rush headlong into marketing campaigns without regard for the strategic implications. Because marketing challenges often reflect a heat-of-the-moment situation, the tendency is to address immediate marketing needs without concern for the broader implications of these actions. This all-too-common situation underscores the need for a strategic orientation at all levels of the organization.

The Strategic Planning Process

The various steps in the strategic planning process are outlined below in general form. Ample additional sources of information on the details of the strategic planning process exist (see, e.g., Thomas 2003).

Planning for Planning

Although different authors have different perspectives on the steps and sequencing of the planning process, the approach here is a typical one. (Chapter 15 provides more detail on the planning process.) The first step in the strategic planning process involves planning for planning, and a good starting point for this phase is a review of the organization's mission statement and any existing corporate goal(s). Much of the activity at this point is organizational in nature and focuses on identifying the key stakeholders, decision makers, and resource persons who must be taken into consideration in the process. This knowledge should inform, and the establishment of a planning team should guide, the process. The planning team should include representatives of the various stakeholders, key decision makers, opinion leaders, and representatives of all constituent groups as well as those representing various substantive areas within the organization.

Stating Assumptions

One of the critical early steps is the stating of assumptions. Assumptions may be stated relative to the players involved in the local healthcare arena or in regard to certain healthcare facts of life. Assumptions also may be stated in regard to the nature of the market (and its population), the political climate, the position of other providers, and any other factors that may affect the strategic-development process. Many assumptions ultimately involve a marketing dimension. Assumptions stated during the strategy-development process are likely to relate to the organization's position within the market, nature of competition, distribution of the organization's facilities, and so forth. Although assumptions will undoubtedly be refined as the planning process continues, it is important to begin with some general assumptions—for example, "Managed care will continue to exert a major influence on the local market" or "We're number four in market share, and there is no way we will ever be number one."

Initial Information Gathering

The data-collection process begins with the gathering of general background information on the organization. This will include a review of any available organizational materials such as publications produced by the organization (e.g., annual reports), press releases, and marketing materials. Other potential sources of information include reports filed with regulatory agencies, business plans that have been presented to funding sources, grant applications, and certificate-of-need applications. Certain internal documents, such as executive committee minutes, planning retreat summaries, and evaluation studies, may also be useful. This step should include an inventory and assessment of existing marketing activities.

Initial information gathering should include interviews with knowledgeable individuals within the organization who represent different functional areas, vested interests, and perspectives. For large organizations these interviews may be restricted to key administrators and medical staff and perhaps one or more individuals with a handle on institutional history. Within a smaller organization, such as a physician's practice, it may be possible to conduct interviews with medical staff, administrative staff, and perhaps other key individuals during initial information gathering.

This stage of the process should also identify the key constituents of the organization. Who, in effect, must the organization report to? Who does it have to satisfy? For a tightly held private organization few outside the organization may matter. On the other hand, a private, not-for-profit entity is likely to be accountable to board members, regulators, and others. In a publicly held company the board of directors and its shareholders represent constituents of some importance as well. Other constituents to consider include patient groups, referring physicians, employee benefits managers, insurance plan representatives, and political officials. The list should include consumers (who must have their awareness raised), existing customers (whose loyalty needs to be strengthened), medical staff (whose continued support must be ensured), and the media (who must be kept up-to-date on the organization's activities).

Much of what is gleaned during initial information gathering could be considered to reflect the *corporate culture* of the organization, the character of the organization's internal environment. There is now ample documentation of the manner in which the corporate culture affects the operation of an organization and determines the extent to which its environment is amenable to the planning process. The culture of the organization will typically influence the extent to which a marketing mind-set is in place.

The planning team is unlikely to have the complete answers to all of the questions raised above at this point, and typically more questions than answers will have been generated. Nevertheless, knowledge will begin to accumulate, and an appreciation of potential roadblocks should emerge as background information is compiled.

Profiling the Organization

These initial information-gathering activities should generate a sense of what the organization is and what business it is in. This will involve examining its existing mission statement and goals in light of the information compiled. One real turning point for any healthcare organization occurs when it comes to grips with what business it is in. Hospitals that continued to think they were in the hospital business rather than the healthcare business found themselves at a competitive disadvantage with hospitals that realized they had a broader mission. In fact, the redefinition of healthcare organizations during the last quarter of the twentieth century was a major contributor to the emergence of marketing as an essential healthcare function.

In profiling the organization a couple of important questions must be addressed during the early stages of research. First, "What is our product or products?" This may appear to be an easy question, but it is one that few healthcare organizations can readily answer. This is partly because healthcare organizations have not historically thought in terms of discrete products, but also because of the complexity of healthcare. Unless the organization's sole business is selling a healthcare "widget," the goods and services offered are likely to be complex and not easily classified. How does one conceptualize public health or occupational medicine, as examples, in terms of goods and services? Regardless of the complexity involved, specifying the organization's products is an important step in developing both general strategies and marketing-specific strategies. (The nature of healthcare products is discussed in more detail in Chapter 8.)

The second question is, "Who are our customers?" or "Who do we have to convince to purchase our services?" The more multipurpose an organization, the broader the range of customers it will have. For a hospital it could be argued that the list of customers includes patients who receive services, family members and other decision makers who influence patient behavior, staff physicians and referring physicians, major employers and business coalitions, and insurance companies and managed care plans. In many cases other providers of care may be customers, especially with the emergence of provider networks and integrated delivery systems. The list does not stop here, particularly if the hospital is tax exempt as a result of its not-for-profit status. In this case other customers may include consumer advocacy groups, policymakers, legislators, regulators, and the press.

Collecting Baseline Data

The initial information-gathering process provides the basis for the establishment of a more intensive data-collection agenda involving both internal and external audits. Although the primary driver for strategic development is the external environment, the process begins with a thorough organizational self-analysis. The intent of the internal audit is to determine who does what within the organization, when and where they do it, how they do it, and even why and how well they do it.

The internal audit covers a wide variety of organizational features and can be incredibly detailed and thorough. The following list illustrates the aspects of the organization that may be addressed by means of an internal audit:

- Policies and procedures
- Existing services and products
- Nature, number, and characteristics of customers
- Utilization patterns for services
- Sales volume
- Staffing levels and personnel characteristics
- Management processes
- Financial situation
- Fee or pricing structure
- Billing and collections practices
- Marketing arrangements
- Location of service outlets
- Referral relationships

The internal audit for a strategic plan will typically involve some type of operational analysis, including, at a minimum, analyses of patient flow, paper flow, and information flow. The operational analysis may also examine staffing patterns, physical space considerations, and productivity. While this information may not apply directly to most marketing initiatives, it is critical for any internal marketing activities carried out.

The scope of the external audit will be determined by the nature of the organization and the issues being considered. Macrolevel trends are obviously more important for organizations involved in regional or national marketing initiatives. For most healthcare organizations this analysis is carried down to the local market level, as this is the level at which most marketing takes place. The climate of the market area must be considered and the ability to take the "pulse" of the community taken.

Perhaps the component of the strategic analysis that has the most salience for marketers is dealing with the identification and description of the market. The market for the organization can be defined in a number of different ways. The definition used depends on the purpose of the analysis, good or service being considered, competitive environment, and even type of organization involved in marketing. Markets may be defined based on geography, demographics, consumer demand, disease prevalence, and so forth. (Issues related to the identification of markets are discussed in Chapter 6.)

In the typical strategy-development initiative a profile of the market-area population is the first task. The first type of data typically compiled involve demographic traits, including biosocial and sociocultural attributes. At a minimum the analyst would examine the population in terms of age, gender, race/ethnicity, marital status/family structure, income, and education. The insurance coverage situation is typically assessed. Furthermore, the migration process has taken on increasing importance in community analysis, and information on both the volume and traits of in-migrants and out-migrants is required.

The demographic analysis is often accompanied by an assessment of the psychographic, or lifestyle, characteristics of the market-area population. Information on the lifestyle categories of the target audience can be used to determine the likely health-related priorities and behaviors of a population subgroup. Consumer attitudes are often a reflection of lifestyles and are typically considered at this point. The attitudes displayed by consumers in a market area are likely to have considerable influence on the demand for almost all types of health services. The attitudes of a wide variety of constituents besides direct consumers must be taken into consideration by the marketer.

Identifying Health Characteristics

The salient health characteristics of the target market are identified through the external audit and invariably include the fertility, morbidity, and mortality characteristics of the population. Information on these processes provides insights into the health status of the population and, ultimately, into the types of health services required.

Historical patterns of *fertility* exert a major influence on current patterns of health services demand, and a wide range of product needs revolve around childbearing. Childbearing also triggers the need for such down-the-road services as pediatrics for children and gynecological services for their mothers. The demand for treatment of male and female reproductive system conditions and the heightened interest in infertility treatment reflect issues related to the reproductive process.

The level of *morbidity* within a population is a major consideration in strategic planning. The incidence and prevalence rates that characterize a population provide a context for strategic development. To the extent possible, analysts must project incidence and prevalence rates into the future to anticipate down-the-road service needs. Disability data should also be considered under the morbidity heading.

The level of *mortality* and the leading causes of death for the population of the market area should be determined. Market researchers typically have less interest in mortality than in morbidity, as the latter is more closely linked to service demand. Nevertheless, mortality data are almost always examined to determine what they can tell us about the health status of the community.

Once the health conditions of the population have been identified, a determination of the required health services and products is possible. These healthcare needs can be conceptualized in terms of the utilization of services (e.g., inpatient services, ambulatory care), performance of diagnostic and therapeutic procedures, prescribing of drugs, and a variety of other goods and services required based on the existing level of health conditions within the population. This step should determine the range of goods and services needed by the target population.

While the second step determines the level of need that technically characterizes the population, the amount of goods and services actually consumed will be determined by a variety of factors. For this reason the actual health behavior of the target population needs to be considered. *Health behavior* refers to any action aimed at restoring, preserving, or enhancing health status. It involves such formal activities as physician visits, hospital admissions, and drug prescriptions as well as informal actions on the part of individuals designed to prevent health problems and maintain, enhance, or promote health. Healthcare organizations focus on those indicators of health behavior most relevant for their operations. Hospitals require information on almost all of the indicators described throughout this book. Other organizations with operations of more limited scope focus on a narrower range of indicators of utilization in their analyses.

The following indicators of health behavior are likely to be considered, depending on the type of organization involved:

- Inpatient admissions
- Outpatient visits
- Other service utilization
- Procedures performed
- Prescriptions written

Strategy-development initiatives require information on the informal aspects of health behavior as well. It may be important to determine the extent to which the market-area population pursues self-care, is involved in healthy lifestyles, or practices risky health behavior. Organizations involved in social marketing, for example, are likely to require information on the extent of unhealthy lifestyles or risky behavior inherent in the population.

Resource Inventory

The resource-identification process establishes an inventory of the facilities, personnel, and other resources available to meet the healthcare needs of the target population. While the full range of available health services within the market area must be identified in some situations, the focus will typically be on the organizations or services likely to be in competition with the entity involved in marketing. Given the role of marketing in countering the competition, the resource inventory is a critical piece of the strategy-development process.

Options to consider for the resource inventory include the following:

- Healthcare facilities
- Healthcare equipment
- Health personnel
- Programs and services
- Funding sources
- Networks and relationships

The final category—networks and relationships—has become increasingly important in the contemporary healthcare environment. In an era of managed care and negotiated contracts for health services the existence of networks and relationships has taken on added importance. The significance of such situations cannot be overestimated, and many organizations have come to view these arrangements as the responsibility of the marketing department.

An important aspect of this analysis involves referral relationships. As relationships have become more important, they are being increasingly emphasized in the strategy-development process. In fact, it can be argued that in the future, patients will utilize a provider because of existing relationships, rather than the traditional approach involving relationship development *following* utilization. The existence of networks, integrated delivery systems, and other relationships within the community should be fully addressed during the strategic planning process. Marketers are increasingly being given responsibility for relationship building and the management of customer relations.

By this stage of the strategy-development process a great deal of data of value to the marketer have been compiled. Based on the information available at this point the marketer should be able to determine the following:

- Overall societal, healthcare, and service trends
- Market-area delineation
- Market-area population profile
- Market-area population health characteristics
- Current position of the organization or product
- Customer profile(s)
- Resources available in the service area
- Likely future developments affecting the organization

A major component of the external audit is likely to be the competitive analysis. Strategy development does not occur in a vacuum but rather must consider the healthcare environment and other players in that arena. Any strategy development must reflect the organization's position relative to its competitors.

The summary of accumulated knowledge at this point represents an opportunity to frankly describe the state of the organization and assess its position vis-à-vis the market. It also allows all parties to get on the "same page" and develop consensus with regard to the assumptions that will underlie the strategy-development process.

Developing the Strategic Plan

The effort expended up to this point provides the foundation for strategy formulation. Different strategists may sequence the actual development of strategy at various points within the process. From this author's perspective the development of marketing strategy should occur at the point at which adequate baseline data have been acquired and analyzed. The sequencing of the strategy-development process as described below will ultimately depend on the nature of the organization and the particular circumstances. The actual process of specifying a strategy is discussed in the next section.

Setting the Goal(s)

The goal or goals established in the strategic plan should reflect the information compiled to date and should be in keeping with the organization's mission statement. The goal depicts an ideal state that will serve as the target for future development. For a national medical-products company, for example, the goal may be to establish the firm as the low-cost provider of a certain product. For a local health services provider, the goal may involve positioning the organization as a niche player to take advantage of certain market opportunities. For the purveyor of a specific service, the goal may be to become recognized as the provider of choice for a certain segment of the market.

Setting Objectives

Objectives should be established in support of the stated goal or goals. To many, objectives represent the tactics that support the strategic initiatives. Objectives for a strategic plan are stated in such terms as, "The hospital's orthopedic practice will recruit a sports medicine specialist within the next 12 months" (in support of the stated goal of expanding the organization's orthopedic product lines).

For every goal a number of objectives are likely to be specified. Multiple objectives are common because action will likely be required on a number of different fronts. As the planning team establishes objectives, any barriers to accomplishing the stated objectives should be considered, identified, and assessed.

The possibility of unanticipated consequences arising from the meeting of any of the objectives should also be considered. For example, a successful marketing campaign may overwhelm the service providers or otherwise overstretch resources. If the organization cannot deliver on the marketer's promises, negative consequences are likely. A marketing campaign may serve to alert competitors to the strategic direction of the organization, or the campaign may alienate an organization that has been a strong supporter of the entity involved in marketing. While negative consequences cannot be totally eliminated, conceding their existence is the first step toward minimizing their impact.

Strategic Options

A number of factors must be considered in the selection of a strategy. Analysts must consider the nature of the organization and its mission, characteristics of the market (and more specifically the organization's customers), and nature of the competition. The strategy chosen will ultimately determine how the public perceives the organization. The approach taken will have long-term implications for the organization.

The SWOT Analysis

Unfortunately, there is no standard list of strategies from which the organization can choose; each situation is likely to be unique and call for creativity. One analytical approach that can be pursued in determining the appropriate strategy is the *SWOT analysis,* which examines for a particular market, organization, or product its strengths, weaknesses, opportunities, and threats (see Box 10.1). The SWOT analysis should provide a basis for subsequent development, as it simultaneously considers several dimensions of the situation.

The assessment of the strengths of the organization will indicate the attributes on which the strategist should capitalize. Weaknesses indicate aspects of the organization that should be minimized or ameliorated. Threats indicate aspects of the organization or environment that should be neutralized by means of the strategic thrust. Of the four dimensions, opportunities have perhaps the most salience for strategy development, as an

Box 10.1: SWOT Analysis

SWOT analysis has become an increasingly common technique for assessing the position of a healthcare organization within its market. It involves an examination of the organization, the environment, and the way the organization and environment interact. SWOT analysis is an important tool for strategists and marketers, one with numerous applications in healthcare. It can be done for departments within organizations as well as for total organizations. SWOT analysis involves an examination of the strengths, weaknesses, opportunities, and threats relative to the community or organization.

A strength can be thought of as a resource, particular skill, or distinctive competence the organization possesses that will aid it in achieving its stated objectives. These would include marketing capabilities, management skills, the organization's image, financial resources, and any number of other assets. The strategy chosen should be designed to capitalize on the strengths of the organization and focus on leveraging them into a strategic advantage.

A weakness refers to any aspect of the organization that may hinder the achievement of specific objectives, such as inadequate working capital, poor management skills, a lack of certain services, or personnel shortages. The organization needs to address any identified weaknesses through eliminating the deficiency (e.g., improving outcome indicators), stabilizing the condition (e.g., replacing aging medical staff members with younger counterparts), or minimizing the impact (e.g., damage control of adverse events). To the extent that weaknesses cannot be eliminated marketing may be used to counter any negative effects.

An opportunity is simply any feature of the external environment that creates conditions advantageous to the firm in relation to a particular objective or set of objectives. Opportunities may take a variety of forms such as gaps in the market, new sources of reimbursement, demographic changes, and weaknesses among competitors. Organizations should capitalize on opportunities by marshaling resources, reallocating funds, and otherwise focusing effort to take advantage of such situations.

A threat is any environmental development that may present problems and hinder the achievement of organizational objectives. Threats may come in the form of competitive activity, unfavorable demographic changes, or anticipated reimbursement changes. Some threats (e.g., reduced Medicare reimbursement) are obviously beyond the control of the organization. However, responses can be developed to most threats, even if the response only involves a marketing initiative to counter the impact. Threats often arise as a result of changing market conditions, managed care developments, or actions of competitors. Threats of these types can usually be addressed through aggressive action.

SWOT analysis should include input from the quantitative research being conducted as well as from the interviews administered. Because the strengths, weaknesses, opportunities, and threats identified will guide further development of the plan, consensus must be reached on these attributes before proceeding with the planning process.

implicit goal of the strategy chosen should be to exploit opportunities that exist in the marketplace.

Ideally, the strategy employed for any marketing initiative will support the organization's mission statement and reflect the strategies embodied in the organization's strategic plan. Thus, if the organization's strategy involves positioning itself as a caring organization, the organization's marketing initiatives should support this approach. Of course, a particular marketing situation may call for a departure from the established approach. For example, a hospital that has been content to live in the shadow of a more powerful competitor while adopting a "We're number two" approach may develop a world-class program in a particular clinical area and decide to be much more aggressive in the marketing of this service. Thus, a "second fiddle" strategy may be displaced by a "flanking" strategy in light of the new developments.

Market-Oriented Strategies

Other approaches to strategy development may focus on the market and generate market-oriented strategies. Others may focus on a product or service line and emphasize a product-oriented strategy. Another approach may address an aspect of the marketing mix, as in the case of a pricing strategy, or may cut across the marketing mix and be broader in scope.

A *market-penetration strategy* (existing market/existing product) would involve efforts to extract more sales and greater usage out of existing customers, acquire customers from competitors, and convert nonusers into users. A *market-development strategy* (new market/existing product) would involve identifying new market sectors based on different benefit profiles, establishing new distribution channels, determining new marketing approaches, and identifying underserved geographic areas. For example, a market niche strategy may be pursued by a healthcare organization that serves small segments of the market that other firms overlook or ignore.

A *new-product or service-development strategy* (existing market/new product) would call for modifying existing services, introducing differing quality levels, or developing entirely new products. A *diversification strategy* (new market/new product) would involve actions such as horizontal or vertical integration, concentric diversification, and conglomerate diversification.

Looked at differently, the market-product relationship can be depicted in five distinct configurations: (1) full service, (2) product/market specialization, (3) product specialization, (4) market specialization, and (5) selective specialization (see Box 10.2).

Examples of each of these relationships can be drawn from the health-care field, with the term *service* substituted for *product* in most cases. The *full service approach* was typical of most hospitals in the past, particularly during the production era. General hospitals attempted to be all things to all people, and their strategies reflected this orientation. Thus, all products are marketed to all markets when employing this strategy. A *product/market specialization strategy* would be adopted by an organization that supports a single service or service line for a defined market, as in the case of a home infusion company that provides a discrete set of services to a narrowly defined market.

An example of *product specialization* may be provided by a firm specializing in assistive equipment such as wheelchairs, walkers, home monitoring devices, and so forth. This firm offers a distinct set of products that can be promoted to a number of markets with one characteristic in common—physical limitations that require assistive equipment. This firm's market would include the frail elderly, individuals suffering from birth defects, injury victims, and those undergoing rehabilitation from surgery.

Organizations emphasizing *market specialization* typically develop a range of products geared to a certain market—for example, an organization that offers senior services or one that specializes in women's health-care goods and services. This approach assumes that a particular market is open to a range of different products. Pharmaceutical companies are probably the best-known example of *selective specialization*. Each drug constitutes a product line targeted to a specific market. Thus, ABC Pharmaceuticals's hypertension drug is marketed to the hypertensive market, its diabetes drug to the population affected by diabetes, and its arthritis drug to the population of rheumatics.

Another approach to strategy development examines the combination of *market attractiveness* and *competitiveness* found in the situation under study. For example, an area characterized by high market attractiveness and high competitiveness may call for a strategy involving investment and growth or, more likely, a strategy emphasizing selective growth that focuses on vulnerable areas. Different combinations of market attractiveness and competitiveness call for different strategies.

A number of examples of market-oriented strategies used in health-care can be identified:

- *Dominance strategy:* the number-one player in the market opts to focus on maintaining this position
- *Second-fiddle strategy:* the runner-up in the market concedes its second fiddle status and acts accordingly, adopting what may also be called a *market-follower strategy*

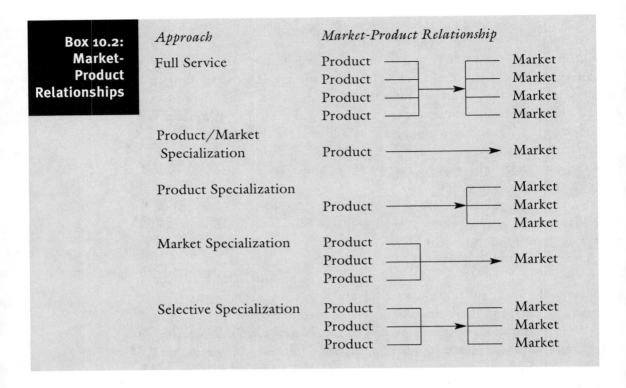

Approach

Market-Product Relationship

Full Service

Product —— Market
Product —— Market
Product —— Market
Product —— Market

Product/Market
Specialization

Product ————————→ Market

Product Specialization

Market
Product ————→ Market
Market

Market Specialization

Product
Product ————————→ Market
Product

Selective Specialization

Product —— Market
Product ——→ Market
Product —— Market

- *Frontal-attack strategy:* the organization decides to confront the market leader or major competitors head on
- *Niche strategy:* the organization concedes that it cannot successfully compete for the mainstream market but instead concentrates on niche markets based on geography, population groups, or selected services
- *Flanking strategy:* the organization outflanks the competition by entering new markets, cultivating new populations, or offering fringe products

Strategy Development and the Four Ps

One approach to selecting a strategy reflects the role of the marketing mix in establishing direction. The *marketing mix* is the set of controllable variables that the organization uses to influence the target market. The mix includes product, price, place, and promotion. The strategy could focus on any dimension of the four Ps or cut across all four. Approaches to the four different components of the marketing mix are addressed below.

Product Strategies

As the name implies, product strategies focus on a good (or product line) or service (or service line) of the organization. The strategy is built around the qualities of the product, and the marketing approach attempts to capitalize on this. Some product strategies were previously discussed within the context of market/product strategies.

An example of a product strategy would be a *preemptive strategy,* used where only limited differences exist between the products within a given product class. A preemptive strike attempts to say something about a product that competitors would be reluctant to repeat on the risk of being labeled as blatant imitators. Another product-oriented approach focuses on a *unique selling proposition* and relates to the ability of the organization to establish and communicate a distinct product benefit that competitors cannot make or refuse to make. Marketers may also adopt a *brand-image strategy* concerned more with psychological than physical differences between products. The aim is to associate the product with symbols and characters to which the potential target audience relates.

A *positioning strategy* attempts to heighten in the consumer's mind the differences between one product and another. The task is to identify weaknesses in competing products and strengths in one's product that can be reinforced to gain a competitive edge. A positioning strategy can be created by (1) identifying alternative competitors and competing products within a defined product category, (2) establishing consumers' perceptions of competing products, (3) determining the relative position of competing products using a perceptional positioning map, (4) identifying the gap within the market by assessing customer needs with regard to existing product offerings, (5) selecting the desired positioning, (6) implementing the marketing and promotional strategy, and (7) monitoring and controlling the process. (See Berkowitz 1996 for additional examples of strategic approaches.) An example of strategy development is presented in Case Study 10.1.

Pricing Strategies

Healthcare providers have seldom employed pricing strategies in the past. End users of health services historically have not known the prices of the services provided before they were received, and the primary decision maker with regard to purchasing decisions—the physician—seldom took pricing into consideration in determining the therapy. Furthermore, the amount of reimbursement for services from third-party payers was often established independent of the price set by the provider.

For these reasons healthcare has provided few opportunities for organizations providing patient care to compete in terms of price. On the other hand, more retail-oriented healthcare businesses, such as personal-health product manufacturers, are likely to employ pricing strategies in much the same manner as producers of other consumer goods.

Another sector of the industry where price may be a factor is the insurance industry. While insurance premiums have historically been established based on the perceived risk to the insurer, the emergence of managed care plans resulted in a situation of unprecedented competition. By the 1990s managed care plans had become more standardized and were forced to compete in terms of price. Because the products were essentially undifferentiated, price became a rational basis for competition.

A major drawback to the use of pricing strategies in healthcare is the fact that healthcare providers have not historically been able to determine the cost of producing a service. The development of an intelligent pricing strategy requires some objective basis for establishing a price. Furthermore, restrictions related to price fixing have prevented healthcare providers from using the fee schedules of other organizations as models.

Despite these barriers to the use of pricing strategies, growing numbers of providers are competing on price, primarily reflecting the growing importance of elective procedures in the industry. Price can be used as a basis for competition for services that are discretionary and typically paid for out of pocket. Most cosmetic surgery falls into this category, and, as competition has increased among ophthalmic surgeons, ophthalmologists performing laser eye surgery have begun to compete on the basis of price.

Place Strategies

Place focuses on the manner of distribution for a good or service; in healthcare this typically refers to the place where services are rendered. An important aspect of place is the channel of distribution—the path a good or service takes as it travels from the producer to the consumer. While this concept has traditionally applied to consumer goods, it also applies to health services.

A variety of distribution channels are used to deliver health services. Primary care centers are typically located near potential patients (e.g., in neighborhoods, in heavily populated residential areas), whereas tertiary services are concentrated in medical centers regardless of the proximity to population centers. (Indeed, one of the major considerations of the last years of the twentieth century was the movement of populations away from inner-city medical centers.) Emergency services represent a combination of distribution methods because ambulances travel to the individual but then take the individual to the hospital for treatment.

During the production era in healthcare little emphasis was placed on the location of service outlets. The bulk of the care was provided by hospitals, and patients were expected to travel to wherever the hospital was located. The same attitude was evinced on the part of physicians, especially specialists. While primary care providers may have sought out locations in the community that were close to patient populations, the overriding attitude was, "If you build it, they will come."

The actions of some hospitals in the 1990s provide an example of channel-management efforts. In the early 1990s hospitals attempted to control the distribution of their primary care providers by purchasing and controlling physicians. However, hospital administrators failed to consider that the product—physician practice patterns—could not be easily controlled. As a result these attempts at controlling distribution channels largely failed. Although the distribution of the practices was controlled by the hospitals, hospitals were unable to control the product or price of these same physician practices, thereby failing to benefit from their control of the distribution outlets.

As the focus of healthcare shifted from the inpatient to outpatient setting healthcare providers were forced to pay more attention to the location of services. While hospitals were effectively immobile, outpatient services could be established potentially anywhere. Those who sought to compete with hospitals took advantage of their relative immobility and established facilities in proximity to target markets.

Furthermore, a new generation of healthcare consumers with different expectations of healthcare providers emerged. Led by the baby boom cohort, these patients brought a consumer orientation that demanded convenience of location and easy access to services. They placed a high value on their time and expected the same of service providers. The healthcare industry responded to this emerging consumerism by offering urgent care centers and freestanding diagnostic and surgery centers as convenient alternatives to traditional sources of care.

This new emphasis on place has also been encouraged by the employers and business coalitions that pay a large share of the healthcare bill. Employers want their employees to have convenient access to services, not only to ensure patient satisfaction but also to limit the time lost from work. In addition, one of the bases for competition among managed care plans has been the convenience they provide their enrollees. Health maintenance organizations and other health plans found it necessary to establish networks of providers distributed in a manner that would meet the needs of their enrollee populations.

The combined influence of these developments has encouraged healthcare providers to take healthcare to the community. It is no longer a viable approach to expect patients to come to the source of care. The contemporary consumer demands convenient locations, and, in cases where locations cannot be changed, healthcare providers are attempting to enhance effective access through more efficient patient-processing methods and more appealing facilities.

Promotional Strategies

The most visible type of strategy employed by healthcare organizations is likely to be one that relates to the promotion of the organization or its services. Much of the marketing effort on the part of healthcare providers over the past two decades has focused on advertising, direct mail, and other promotional strategies. The limitations on competition based on product, price, and place have encouraged healthcare providers to attempt to differentiate themselves through promotional strategies.

Promotional strategies should reflect the overriding strategic orientation of the organization. If, for example, a hospital adopts a niche strategy, its promotional efforts will be highly focused on a narrow range of services or a highly targeted population. On the other hand, a hospital pursuing a full-service strategy is likely to employ a strategy that promotes the organization as the source of virtually any service.

Similarly, the promotional strategy should reflect the approach to the market that the organization has chosen. If the organization has adopted an aggressive, hard-sell approach to the market, the promotional strategy should reflect this. Conversely, the organization may have adopted a soft-sell approach that would be reflected in initiatives meant to educate the market.

A promotions-oriented strategy can take a variety of forms. For example, a *resonance strategy* is one that strikes a chord with the consumer. The intention is to portray a lifestyle orientation synonymous with the target group and easily recognizable. Such an approach may be advocated for the promotion of a hospital-based fitness center. An *emotional strategy* may be adopted by healthcare organizations wishing to play on, as well as play to, the emotions of the consumer, as in the case of children's health services.

In the contemporary healthcare arena promotional strategies involve far more than advertising. Increasingly, healthcare providers are turning to personal selling and sales promotions in an effort to compete more effectively (Berkowitz 1996). An effective promotional strategy requires an understanding of the various media available and the ability to craft a message with appropriate content and tone. Promotional strategies are addressed frequently throughout the remainder of this book.

Branding as a Strategy

Corporate identity refers to a company's name, logo, or tagline. *Corporate image* is the public's perception of a company, whether that perception is intended or not. By contrast, *corporate branding* is a business process that is planned, strategically focused, and integrated throughout the organization to establish the direction, leadership, clarity of purpose, and energy of a company's corporate brand. Thus, a brand identity is the visual, emotional, rational, and cultural image a consumer associates with a company or product. These features include the brand's name, image, typography, color, package design, and slogans (Mangini 2002).

An effective brand name evokes positive associations with the brand. The brand image indicates what business the company is in, what benefit it provides, and why it is better than the competition. Brand associations are the attributes consumers think of when they hear or see the brand name. Therefore, the logic behind branding is simple: If consumers are more familiar with a company's brand, they are more likely to purchase the company's products.

A company's brand also has significant internal value. A strong corporate brand generates and sustains internal momentum. Employees have proven to be more committed to the brand's promise if every key player understands and follows it. Thus, to maximize the effectiveness of the company's brand all relevant audiences—consumers, prospects, business partners, the media, and employees—must understand it. Corporate communications should be coordinated to reinforce the branding effort.

Branding has been relatively uncommon among healthcare providers in the past, although some notable exceptions exist: the Mayo Clinic and the Cleveland Clinic, for example, have established national brands (see Case Study 10.2). This is a reflection of the particular characteristics of healthcare. Branding is most effective for products that command a mass market, can benefit from advertising, and can be effectively evaluated by consumers. Few healthcare services display these characteristics.

The lag in the adoption of branding strategies in healthcare has had both negative and positive consequences for healthcare marketing. The negative consequences include the lack of expertise in and success for today's healthcare branding strategies. The positive consequences, however, focus on the various branding techniques and lessons that have developed in other industries that healthcare can adopt. The emergence of the new healthcare consumer has raised the interest in branding among healthcare providers. This revitalized consumerism is being driven by well-informed consumers who are demanding choices.

For established retailers of healthcare products (e.g., pharmaceuticals, personal-health products), branding has been an inherent part of their strategy. In those cases consumers are more likely to be familiar with the brand (e.g., Claritin, Band Aids) than with the corporation that produces the product. The development of branding strategies in this segment of the industry reflects the appropriateness of these products for this approach.

According to Mangini (2002) establishing a brand identity requires several steps. First, an institution must decide what to brand. This requires careful consideration of the services the organization offers, the people who provide the service, the competition's services, and the population the organization serves. Branding can focus on the entire health system, outpatient services, a prominent department, or a particular medical group. In addition, an institution may choose to focus on products and services that have a high demand but are difficult to emulate. No matter what area a healthcare organization decides to brand, effective brands in healthcare have almost always been linked to a specific target audience such as women or senior citizens.

Second, a healthcare institution must define the brand message it wants to communicate about the service it has decided to brand. For example, an institution may choose to focus on quality of care, convenience, or its technological capabilities. Each of these aspects can be effective if the brand message relates to the target audience and the service being branded.

Third, the brand must be communicated both internally and externally. Internal communication is important to ensure both staff acceptance and enthusiasm, which are necessary for brand success. This can be accomplished through establishing staff ownership of branding communications and rewards for staff involvement in the campaign. External communication can take place through various channels such as business documentation and advertising. The most important aspect, however, is that the overall message is clear, consistent, and continuous.

The true test of an institution's brand is performance. An institution must be confident that it will be able to fulfill the promise its brand portrays. Every consumer interaction must reinforce the brand identity and be used to establish a relationship with that consumer. If consumers have a positive interaction with the organization and are satisfied, they have the potential to be sources of new business. Thus, information will be key in determining the performance of an institution's brand. The healthcare institution must develop a systemwide computerized data collection, analysis, and reporting network. This information will allow the institution to continually assess the success of its brand and make necessary changes.

Once a brand is built, it must be continually updated and revitalized. Brand revitalization does not simply encompass a new product, service logo, or repackaging but must also focus on the company's true point of differentiation. A successful branding process provides a framework for the organization that links the branding and business strategies. This linkage is essential, as a key component of a successful branding strategy deals with the commitment and involvement of executive management. Finally, once the institution's brand identity and framework is understood by all key players, documentation of the branding system can begin.

Summary

A well-thought-out marketing strategy is essential for any healthcare organization that hopes to compete in today's environment. Strategies set the tone for marketing activities and establish the parameters within which the marketer must operate. The strategy chosen will influence the nature of the marketing plan that is ultimately developed and will guide any subsequent marketing initiatives. A strategy performs a number of functions for an organization, and de facto strategies emerge in the absence of a formal strategy. Strategies may be developed at different levels, from an overall corporate strategy to a specific marketing initiative.

Strategies should be developed during the strategic planning process and be imposed on any marketing activities. A number of steps should be followed in developing the strategic direction of the organization, from initial data collection through data analysis to the identification of strategic options. All key stakeholders should participate in the strategy-development process.

Strategies often reflect the importance of the four Ps of the marketing mix—product, price, place, and promotion. A SWOT analysis may be used to provide direction to strategy development.

A number of different strategy options are available to healthcare organizations, and the particular type of organization and circumstances related to the environment will determine the best option. The strategy chosen should reflect the organization's positioning within the market. Most strategies involve some consideration of the product-market relationship, with options ranging from matching a specific product to a narrowly defined market to "shotgunning" a range of products to a broad market. Branding as a strategy has become increasingly important in healthcare.

Discussion Questions

- What are some of the different functions that a strategy performs for an organization?

- What is meant when it is said that the lack of a strategy represents a strategic statement on the part of the organization?
- What are the steps involved in the strategic planning process?
- In what way should an organization's marketing strategy link to its strategic plan?
- What are some of the types of strategies that may be formulated, and what determines the best type of strategy for a particular situation?
- What are some ways in which the product and market interface during strategy development?
- What is the relationship between strategy development and the four Ps of the marketing mix?
- What determines which of the four Ps is most relevant to strategy in a particular case?
- Why is a branding strategy not universally accepted by all healthcare organizations?
- Under what circumstances does a branding strategy appear to work best?

References

Berkowitz, E. N. 1996. *Essentials of Health Care Marketing.* Gaithersburg, MD: Aspen.

Mangini, M. K. 2002. "Branding 101." *Marketing Health Services* 22 (3): 20–23.

Thomas, R. K. 2003. *Health Services Planning, 2nd ed.* New York: Wolters Kluwer.

Additional Resources

Ansoff, H. I. 1957. "Strategies for Diversification." *Harvard Business Review* 35 (5): 113–24.

Bashe, G. 2000. *Branding Health Services: Defining Yourself in the Marketplace.* Sudbury, MA: Jones and Bartlett.

Coddington, D. C., E. A. Fischer, and K. D. Moore. 2001. *Strategies for the New Healthcare Marketplace.* San Francisco: Jossey-Bass.

Mintzberg, H. 1994. *The Rise and Fall of Strategic Planning.* New York: The Free Press.

10.1

STRATEGY DEVELOPMENT

A hospital management company recently acquired a 150-bed general hospital in a medium-sized city in the southeastern United States. Although it acquired the facility with relatively limited knowledge of the local market, the organization's first thought was to continue to run the facility as a general hospital. However, given that the hospital had not been particularly profitable offering general care and faced competition from three large facilities that had access to almost unlimited resources, the new managers chose to perform a situational analysis to determine the most appropriate strategic approach to pursue.

The managers commissioned a study of the immediate market area, the five-mile radius of patients who could be attracted to a general hospital. The immediate market area was examined within the context of overall trends for the metropolitan area. The analysts reviewed demographic trends to determine the future size and composition of the population, analyzed trends in service utilization, and developed projections of the likely future demand for health services in the broader community and the immediate market area. Particular attention was paid to the competitive situation to determine the service offerings of various players, existing market shares for various services, and nature of existing managed care contracts and other negotiated relationships.

The analysis determined that the immediate service area was not likely to support a general hospital. The payer mix was not favorable, and other facilities maintained major shares of the local market. Furthermore, most area employers were tied into the provider networks of the two dominant systems in the community. The hospital did not have a large or strong medical staff, and it would be difficult to attract additional physicians to the facility.

Having conceded that it was not possible to operate effectively as a general community hospital nor confront large, established competitors head on, other types of strategies were given consideration. After an analysis of the data it was decided that under the circumstances a niche strategy was appropriate for the hospital. Specific niche services would be identified, and corporate efforts would be focused on exploiting these niches.

The hospital had previously developed an occupational health program that catered to the numerous employers proximate to the area. Facilities were available, a basic program was in place, and adequate personnel were available to provide the basis for expansion of this program. Given the void in this service in the community, this appeared to be a logical direction to take. In addition, the hospital had long had a behavioral health program that had experienced some success in attracting patients. Some of the area's leading substance abuse experts were also affiliated with the hospital. Because a fledgling program was already in place, key personnel were available, and the market was underserved, behavioral health (including substance abuse treatment) was identified as a high priority for the hospital. In view of the large Medicaid population in the general area and the lack of geropsychiatric services in the community, it was decided to add geropsychiatric services to the behavioral health component.

This niche strategy focused on services that were not being adequately provided to the community, and another niche initiative was considered but eventually rejected. Market research had indicated that the community contained a large proportion of minority group members, primarily African Americans, and that the Hispanic population in the area was growing rapidly. Furthermore, these populations had historically been neglected by mainstream providers. A niche strategy focusing on these target populations was considered to essentially convert the hospital into a facility specializing in minority care. Because of the many unknowns surrounding this concept and the potential controversy such a strategy might arouse, this idea was rejected.

After carefully assessing the situation the hospital chose a niche strategy from among the various strategic alternatives. The managers conceded that the facility could not successfully operate as a general hospital and chose to pursue a narrower strategy. The approach has, in the short run at least, been relatively successful, with this hospital maintaining a significant share of the occupational health and behavioral health markets in the city and earning a reputation as a facility that does not do a lot of things but does a few things well.

10.2

ESTABLISHING A BRAND

The healthcare industry has not adopted branding as a strategy to the extent that other industries have, and healthcare organizations have experienced both successes and failures with regard to their branding initiatives. One example of a successful branding initiative is that developed by the Cleveland Clinic Foundation in Cleveland, Ohio. The Cleveland Clinic exemplifies the potential of branding for healthcare organizations and provides an illustration of how a small outpatient practice can be transformed into a national brand. The Cleveland Clinic was founded in 1921 by four veterans of World War I medical units and is now a leading U.S. healthcare organization. From its start the clinic was highly regarded for the quality of its specialty care, basic science achievements, and medical research. The clinic's initial marketing approach, typical of healthcare organizations in the premarketing era, directed all efforts toward the physician audience in an effort to increase patient referrals. Promotional activities consisted of the development of fundraising brochures and dissemination of press releases to the media.

In the 1990s the clinic, realizing that healthcare consumers were looking for a trusted brand name, expanded its market research. The research indicated that the name "Cleveland Clinic" was highly respected by local consumers; as a result the clinic focused on the maintenance and protection of its brand through an integrated marketing effort.

The 1990s also marked a period of hospital mergers and acquisitions in the healthcare industry, and the clinic played a significant role in this development. Over a two-year period the Cleveland Clinic Health System was formed, building on the clinic's merger with ten local community hospitals. The formation of this system presented a challenge in that the clinic had to decide how much it could share its brand identity without causing brand dilution.

To address this challenge the clinic established a four-tiered marketing approach that applies to all organizations using the Cleveland Clinic brand. Tier 1 members represent the core organizations and the essence of the Cleveland Clinic. These core organizations are seen as the conservators of the brand, and all marketing efforts are directed out of Tier 1. Tier 2 members include entities owned by the Cleveland Clinic. These entities have their own brand equity and in their advertisements are allowed to use only the words "Cleveland Clinic Health System," in half size under their own hospital names. Tier 3 includes Cleveland Clinic departments in nonowned hospitals. Tier 3 entities are not part of the Cleveland Clinic Foundation or Cleveland Clinic Health System, and the appropriate relationships are outlined in their advertising. The use of the Cleveland Clinic name, logo, or tagline is prohibited in this tier. Finally, Tier 4 includes organizations to which the Cleveland Clinic belongs. In these relationships the Cleveland Clinic logo may be used, but only in visual arrangements with the logos of the other participating hospitals.

The Cleveland Clinic has been successful in its branding initiatives to support the integrity of the Cleveland Clinic brand while extending the positive image of the brand to other entities and avoiding dilution of existing brand equity. While not all healthcare organizations can be expected to have the same success as the Cleveland Clinic, this case illustrates how, with sound market intelligence and thoughtful planning, a successful branding initiative can be implemented.

PROMOTIONS, ADVERTISING, AND SALES

T his chapter provides an overview of the traditional promotional techniques used by marketers. A discussion of established approaches like public relations, advertising, personal sales, and sales promotion will be accompanied by a discussion of direct-marketing techniques. The communication model that underlies all promotions is described, and the rationale for the use of various techniques is presented.

Promotional Mix

The promotional component of the marketing mix could be considered the "action" component in that the marketing plan is implemented through promotions. *Promotions* refers to the variety of techniques used to communicate with customers and potential customers with the purpose of promoting an idea, organization, or product. The range of traditional promotional activities include public relations (PR), advertising, sales promotion, and personal selling. For our purposes we will also include direct marketing. Each of these categories include a number of specific techniques. The *promotional mix* refers to the combination of these elements that constitute the chosen promotional strategy.

Promotional Categories

Publicity

Publicity refers to any promotion that draws attention to the organization in a general way without specifically targeting any audience. This traditional activity of healthcare organizations predates the more recent emphasis on advertising and other promotional techniques. The core activity for generating publicity is embodied in the PR function.

As noted earlier, PR is a form of communication management that seeks to make use of publicity and other nonpaid forms of promotion and information to influence feelings, opinions, or beliefs about the organization and its offerings. PR includes press releases, press conferences, distribution of feature stories to the media, and other publicity-oriented activities. Core functions include the gathering of media representatives for announcements and distributing news releases describing some newsworthy event or activity with the hope of getting press coverage.

The public service announcement (PSA) may also be considered a vehicle for publicity. The PSA is an advertisement or commercial carried by an advertising vehicle at no cost as a public service to its readers, viewers, or listeners. PSAs could be carried on radio or television or be printed in a newspaper or magazine. Billboards are also used for PSAs. While the no-cost aspect is appealing, the downside is that the organization has no control over the placement or timing of PSA presentations.

Various forms of communication may also be considered under the publicity heading. Healthcare organizations typically establish mechanisms for communicating with their various publics (both internal and external). Communications staff develop materials for dissemination to the public and employees of the organization. Internal newsletters and publications geared to relevant customer groups (e.g., patients, enrollees) are generated, and patient education materials are frequently developed by communications staff. Separate communications departments may be established, or this function may overlap with the PR or community outreach functions.

Another form of publicity may involve sponsorships on the part of the organization. This may involve corporate financial backing for a project or event in return for public exposure and goodwill. The sponsor typically does not run an advertisement but may be mentioned in terms of "brought to you by. . . ." A sponsorship can be defined as the process through which an organization supports a beneficiary for altruistic reasons or purposes of gaining favorable attention and publicity. A sponsorship has two main advantages for the sponsor: (1) it provides the sponsor with potentially substantial media coverage, and (2) it can have the internal benefit of helping to improve employee morale.

Publicity may also be generated by means of campaign spokespersons, who often include national or local celebrities, depending on the nature of the organization. Spokespersons could be athletes, entertainers, community leaders, or others thought to influence the public mind-set. They could be animated characters known to the public or characters created specifically for a promotion. By associating itself with a recognizable person or character, the organization benefits from the goodwill generated by the spokesperson.

Community outreach programs may also be considered under the heading of publicity. Community outreach is a form of marketing that seeks to present the programs of the organization to the community and establish relationships with community organizations. Community outreach may involve episodic activities such as health fairs or educational programs for community residents. This function may also include ongoing initiatives involving outreach workers who are visible within the community on a recurring basis. This aspect of marketing emphasizes the organization's commitment to the community and its support of community organizations. While the benefits of community outreach activities are not as easily measured as some more direct marketing activities, the organization often gains customers as a result of its health-screening activities, follow-up from educational seminars, or outreach-worker referrals.

Also included under publicity may be the basic informational materials that would be developed for any organization, program, or product. These include informational brochures, letterhead, business cards, e-mail addresses, and increasingly web sites. Every organization needs these basic materials to promote itself or its particular product.

This approach is typically low cost and easily implemented and is particularly useful for helping maintain visibility and keeping the public informed of the organization's activities. On the other hand, there is always a lot of competition for attention from the press, and the organization is often at the mercy of other parties in terms of getting the word out. This approach involves a relatively soft sell, does not allow for repeated exposures to the same product, and is diffuse in its impact.

Advertising

Advertising refers to any paid form of nonpersonal presentation for the promotion of ideas, goods, or services by an identifiable sponsor, typically using mass media as the communication vehicle. The advertising objectives are similar to those outlined for publicity, although advertising is often more focused. The objectives of advertising include the following:

1. Promoting products, services, organizations, and causes
2. Increasing product usage
3. Reinforcing and reminding consumers of the organization or product
4. Building customer loyalty
5. Introducing new products
6. Offsetting competitors' advertising
7. Assisting sales personnel

8. Alleviating sales fluctuations
9. Educating consumers
10. Maintaining visibility

Not all of these objectives apply directly to healthcare marketing, and they are likely to be applied selectively in response to the type of marketing being undertaken. Many types of healthcare organizations would find some of these objectives irrelevant.

Advertising may be classified as institutional (or corporate) advertising or product advertising. *Institutional advertising* promotes an organization's images, people, ideas, or political issues and anything that the advertiser wants to publicize. *Product advertising* promotes specific goods and services.

Institutional advertising has several variations and can focus on the introduction or announcement of a new service, product or facility, comparative advertising, or the presentation of a public policy stance. Product advertising can take one of three forms or a mixture of the three; it can (1) be informational in nature, (2) be competitive in nature, or (3) serve as a reminder. Informational advertising promotes the attributes of the organization independent of any other market factors, whereas competitive advertising compares one brand directly or indirectly to one or more other brands.

Professional advertising targets members of a profession such as law, medicine, engineering, or architecture. Much of the advertising that occurs in healthcare is aimed at physicians, with other health professions also attracting a certain amount of advertising attention. Pharmaceutical companies are notorious for their advertising campaigns toward physicians, with advertising inserts in professional journals and trade publications and the production and distribution of a wide range of advertising gimmicks to physicians.

Specialty advertising involves the placement of advertising messages on a wide variety of items of interest to the target markets such as calendars, coffee cups, pens, hats, note paper, or t-shirts. While this is technically advertising, the distribution of such items probably is more appropriately classified under sales promotion.

An understanding of the various media that serve as vehicles for advertising is important to healthcare marketers, and this topic is addressed in a separate section below.

Personal Selling

A major tool of the promotional mix is *personal selling,* which involves the oral presentation of information through a conversation with one or more prospective purchasers for the purpose of making sales. The primary difference between personal selling and advertising is that the former involves a personal form of communication.

The primary purposes of personal selling are to (1) find prospects, (2) convince prospects to buy the product, and (3) keep existing customers satisfied. The functions of personal selling at the prenegotiatory stage include finding potential buyers, discovering their latent needs, and producing feedback related to the products. At the negotiatory stage the functions include persuasively presenting the product and negotiating mutually agreeable prices and terms of sale, administrating sales efficiently, and providing technical backup service. At the postnegotiatory stage the functions involve providing after-sales service, forecasting future sales, and maintaining relationships. Thus, the role of the salesperson involves more than merely selling; it includes communicating with customers in the wider sense and performing market research.

An advantage of personal selling is that it allows for direct feedback from the receiver. The message can then be refined or explained in greater detail to correct any misunderstandings or difficulties that the receiver had in interpretation. Personal selling also has an advantage over advertising in that it provides more direct control over who receives the message. With personal selling, a company can directly target the audience to communicate. Hospitals that incorporate personal selling into their promotional mixes report several benefits, including increased facility occupancy, improved medical staff relations, higher profitability, and increased market share (Berkowitz 1996).

Well-established personal selling activities in healthcare include calls on physicians by pharmaceutical and medical supplier representatives, calls on consumers by insurance salespeople, and calls on hospitals by biomedical equipment representatives. More recently healthcare providers have become active in personal sales, with hospital representatives calling on referring physicians, employers, and other organizations to promote the hospital's emergency room, sports medicine program, or a particular service line. These activities have become increasingly important as interaction between individual physicians and patients has been displaced by interfaces between groups of providers and groups of purchasers.

As with any promotional tool, however, personal selling also has limitations. A major limitation of personal selling is its cost. Costs for a sales staff also include individual benefits, travel costs, and technical and equipment support, in addition to salaries. The number of sales calls a person can make in one day is limited, and in healthcare sales calls to referring physician offices or companies can be time consuming. Another limitation to personal selling is related directly to the strength of the interpersonal communication. Because sales involves a person, the message may vary as a function of the individual's training, disposition, or style (Berkowitz 1996).

The more technologically sophisticated the service, the greater the need for personal selling. A salesperson may be needed to explain the intricacies of a particular diagnostic technique or program. A health system may use a sales representative to call on potential referring physicians to introduce new diagnostic technology, for example. Personal sales are also important when a variety of decision makers (perhaps coming from differing perspectives) are involved or when the decision carries an element of risk (such as committing to a managed care contract).

While healthcare-product companies are expected to continue to rely on sales staff to promote their goods and equipment, healthcare providers are likely to rely more on advertising than on personal sales. This reflects the fact that in a consumer-choice environment the necessity of gaining exposure to thousands of prospective customers makes promotional efforts rather than personal selling more practical.

The personal selling mix can involve a combination of sales presentations, sales meetings, incentive programs, distribution of samples, and participation in fairs and trade shows. Regardless of the personal selling mix, certain steps are followed in the selling process (see Box 11.1).

An aspect of personal sales that characterizes many not-for-profit healthcare organizations is fundraising. Many healthcare organizations rely on donations to support their operations or fund capital improvements. These organizations must market themselves to potential donors to secure contributions. While much of this effort may involve direct marketing in the form of direct mail or telemarketing, major contributors typically must be contacted in person. Thus, many larger not-for-profit healthcare organizations maintain a sales staff dedicated to the solicitation of large donors.

Sales Promotion

Sales promotion refers to any activity or material that acts as a direct inducement by offering added value or incentive to the product for resellers, salespersons, or consumers to achieve a specific sales and marketing objective. The sales promotion mix includes (1) health fairs and trade shows, (2) exhibits, (3) demonstrations, (4) contests and games, (5) premiums and gifts, (6) rebates, (7) low-interest financing, and (8) trade-in allowances.

Consumer-sales promotion methods have less application to healthcare than to most other industries, although both "pull" and "push" incentives are used at various times within the industry. Some *pull incentives* used with consumer goods may also apply to personal healthcare products and include money off next purchase, cash refunds, discount coupons, buy-

**Box 11.1:
Steps in
the Selling
Process**
The selling process is divided into a number of separate steps that the salesperson follows when promoting an organization or product. These steps and some examples of the activities involved are presented below.

Prospecting and Qualifying

The first step in the selling process involves the identification of qualified potential customers. In healthcare this may mean identifying potential referring physicians, organ donors, or purchasers of biomedical equipment. In the case of a pharmaceutical representative this would involve identifying the physicians who practice in the relevant specialties.

Preapproach

At this step in the process the salesperson learns as much as possible about a prospective customer before making a sales call. If supplies are being marketed to hospitals, it is important to determine the level of usage and current source of supplies. A pharmaceutical representative must know something about a physician's prescribing practices and the drugs she typically prescribes.

Approach

At this step the salesperson meets the buyer establish a relationship. Healthcare sales are typically not characterized by the wining and dining that often accompany promotional activities in other industries; in fact, defining the appropriate approach for use in healthcare sales is difficult because of the wide variation in situations. This step is carried out by the pharmaceutical representative at the physician's office.

Presentation and Demonstration

At this step in the selling process the salesperson tells the product story to the buyer, indicating its attributes and benefits for the customer. Healthcare providers are not necessarily used to being marketed to, and even getting in front of the right person is often a challenge in a large healthcare organization. The pharmaceutical representative will be allotted a few minutes of the physician's time in order to tell his product story.

Handling Objections

At this step the salesperson seeks out, clarifies, and overcomes customer objections to buying. Because of the nature of healthcare, the process is likely to take on more of a consultative aspect rather than a hard-sell approach. Objections are likely to be addressed in a collaborative rather than a negotiatory manner. The pharmaceutical representative will presumably have cost and effectiveness data to provide the physician to counter any objections.

Closing

This is the step in the selling process at which the salesperson asks the customer for an order or otherwise consummates the sale. This is often less straightforward in healthcare than in other industries because so many parties may have to participate in the decision-making process. The pharmaceutical representative would close the deal by receiving assurance from the physician that she will prescribe his drugs, or at least accept some samples for distribution to patients.

Follow-up

The last step involves the salesperson following up after the sale to ensure customer satisfaction and repeat business. In healthcare relationship management is likely to be more important than in other industries, and continued customer support is often required. The pharmaceutical representative will follow-up to determine the extent to which his drug has been prescribed and the feedback the physician has received from her patients.

one-get-more-free promotions, consumer contests, loyalty cards, free trials (i.e., samples), free products, price reductions, merchandising and point-of-sale displays, and advertising in stores.

A *push incentive* is implemented when the manufacturer or provider of services influences intermediaries to carry or deliver the product. Pharmaceutical companies use this strategy when they leave samples at physicians' offices and clinics. The push strategy is used so that physicians and nurse practitioners will give patients samples and write prescriptions, pushing the product through the channel to the end consumer.

Pharmaceutical companies use both pull and push strategies in promoting drugs to their target audiences. By using a pull strategy pharmaceutical companies appeal directly to the consumer, realizing that the consumer will create the demand for the product and pull the product through the channel. Stated differently, the consumer demands that the physician write a prescription for the product, ensuring that at least one intermediary is distributing the product. When the consumer requests the prescription to be filled by the pharmacy, the consumer is again pulling the product through the supply chain, as the pharmacy must order the pharmaceutical from the manufacturer to fill the prescription. At the same time these pharmaceutical companies use samples and sales calls on physicians (push strategy).

Participation in health fairs may be thought of as a form of sales promotions for many healthcare provider organizations. Providers may offer a range of diagnostic tests and distribute health education materials. These fairs provide visibility to the organization and an opportunity to gain exposure to patients who may not otherwise interface with the organization. Participants can be enrolled in patient education or wellness programs, and individuals who test positive in various screening tests can be referred for additional diagnosis or treatment.

Exhibiting at trade shows, professional meetings, and conferences is also a method of sales promotion. This provides an opportunity to expose the organization or product to hard-to-reach prospects such as physicians or hospital administrators. While it may be almost impossible to get past the gatekeepers at the doctor's office to make a pitch, the exhibition hall delivers the doctor to the booth. The decision to exhibit and the type of exhibit developed depend on the nature of the organization and the product as well as the characteristics of the target audience.

An effective exhibit can serve to increase visibility, allow improved market penetration, boost sales, and help maintain market share. Furthermore, exhibits represent a unique opportunity for conducting market research, with many of the best prospects assembled in one location. Many healthcare organizations are not accustomed to exhibiting at trade shows and professional meetings, but this form of sales promotion is likely to become more common in the future. There are a number of caveats to consider when participating in an exhibition (see Box 11.2).

Direct Marketing

The final type of promotion discussed in this chapter is direct marketing. Direct marketing involves an interactive system of marketing that uses one or more advertising media to effect a measurable response or transaction at any location. The categories of direct marketing of interest here are direct mail, direct response advertising, mail order, telemarketing, computerized marketing, and home shopping television. Not all will be given equal attention, but all have a role to play in healthcare marketing.

Direct mail is a means of promotion whereby selected customers are sent advertising material addressed specifically to them. This has been traditionally done through the postal service, but more contemporary approaches use fax or e-mail transmission. Everyone is familiar with the junk mail that regularly turns up in the mailbox. This is now being joined by unsolicited faxes and "spam" e-mail messages.

Despite the annoyance these types of solicitations cause for many people, they are nevertheless considered effective marketing tools. Marketers like direct mail because it can be highly targeted and personalized and can make use of creative designs and formats. Even with a 2 percent response rate, marketers find direct mail to be reasonably cost effective. Research has shown that certain segments of the population are actually relatively responsive to mailed solicitations, and documents related to healthcare are less likely to be summarily discarded than others. Healthcare marketers find that direct mail works best when promoting a specific event (e.g., patient

<table>
<tr>
<td>

Box 11.2: Keys to Exhibit-Marketing Success

</td>
<td>

Organizations that provide healthcare products and services frequently find themselves exhibiting at conferences, professional meetings, and trade shows, but little guidance is available for would-be healthcare exhibitors. Providing such guidance is a challenge given the wide variety of organizations involved in healthcare marketing. Nevertheless, some considerations are relevant for any healthcare organization that plans to exhibit. Following are ten of the most common marketing

</td>
</tr>
</table>

mistakes exhibitors make.

Have a Proper Exhibit Marketing Plan

Having both a strategic exhibit marketing and tactical plan of action is a critical starting point. To make trade shows a powerful dimension of your organization's overall marketing operation total alignment between the strategic marketing and your exhibit marketing plan is essential. Trade shows should not be a stand-alone venture. Know and understand exactly what you wish to achieve (e.g., increasing market share with existing users, introducing new products or services into existing markets or new markets, introducing new products or services into existing or new markets).

Have a Well-Defined Promotional Plan

An important component of exhibiting is promotion, including preshow, show, and post-show activities. Most exhibitors fail to have a plan that encompasses all three areas. The budget plays a major role in deciding what and how much promotional activity is possible. Developing a meaningful theme or message that ties into your strategic marketing plan will help guide promotional decisions. Know whom you want to target and consider having different promotional programs aimed at the different groups of interest. Include direct mail, broadcast faxes, advertising, PR, sponsorship, and the Internet as possible ways to reach your target audience.

Use Direct Mail Effectively

Direct mail is still one of the most popular promotional vehicles exhibitors use. From postcards to multipiece mailings, attendees are deluged with invitations to visit booths. Many mailings come from lists of registrants; as a result everyone gets everything. To target the people you want to visit your booth use your own list of customers and prospects— it is the best one available. Design a benefits-oriented piece that makes an impact. Mail three pieces at regular intervals prior to the show, starting about four weeks out, to help ensure your invitation is seen. Wherever possible use first-class mail; nothing is worse than a mailing that arrives after the show is over.

Give Visitors an Incentive to Visit Your Booth

Whatever promotional vehicles you use, make sure you give visitors a reason to come and visit you. A hall overflowing with fascinating products and services, combined with time constraints, means that people need an incentive to visit your booth. People's primary interest is in whatever is new. They are eager to learn about the latest technologies, new applications, or anything that will help save time or money. Even if you do not have a new product or service to introduce, think about a new angle to promote your offerings.

Have Giveaways that Work

Encourage visits to your booth by offering a premium item that will entice them. The giveaway item(s) should be designed to increase your memorability, communicate, motivate, promote, or increase recognition of your company. Developing a dynamite giveaway takes thought and creativity. Consider items that are desired by the target audience, are helpful to potential customers, are unavailable any place else, and are educational. Think about having different gifts for different types of visitors. Use your web site to make an offer for visitors to collect important information, such as an executive report, when they visit your booth. Giveaways should be used as a reward or token of appreciation for visitors participating in a demonstration, presentation, or contest or as thanks for providing information about specific needs.

Use Press Relations Effectively

PR is one of the most-cost effective and successful methods for generating large volumes of direct inquiries and sales. Before the show, ask show-exhibit management for a comprehensive media list, and find out which publications are planning a special show edition. Send out newsworthy press releases focusing on what is new about your product or service or highlighting a new application or market venture. Compile press kits for the press office that include information about industry trends, statistics, new technology, or production. Also include good product photos and key company contacts. Specifically assign staff members at the booth to interact with the media.

Differentiate Your Products or Services

Too many exhibitors are happy to use the me-too marketing approach—that is, examine their marketing plans and you will find an underlying sameness. With shows that attract hundreds of exhibitors, few of them stand out from the crowd. Because memorability is an integral part of a visitor's show experience, you should be looking at what makes you different and why a prospect should buy from you. This is of particular concern with standardized products and services. Every aspect of your exhibit marketing plan, including your promotions, booth, and people, should be aimed at making an impact and creating curiosity.

Use the Booth as an Effective Marketing Tool

On the show floor your exhibit makes a strong statement about who your organization is, what it does, and how it does it. The purpose of your exhibit is to attract visitors so that you can achieve your marketing objectives. In addition to the exhibit being an open, welcoming, and friendly space, it must have a focal point and a strong key message that communicates a significant benefit to your prospect. Opt for large graphics rather than reams of copy; pictures paint a thousand words, whereas few attendees will take the time to read. Your presentations or demonstrations are a critical part of your exhibit marketing. Create an experience that allows visitors to use as many of their senses as possible. This will help to enhance memorability.

Realize that Your People Are Your Marketing Team

Your people are your ambassadors. They represent everything your company stands for, so choose them well. Brief them beforehand, and make sure they know why you are exhibiting, what you are exhibiting, and what you expect from them. Exhibit staff training is essential for a unified and professional image. The objectives of the exhibit personnel should reflect the marketing plan, and staff should know how to close the interaction with a commitment to follow up. Avoid overcrowding the booth with company representatives, and assign specific tasks for company executives working the show.

Follow up Promptly

The key to trade show success is effective lead management. The best time to plan for follow-up is before the show. Show leads often take second place to other management activities that occur after being out of the office for several days. The longer leads are left unattended, the colder they become. It is to your advantage to develop an organized, systematic approach to follow-up. Establish a lead handling system, set timelines for follow-up, use a computerized database for tracking, make sales representatives accountable for leads given to them, and then measure your results.

Source: Susan A. Friedmann, CSP, president, The Tradeshow Coach, Lake Placid, New York.

education program, open house). This approach probably does not work as well to stimulate action with regard to something not limited by time, although marketers of some elective procedures (e.g., laser eye surgery) have had reasonable success with direct mail.

Direct response advertising involves promotions via print or electronic media that provide a call-in number for potential customers. Typically, a toll-free number is provided, and individuals who want to order a product or service or obtain more information are instructed to call this number. This approach has been used successfully in other industries and is now being tried in healthcare. Physicians performing elective procedures, for example, may have an answering service established to field such calls and provide information on laser eye surgery, hair transplants, or weight-loss programs. This approach has also been used for selling fitness equipment through television ads and demonstrations and for attracting attention to pharmaceutical products.

Telemarketing is the form of direct marketing with which most people are familiar, and the approach has generated considerable backlash among consumers. Direct response marketing as discussed above is a form of telemarketing that involves inbound calls. Most people are more familiar with outbound telemarketing, in which individuals operating from a bank of telephone sets, often equipped with computer-assisted interviewing software, call individuals from a prospect list to offer a good or service. Some telemarketing involves cold calls to individuals or households for which the demand for goods and services is unknown. More likely, the telephone numbers that are used as a sampling frame or are randomly generated relate to areas with the approximate characteristics of the target audience.

A more benign form of telemarketing in healthcare involves periodic contacts with individuals who have expressed an interest to the healthcare organization with regard to a particular program or topic. It is assumed that the individual is willing to receive calls describing such programs and will not consider them an imposition because of their implied previous interest. Hospital call centers frequently use this approach to contact prospects for various services and programs.

Telemarketing is more expensive than direct-mail initiatives, but the costs are not unreasonable. Wages for telemarketers are relatively low, and the benefits to a healthcare organization of each new patient attracted are likely to be significant. Obviously, not all healthcare products lend themselves to this approach, but a surprising number do.

Mail-order catalogs have been a traditional shopping mechanism for Americans since early in the country's history. However, they have not been a traditional means of promoting healthcare goods and services. In recent years, however, as the market for alternative therapies and do-it-yourself healthcare tests and treatments has grown, mail-order catalogs have become an increasingly important vehicle for the distribution of certain healthcare products. In many parts of the country if a consumer wants to purchase herbal potions, natural remedies, or a variety of other nonconventional treatments, mail order may be the way to obtain them. Increasingly, individuals requiring conventional prescription drugs are turning to such sources in search of better prices.

While mail-order catalogs will never become mainstream healthcare-advertising material, this approach does have advantages. It puts product exposure directly in the hands of targeted consumers and can be relatively cost effective with economies of scale. As discussed below, the web site is becoming the modern-day incarnation of the mail-order catalog.

Two other venues for electronic marketing include computerized marketing and home shopping television channels. The Internet has become a virtual marketplace, attracting a wide range of buyers and sellers. A variety of healthcare products are now available via the Internet, and aggressive e-mail marketing techniques have carried these messages to the desktops of everyone online. Healthcare consumers frequently turn to the Internet as a first resort for locating and pricing consumer-health products.

Home shopping channels primarily sell shopping goods and consumer goods. However, they have tried to capitalize on the fitness and wellness movement by offering fitness equipment, workout supplies, and skin treatments via television. Home shopping programs and even entire cable channels are often given over to healthcare products.

Media Options

Because advertising and certain other promotional opportunities typically use the media as their means of communication, attention must be paid to the media options available. A critical part of any marketing plan will be a *media plan,* which specifies campaign objectives, the target audience, and the specific media vehicles that will be used to reach that audience. *Media* refers to any nonpersonal form of promotions. For our discussion the media are divided into the categories of print media, electronic media, and display advertising.

In many ways these are the best of times for marketers in terms of promotional options. There have never been a wider variety of outlets for published material, and electronic publishing has added an entirely new dimension to the information-dissemination process. Marketers are presented with a wide variety of magazines, journals, and newsletters, and changes in publishing technology have introduced unprecedented efficiencies and reduced barriers to entry. The advent of cable and satellite television allows the marketer access to virtually unlimited transmission outlets. The Internet links millions of computers worldwide via telecommunication, creating an enormous potential for interaction with customers. These technological innovations and the expansion of distribution channels for promotions are supported by a vast database of information on consumers for use in profiling markets and targeting specific consumers.

Print Media

Print media are the most traditional of the media and can take a variety of forms. Magazines include periodical publications aimed at the general public as well as trade publications geared to the interests of health professionals. A number of consumer-oriented health-related publications are produced today. The advantages of magazines include (1) opportunity for color reproduction, (2) suitable editorial environment, (3) support target marketing, (4) advertisements are expected by readers, (5) long life spans, (6) read at leisure, and (7) potentially high readership. The disadvantages of magazine advertising include (1) ads may be in "desert" areas seldom noticed by readers, (2) ads may be lost in the clutter of the magazine, and (3) ads appear infrequently because of magazines' publication schedules. Magazine advertising has the potential to be cost effective, depending on the audience served.

Newspapers include weekly or daily news publications that can be national, regional, or local in distribution. In many newspapers, the majority of the space is devoted to advertising. Newspaper advertising has the advantages of (1) extensive audience coverage, (2) flexibility in terms of timing, and (3) the use of illustrations. The disadvantages include (1) an untargeted method for reaching the intended audience and (2) difficulty in getting people to notice the advertising content. Depending on the market, newspaper advertising can be relatively expensive, making it important to match the marketing objectives with the benefits of this medium.

Most cities now have "alternative" newspapers, usually weeklies that have emerged to cover aspects of the news thought to be neglected by the mainstream press. In some communities readership of alternative newspapers approximates that of the conventional press, making them appropriate vehicles for the advertising of many healthcare products. Alternative newspapers are particularly suited for the promotion of progressive or innovative healthcare services likely to appeal to a population interested in holistic medicine or alternative therapies.

Many communities have spawned special-interest newspapers devoted to some aspect of health. Some areas produce regular healthcare newspapers that chronicle developments in the local healthcare arena. Other types of newspapers that deal with fitness and wellness, sports, and alternative therapies have become increasingly common; these could represent advertising venues for a range of goods and services. Newspapers targeted to doctors or other healthcare providers are common—some national and some local—that may accept advertising, public service announcements, or feature articles on products or organizations.

Professional journals are possibly more ubiquitous in healthcare than in any other industry. Physicians and other health professionals are exposed to a wide range of journals. Every medical specialty and all allied health fields generate one or more journals; major associations also publish regular journals. Some of these are academically oriented and typically do not carry advertisements. However, even mainstream medical journals like the *Journal of the American Medical Association* and the *New England Journal of Medicine* carry advertisements.

These vehicles serve the purpose of professional advertising because they are geared to health professionals, not the general public. Pharmaceutical companies are heavy advertisers in these publications, as are medical supply, equipment, and information technology vendors. Professional journals also serve as vehicles for the promotion of a service through the publication of descriptive and research-oriented articles.

Newsletters have also become a common source of information in healthcare. Because of the rapid changes that occur in the industry, the lead time required for more traditional publications means they cannot accommodate the needs of an industry in transition. Newsletters have thus become a valuable source of current information. While advertising opportunities are rare in newsletters, they do provide a venue for publicizing new programs, services, or organizational changes.

Most areas support one or more shoppers' magazines typically distributed without cost to local consumers. These may provide opportunities for the promotion of various healthcare consumer goods and services. Advertisements are relatively inexpensive for these publications, but there may be a downside for some products if they are advertised in a throwaway publication of this type.

Directories have become an increasingly important means of gaining visibility for healthcare organizations. Some directories are compiled for bureaucratic record-keeping purposes, such as state physician directories or a hospital association's hospital directory; these are not generally intended for commercial use, and an organization's inclusion may or may not be mandatory. Some directories are compiled for administrative purposes but are shared with a larger audience. The provider directory made available by a health plan or provider network includes only practitioners who can be seen under that health plan.

Another category of directories is those commercially produced for distribution. One of their functions is to provide visibility to the organizations listed. Fees may be charged for listing the organization in these directories, which are typically sold to customers who need the information. Directories may list physicians, hospitals, information technology vendors, and so forth. A number of publishers compile and distribute directories as their primary business activity. An increasing number of directories are being posted on the Internet.

Electronic Media

Electronic media have arisen to supplement traditional advertising. Obviously a more contemporary format than traditional print media, electronic media include television (and its derivatives), radio, cinema, and now the Internet. Television is often the first advertising medium that comes to mind, and it does have several advantages, including (1) ability to build a high level of awareness, (2) access to large audiences, (3) ability to demonstrate a product (using sound and vision), (4) potential for impulsive purchase decisions, and (5) home viewing in a casual atmosphere. Television's disadvantages include the fact that commercial breaks may be seen as irritating, the medium is considered transient, and the audience cannot be very targeted. In addition, television advertising time is expensive.

Historically, television advertising concentrated on the national networks (ABC, NBC, CBS, and Fox). However, with the advent of cable television and satellite broadcasting the situation has changed. The fragmentation of viewers has resulted in the development of homogenous groups that support particular cable channels. This makes it possible to target the television audience much more precisely. Furthermore, satellite television subscribers are likely to be upscale innovators (if that is the type of population being sought). Advertising time is much less expensive in these venues than on network television.

Radio is a long-standing advertising medium with a lot of advantages. Radios are often considered "companions," more so than television and other electronic forms. The most important attribute is the ability to target the audience fairly precisely, not only with regard to the station but also even with time of day. On the other hand, radio has the disadvantages of lacking visual attributes, being a transient medium, and having a small audience. Radio advertising time is relatively inexpensive, especially compared to television advertising, and production costs are certainly lower.

Over the past several years an explosion in Internet advertising has occurred. This does not refer to marketing web sites (to be discussed later) but to the online placement of banners and pop-up advertisements. Since the advent of the Internet age, growing numbers of healthcare organizations have begun advertising on web sites. The majority of these have been consumer-health-product companies, but some providers are also advertising on the World Wide Web. In addition to banners and pop-up ads many healthcare organizations pay a fee to be listed on various Internet-based directories of physicians, hospitals, or other providers. Although the effectiveness of this form of marketing has not been thoroughly documented, healthcare organizations appear to have an ongoing interest in maintaining some advertising on Internet sites.

The cinema setting is sometimes used as an electronic form of advertising, although seldom for healthcare advertising. However, as healthcare becomes more consumer driven cinema advertising will likely find a place in healthcare. Movies themselves are increasingly becoming vehicles for the advertising of a variety of products through "placement" of the product within the movie. This is not likely to become a regular venue for healthcare advertising but certainly could be utilized for certain products or even organizations.

The growth of electronic media has spawned a new form of advertisement often favored by healthcare organizations—the *infomercial*. Infomercials may take the form of 15- to 60-minute television or radio commercials typically presented in a casual talk show format designed to look like an ordinary television program. They may also be presented in a standard 30- to 60-second commercial format. The infomercial is framed as an educational piece, and the sponsor is only subtly noted. The intent is to soft sell the organization or service by giving the impression that the sponsor is the authority on that topic, thus attracting customers without having to overtly solicit them.

Display Advertising

Another form of media involves display advertising that typically takes the form of outdoor advertising, transportation advertising, and posters. Outdoor advertising primarily involves billboards, although other types of signage (e.g., banners, portable signs) may be used. While billboard advertising has its critics, it appears to be surprisingly popular with healthcare organizations such as hospitals, health plans, and voluntary associations. Transportation or transit advertising involves ads placed on buses, taxis, and other commercial vehicles (e.g., trucks, business cars). Posters are signs displayed in public places to attract attention to the organization, service, or event.

The advantages of this type of display advertising are its (1) ability to build high awareness levels, (2) exposure to large numbers of people, (3) relatively low costs, (4) short- and long-term possibilities, (5) opportunity for national campaigns, and (6) segmentation possibilities. The disadvantages of display advertising include (1) it may be subject to the effect of weather, (2) some sites are subject to environmental criticism, and (3) the general low regard for outdoor advertising held by much of the public.

Integrated Marketing

Given the variety of promotional techniques available and the seeming fragmentation of marketing approaches, determining the type of approach most appropriate for a particular campaign is often difficult. One approach that may help tie some of the parts together is integrated marketing. *Integrated marketing* or *integrated marketing communications* emphasizes the development of consistency within the promotional strategy of an organization. Its ultimate aim is to achieve synergy between its component parts to generate a more effective approach to communications.

Integrated marketing communications involve the strategic choice of elements of marketing communications that effectively and economically influence transactions between an organization and its existing and potential customers, clients, and consumers; management and control of all marketing communication elements; and ensuring that the brand positioning, proposition, personality, and messages are delivered synergistically across every element of communication and derived from a single consistent strategy.

Marketers coordinate advertising campaigns across varied media, increasingly supplementing television advertisements with marketing messages communicated via alternative media vehicles. For example, consumers may see print ads that capture a frame from the television spot, with a tag line that summarizes the 15- or 30-second message, or hear a radio airing of an excerpt of the dialog and the announcer's product claims from that television spot.

A variety of factors have encouraged the use of integrated marketing strategies. Tighter marketing budgets have meant a squeeze on available resources, and the fragmentation of the media demands some force for continuity. The shift from mass marketing to target marketing and the rise of electronic media (especially the Internet) have all contributed to this development. Although this appears to be an obvious step toward more effective marketing, some resist integrated marketing because of traditional patterns of behavior, a cumbersome organizational structure, or incompatibility with the capabilities of an external advertising agency.

Assuming that resistance can be overcome, several major advantages are to be derived from the integration process: (1) mutually reinforcing initiatives, (2) consistent messages, (3) synergy derived from integrated strategies, (4) cost savings, (5) consistent creative approach, and (6) sustainable competitive advantage (see Case Study 11.1).

Summary

A variety of established marketing techniques are available to healthcare organizations. These traditional approaches for reaching the organization's constituents include publicity (e.g., public relations, communication, government relations), advertising, sales promotion, and personal selling. In recent years, direct marketing has been added to the arsenal of healthcare marketers. These techniques have long been used in other industries and have been adopted in various degrees by healthcare organizations.

The choice of marketing technique depends on the type of organization involved and the product being marketed, among other factors. Of special importance is the objective of the promotional initiative. Objectives such as increasing visibility, retaining existing customers, changing consumer attitudes, and increasing market share understandably call for differing marketing techniques. An objective common to most forms of promotion is the education of the consumer.

Different types of media may be required for differing circumstances. Marketers have the options of print media, electronic media, and display media. The various forms of print media (e.g., magazines, newspapers) have their advantages and disadvantages, as do the various forms of electronic media (e.g., radio, television). Display media such as billboards have less to offer healthcare than some other promotional techniques. The emergence of the Internet as a marketing vehicle has brought a different dimension to healthcare marketing.

Healthcare organizations are learning the importance of integrated marketing. This systematic approach to the promotion of an idea, organization, or product serves to instill consistency in the marketing initiative and coordinate what could be a wide range of promotional activities.

Discussion Questions

- What role does the nature of the product play in determining the type of promotion used?
- How important is the culture of the community when it comes to the choice of promotional technique?
- Why is public relations often a preferred form of promotion for healthcare organizations?
- Can it be argued that a major function of promotional activities in healthcare is educating the healthcare consumer?
- Why is there continued resistance against the use of advertising by healthcare organizations on the part of both health professionals and many within the general public?
- What are the steps involved in the personal selling process, and under what circumstances is personal sales the most effective promotional technique?
- What is the difference between a *push* approach and a *pull* approach when it comes to sales promotion?
- What developments in healthcare have encouraged the use of more direct marketing techniques?
- What are the pros and cons of various forms of print media?

- What are the advantages (and disadvantages) of electronic media vis-à-vis print media?
- What factors are encouraging the growing emphasis on integrated marketing among healthcare organizations?

Reference

Berkowitz, E. N. 1996. *Essentials of Health Care Marketing.* Gaithersburg, MD: Aspen.

INTEGRATED MARKETING

Many people who may benefit from hearing aids do not wear them. Of adults 18 and older who have impaired hearing, 78 percent do not own a hearing aid. As the population ages the need for hearing-instrument assistance becomes nearly universal, but even among the hearing impaired older than 65, 61 percent do not wear hearing aids. Our research has found that people would readily acquiesce to wearing eyeglasses to help correct their vision, have no problem taking pain relievers to alleviate aches, and even do not mind terribly having to walk with a cane. However, the thought of wearing a hearing aid is a far less positive prospect.

The hearing and speech communications literature hypothesizes that wearing a hearing aid carries a stigma that the wearer is old, feeble, and incompetent. An article in the American Psychological Association's *Monitor* describes the denial and depression people associate with hearing loss. People do not want to admit their hearing loss to themselves because it connotes aging, nor do they want to admit it to others for fear of being viewed as incompetent. In addition, hearing loss, if not assisted with hearing aids, can lead to greater dependence on a spouse and withdrawal from social events.

Given all these considerations, it is perhaps not surprising that when *Business Week* featured a hearing aid manufacturer in its "Annual Design Awards," the product receiving acclaim was tiny and said to "nestle discreetly in the ear canal." Hearing aids saw a surge in sales after President Clinton's public acknowledgment of beginning to wear one. Perhaps the devices were seen as more acceptable when, rather than being associated with the old and feeble, they were associated with the relatively young and purportedly virile.

A product with such a negative image as hearing aids clearly presents a challenge to the marketer interested in stimulating sales, and a campaign was initiated to determine ways to induce more favorable attitudes toward these personal, stigmatized products. This situation appeared to offer an opportunity for integrated marketing communications. In addition, it was felt that a stigmatized product might best be promoted through multi-modality approaches, thereby reinforcing the advertising message.

A panel of respondents was established as a test market. The researchers contacted 4,344 participants at time 1 before the exposure to any marketing communications. At time 2, the attitudes of 3,351 participants were measured after exposure to the persuasive materials. At time 3, the attitudes of 3,049 respondents were remeasured three months after the marketing efforts.

Three advertising themes were tested in this study: "warm and emotional," "educational," and "wedge of doubt." The warm and emotional print advertisement began with text at the top of the page, "Honey, can you pick up some nails?" A response of "Sure" was printed in the middle of the page, with a photograph of a can of escargot. The tag line printed at the bottom of the page inquired, "Is it any wonder hearing loss can frustrate those around you? . . . Have your hearing checked. For you. For them."

The text for the educational message stated, "Use your head once a year," atop a photograph of headphones. The ad's closing text read, "Annual hearing checkups help you spot changes in your hearing. . . . Hear today. Hear tomorrow." The wedge of doubt advertisement began with text that warned, "If you think it's difficult admitting your hearing problem, imagine admitting all the mistakes you've made because of it." At the bottom the ad read, "When you can't hear clearly, it's easy to misunderstand someone. And before you know it, people start thinking you've lost your mental edge."

These advertising messages were delivered via varied media vehicles to simulate a real-world advertising campaign. These included mass media (standard in their appeal), namely print ads and television ads, and private media (customized to appeal to their target), specifically telemarketing phone calls and direct-marketing mailings.

The analysis showed that consistent combinations of media (both private or both public) were indeed more effective than mixed media—the two private media (telemarketing combined with direct marketing) outperformed any two mixed media (telemarketing and print, telemarketing and television, direct marketing and print, or direct marketing and television).

In addition, the private media combination outperformed the public media, which makes sense for the hearing-aid product category. If a stigma or embarrassment is associated with a purchase, even learning more about the product prior to purchase may require some delicacy and privacy.

Finally, it was found that the content of the message affected the preference for a particular class of media (private or public). The integrated private media (telemarketing and direct marketing) performed best, first with the wedge of doubt and then the warm and emotional ad content. Note that two private exposures were not always superior—the combination with the educational advertising message performed poorly. Also note that the wedge of doubt, which did the best when delivered via the two private media, was not uniformly superior either; it performed the worst when delivered via a mass medium.

Marketing health services can be complicated. As this investigation demonstrates, rarely can a marketer choose a medium or advertising message without considering the big picture. Media cannot be simply pasted together to achieve some seemingly critical threshold of ad weight—many mixed media can perform worse than fewer exposures of sensibly integrated media. Similarly, the choice of media outlets depends on both the product and the content of the advertisements themselves. Thoughtful combinations of media and messages appear to facilitate greater influence than haphazard collections of media and messages. Many other product categories similarly carry some stigma and may therefore also yield better adoption under private media.

Source: Iacobucci, D., B. J. Calder, E. Malthouse, and A. Duhachek. 2002. "Did You Hear? Customers Tune in to Multimedia Marketing." *Marketing Health Services* 22 (3): 16–20.

12

EMERGING MARKETING TECHNIQUES

Marketing as a field experienced a number of changes during its evolution, and these developments eventually filtered through to healthcare. The 1990s witnessed the adoption of techniques from other industries and the development of new healthcare-specific approaches. The developments in healthcare over the past two decades that have led to a need for innovative marketing techniques are noted, and some of the new emerging techniques are described. The significance of customer relationship management, direct-to-consumer marketing, and other emerging techniques is discussed, and the relative merit of these techniques is assessed. The shift from mass marketing to micromarketing is reviewed.

Emerging Marketing Techniques

Over the past decade healthcare has experienced a number of trends related to marketing. These include a shift in emphasis from image marketing to service marketing and movement away from a mass marketing approach to a more targeted strategy. Healthcare marketing has experienced a move away from a one-size-fits-all philosophy to one that emphasizes personalization and customization. Emphasis on the specific healthcare episode has shifted to an emphasis on long-term relationships. Healthcare, like other industries, has benefited from the application of information technology to marketing. Finally, emphasis on marketing to organizations rather than individuals has increased during this period, resulting in greater emphasis on business-to-business marketing.

The marketing techniques that appear to be gaining momentum in healthcare can perhaps be divided into techniques that involve organizational changes and those that are technology based. The former implies an innovative approach at a conceptual level, and the latter involves the application of technology to either traditional or innovative marketing techniques.

One factor common to both types of techniques is their emphasis on relationship marketing. Relationship marketing is the process of getting closer to the customer by developing a long-term relationship through careful attention to customer needs and service delivery. Relationship marketing is characterized by (1) focus on customer retention, (2) orientation toward product benefits rather than product features, (3) long-term view of the relationship, (4) maximum emphasis on customer commitment and contact, (5) development of ongoing relationship, (6) multiple employee-customer contacts, (7) emphasis on key account relationship management, and (8) emphasis on trust. All of the techniques discussed below incorporate at least some of these attributes.

Organizational Approaches

Direct-to-Consumer Marketing

The *direct-to-consumer* (DTC) movement is gaining momentum in health-care as the industry becomes more consumer driven and the ability to target narrow population segments becomes better refined. Healthcare marketers are modifying their methodologies to take into consideration the potential represented by 280 million potential prospects.

Toward the end of the twentieth century the consumer was redis-covered by the U.S. healthcare industry. The consumer—the end user of health services and products—had long been written off as a marketing target. For most medical services the physician made the decisions for the patient; for the insured the health plan controlled the choice of provider and range of services that could be obtained from that provider. Choice of drug typically depended on the physician's prescription, and supply channels in general focused on the middleman rather than the end user.

With the rediscovery of the healthcare consumer, all of this is undergoing dramatic change. Aided by access to state-of-the-art technology, consumers are now expressing their preferences for everything from physicians and hospitals to health plans and prescription drugs. As a result, DTC advertising is beginning to emerge as a force in healthcare.

The DTC movement has been given a jump start by the pharmaceutical industry. Once certain restrictions to DTC advertising were removed, the pharmaceutical giants began targeting the consumer through a variety of media. This industry is certainly leading the way in terms of expenditures and visibility, as pharmaceutical interests attempt to attract consumers to their brands.

This trend has been followed, albeit at a safe distance, by various health insurance plans that are beginning to offer their policies via the Internet, thereby causing a resurgence in insurance plans aimed at individuals rather than groups. The accelerating shift from defined benefits to defined contributions is rapidly making the ability to customize health plans to the needs of specific groups—and indeed, individuals—essential for any health plan that hopes to remain competitive.

The reemergence of the consumer has not been lost on practitioners either, as hospitals, physicians, and other providers establish web sites for maintaining contact with existing customers and enticing prospective customers. Now it is possible to bid online on an elective procedure (e.g., a facelift by a plastic surgeon), thereby establishing a direct negotiating link between provider and consumer.

The trend toward DTC advertising has been driven by a number of factors. Changed regulations within the pharmaceutical industry have been a major contributor, at least for pharmaceutical companies. The introduction of defined contributions that allow increased consumer latitude in choice of goods and services has affected health plans, and managed care organizations are attempting to reposition themselves in the eyes of the consumer by offering customizable menus of services. Providers are increasingly chasing discretionary patient dollars (e.g., for laser eye surgery), and product vendors have discovered the Internet as a direct path to the hearts, minds, and pocketbooks of healthcare consumers.

For their part consumers have eagerly accepted this onslaught of direct-marketing attention. Spearheaded by the baby boomers, a better educated, more affluent, and more control-oriented consumer population is eagerly searching for information tailored to its particular needs. Much of the traffic on the Internet is health oriented, and consumers are obtaining much of their health-related information via the World Wide Web.

Although the Internet has served as the impetus for much of the new attention on individual consumers, the DTC movement has affected other media as well. In addition to the Internet, television and print media have experienced a considerable increase in expenditures for this purpose. Direct mail appears to be making a comeback as well. While much of this has been driven by the pharmaceutical industry, there is no reason to expect that other parties chasing these same consumers will not follow suit.

For marketing the most significant changes involve the need to shift away from the traditional channels (and marketing targets) to a much more diverse and dispersed target audience. There is a big difference between a pharmaceutical company targeting 50,000 physicians in its specialty areas and trying to reach 50 million potential consumers. While traditional pharmaceutical marketing approaches will not be abandoned, the drug company representative is being devalued in relation to the television ad agency given this new emphasis. There is also a big difference between a hospital schmoozing with the handful of plastic surgeons located in its ambulatory surgery center and directly approaching thousands of potential cosmetic surgery patients.

Perhaps the major implication of these changes is the fact that, while traditional targets had been essentially known entities, the new targets are not only less well known but also exceedingly diverse. By definition 50,000 physicians have a lot more in common than do 50 million patients, not only in terms of background, demographic attributes, and expectations but also in terms of behavior.

The need to target large numbers of consumers will likely encourage a resurgence of interest in psychographics and other consumer-profiling methodologies. In the past if you knew a couple of things about a patient or potential patient (e.g., referring doctor, health plan), you did not need to know much more. In the future the ability to contact and subsequently cultivate prospective patients will place significant pressure on the marketer (as it already is in the pharmaceutical industry).

This new environment will also likely mean the end of any one-size-fits-all approach in healthcare. The challenges for the marketer will increase by virtue of the need to offer unbundled services to a wide array of potential customers with highly specific needs, rather than offering a bundled program to all customers. Take, for example, the health plan that has historically offered a standard package of benefits to all enrollees. If we move to a defined contributions approach, the marketer has to be able to promote a variety of unbundled services to a variety of consumers with different needs and preferences. In the past Employer A, with a poorly educated, blue-collar workforce, offered the same benefits as Employer B, with a highly educated, professional workforce. In the future the plan being offered to Employer A must reflect the needs of Employer A's employees and necessarily must be different from the plan being sold to Employer B.

This development suggests that the healthcare marketer may have to go back to the drawing board in more ways than one. The marketer must be in closer touch with the end user than at any time in memory, ultimately developing an in-depth understanding of the wants, needs, and preferences of the various categories of potential customers. He must be able to determine who wants particular products and services and the extent to which a population category wants standardization versus customization. This will require the development of an understanding of consumer characteristics and behaviors down to the household level, as is already evidenced in other industries.

Business-to-Business Marketing

Although much of the discussion around healthcare marketing focuses on the patient or other end user, a significant amount of marketing in healthcare involves business-to-business transactions. The increasing corporatization of healthcare means that more and more relationships are between one corporate body and another. The traditional doctor-patient relationship has been supplanted by contractual arrangements between groups of buyers and sellers of health services. Many hospital programs now target corporate customers rather than individual patients. The shift to a more businesslike approach to healthcare delivery has also contributed to the growth of *business-to-business marketing.*

Clearly, business-to-business marketing in healthcare is nothing new. Healthcare organizations are major purchasers of a wide variety of goods, and large organizations do business with hundreds of vendors, but the importance of business-to-business marketing is expected to increase in the future. Business-to-business marketing involves building profitable, value-oriented relationships between two businesses and many individuals within them. Business marketers focus on a few customers with usually much larger, more complex, and technically oriented sales processes. Statistical tools, data mining techniques, and other sorts of research that work so well in the land of consumer marketing must be fine tuned by the business marketer.

The differences between marketing to businesses and marketing to consumers are significant. Business customers and traditional customers do not buy in the same way; they are driven by different impulses and respond to different approaches. Business buyers behave differently and require a different marketing approach.

Business-to-business marketing is a complex discipline that has become integral to selling goods and services to business, industrial, institutional, or government buyers. In past decades innovative products, great engineering, or great salesmanship alone might have been enough to close a business sale, but sellers no longer have the luxury of "build it and they will come" thinking.

While business-to-business product development is driven by technological progress, business-to-consumer development is driven by fashion and trends. Business-to-business purchases are often considered group decisions, whereas business-to-consumer purchases are personal and more impulsive.

Internal Marketing

Internal marketing refers to efforts by a service provider to effectively train and motivate its customer-contact employees and supporting service people to work as a team to generate customer satisfaction. Internal marketing aims to ensure that everybody within an organization is working toward the achievement of common objectives. It recognizes that people who work together stand in exactly the same relationships to one another as customers and suppliers. Internal marketing represents a marketing effort, inside a company's four walls, that targets internal audiences. Its goal is to increase communications among staff members to maximize a marketing campaign's effectiveness.

Internal marketing redefines employees as valued customers. The rationale is that anticipating, identifying, and satisfying employee needs will lead to greater commitment. This in turn will allow the organization to improve the quality of service to its external customers. Internal marketing represents a combination of marketing, human resources, training, and behavioral science.

The marketing department is a logical focal point for internal marketing because of its knowledge of the organization's overall strategy, appreciation of external customers' needs, expertise to deploy these tools with regard to internal customers, and access to the budgets and financial resources to do the job. Internal marketing begins with communication; communication, of course, is the primary responsibility of the marketing staff.

In order for internal marketing to be successful, employees must be made fully aware of the aims and activities of the organization. It is amazing how often employees of large healthcare organizations are unaware of services or programs the organization offers. While this could happen in any organization, it appears to be an inherent characteristic of healthcare organizations. Employees must also be given a basic understanding of the nature of the customer. Employees of healthcare organizations are often isolated from the service delivery aspects of the operation. They may have virtually no knowledge of the customer-interaction process or at best a partial understanding of service delivery.

Investment in internal efforts has always been a fraction of most marketers' budgets, probably more so in healthcare than in other industries, but the process of internal marketing requires a great deal of training to instill the requisite knowledge and ensure that all employees are on the same page. Lack of investment in internal marketing may be the result of corporate distraction. Companies that are frantically trying to boost revenues and cut costs may not see why they should spend money on employees, missing the point that these are the very people who ultimately deliver the brand promises the company makes.

Lack of investment may also reflect a conscious decision by executives who dismiss internal efforts as feel-good pseudoscience, missing the point that research consistently demonstrates that service-quality problems (people problems more than product problems) are what push customers away and into the arms of competitors. Many healthcare administrators may feel they were burned by the quality improvement initiatives of the 1980s, in which a great deal of effort and resources were spent without lasting effects in many cases.

Internal marketing is an important implementation tool. It aids communication and helps to overcome any resistance to change. It informs and involves all staff in new initiatives and strategies. Internal marketing is simple to construct, especially if you are familiar with traditional principles of marketing. (If not, it would be valuable to spend some time considering marketing plans.) Internal marketing obeys the same rules as, and has a similar structure to, external marketing. The main difference is that the customers are staff and colleagues from your own organization.

There is nothing magic about internal marketing; in fact, most of it involves the application of common sense. Among the most common features of internal marketing programs are meetings, special events, company-anniversary celebrations, appreciation dinners, brown-bag lunches, off-site or satellite office visits, internal newsletters, bulletin boards, e-mail newsletters, intranets, and broadcast e-mails.

The first step in the development of an internal marketing initiative is the identification of internal customers. As with external customers, internal customers will have their own buyer behavior, or way of buying into the changes marketing is charged with implementing. The similarities in differing groups of internal customers allow the marketer to segment them. Three different internal customer segments ("supporters," "neutral," and "opposers") should be targeted; each group requires a slightly different internal marketing mix so that internal marketing objectives can be achieved.

Concierge Services

Over the past several years the healthcare field has experienced the emergence of *concierge services,* which primarily involve physician practices designed to meet a broad range of needs for a small, select patient population. These practices—involving usually one or a small number of physicians—accept only a limited number of patients who pay an annual fee above and beyond the cost of any care provided.

The concept behind these types of practices is simple, if somewhat controversial. Participating physicians agree to accept only a small number of patients (e.g., 300 rather than the typical several thousands) in exchange for an annual fee (currently ranging from $1,500 per year for limited services for an individual to $7,500 per year for expanded services for a family). These services include 24-hours-a-day, seven-days-a-week access, immediate telephone response, same-day appointments, longer time spent in office consultation, and even house calls. The physician may even accompany his or her patients to visits with other healthcare providers to serve as an "interpreter." In most cases existing insurance continues to pay for the rendering of covered services.

The number of such practices is still small, but this approach appears to be gaining momentum. Most of these practices have been initiated by the physicians themselves, although hospitals may increasingly become involved in the establishment of concierge practices. These concierge practices have emerged in Florida, Boston, Seattle, and a few other locations where this form of practice is thought to be acceptable. Chains of concierge practices appear to be emerging as the number of sites grows. Case Study 12.1 presents an example of a concierge program.

This approach is not without its critics. Observers inside and outside medicine have condemned this approach as avaricious and likely to contribute to an already serious shortage or maldistribution of physicians. If large numbers of physicians reduce their patient loads from 5,000 to 300, many patients are left without access to physicians. Indeed, established patients of physicians converting to a concierge practice must either be among the first to sign up or face finding another doctor.

This new practice form reflects broader trends affecting society in general and healthcare in particular. Many point to the role of managed care as a factor in creating dissatisfaction and disenchantment among physicians across the country. The need to adopt an assembly-line approach, oversight imposed by nonclinical personnel, limitations on utilization, and all of the other characteristics of managed care have led to some radical approaches by physicians. Already we have seen the emergence of practices that do not participate in managed care and may, in fact, accept no insurance; direct-pay practices only accept out-of-pocket payments, but at half the managed care rate.

Issues with current methods of reimbursement may not be the major factor in the emergence of concierge practices—the baby boomers may be. Born between 1946 and 1964 to parents who survived the Great Depression and World War II, baby boomers were destined to be America's golden children. With doting parents who wanted their children to have what they only dreamed of as youth—a carefree, prosperous life—boomers quickly became the target of mainstream marketing campaigns.

As boomers entered the workforce, new energy was thrust into corporate America. The "need to have it now" attitude, manifested so deeply throughout their youth, became part of the mainstream business culture. A new picture of a technological generation emerged. Boomers were more educated and expected more options from life. Increased salaries made possible the lifestyles to which they quickly became accustomed.

At some point boomers heard that they may not live forever, and fitness joined their list of priorities. Aerobics and jogging became popular mechanisms to stay fit. Then came the unexpected blow of caring for their parents. Healthcare issues became a reality, and a different kind of message began to permeate. With the oldest boomers reaching 55, the healthcare system can expect to experience the onslaught of the aging boomer. Boomers, however, are not going to accept their aging fate without a fight. Their youth taught them the power of consumerism, their college years taught them the power of a collective voice, and their careers taught them the power of money. These lessons, combined with boomers' overall skepticism of the institution, will likely restructure healthcare as we know it.

Technology-based Approaches
Database Marketing

Database marketing is a well-established component of marketing in virtually every industry beside healthcare. Although the concept has been talked about by health professionals for years, healthcare has been slow to adopt this approach. For some obvious reasons healthcare is different from other industries and does not lend itself to the more retail-oriented application of this concept. At the same time, health professionals are increasingly recognizing the ways in which healthcare could benefit from some aspects of database marketing.

This is not to say that components of database marketing do not already exist in healthcare; with DTC marketing picking up momentum, database marketing is being given a closer look. The empowerment of healthcare consumers, emergence of defined contributions, and growing competition for elective surgery patients, among other developments, are creating a healthcare environment that may be more fertile than ever for database marketing.

Database marketing involves the collection, storage, analysis, and use of information regarding customers and their past purchase behaviors for purpose of guiding future marketing decisions. It involves building a comprehensive database of customer profiles and initiating direct marketing based on these profiles. The resulting direct marketing must be responsive and outcome oriented to fit the notion of database marketing.

Database marketing is closely linked to *customer relationship management* (CRM), which involves the creation of a centralized body of knowledge that interfaces internal customer data with external market data. This integrated data set can be analyzed to determine patterns relevant for an understanding of the task at hand. The final step involves converting this knowledge into a communication vehicle that allows the healthcare organization to target relevant prospects and deliver the appropriate message.

A number of constraints are implicit when it comes to database marketing in healthcare. These constraints may be legal or ethical and often relate to issues of privacy, confidentiality, and data security. The potential repercussions from disclosing the medical condition of a customer are much greater than those from disclosing grocery store purchases or even financial transactions. Indeed, the enactment of the Health Insurance Portability and Accountability Act (HIPAA) has focused the spotlight on the issue of patient-data confidentiality. (See Chapter 16.)

Healthcare has historically not been consumer driven (although we are now seeing significant movement in that direction). Furthermore, database marketers have focused primarily on retail-type industries, where the consumer decision-making process is much different from that in healthcare. Products and services must generate adequate margins to be candidates for database marketing, and some health services do not qualify on this score.

From a technical perspective healthcare is much more complex, with numerous data-collection points in the process. The adaptation of database marketing to healthcare requires a certain level of sophistication and for health professionals to buy into a relatively expensive high-tech solution to incorporate database marketing capabilities.

Ultimately, the complexity of healthcare is the issue, not the technology. With convoluted decision making and a complex financing arrangement, conceptualizing the ideal system for database marketing is difficult. Just dealing with the variety of coding systems will bring any application to its knees. Developing a database-marketing initiative is a challenge when many healthcare executives still "don't get it" when it comes to responding to consumer demands.

A database marketing approach cannot be transferred straight from another industry without serious modification, and patients cannot be treated the same way as customers for hamburgers. Yet, the potential CRM applications to healthcare are almost unlimited. The very complexity of healthcare offers opportunities to those who can develop the structure for capitalizing on them. The data mining potential from a well-designed customer marketing information file is considerable.

Any choice-driven program is a natural for database marketing. Such programs could include anything from affinity programs (e.g., seniors programs) for hospitals to interaction with patients for physician practices to fundraising initiatives for healthcare organizations. Pharmaceutical companies are already using a version of database marketing in their DTC campaigns for targeting customers. Health plans are beginning to use this approach for segmenting their enrollee populations.

In other industries database marketing is used for cross-selling, upselling, follow-up sales, and so forth. Healthcare organizations are starting to expand their boundaries and think more broadly about what are appropriate (and potentially profitable) products and services.

Overt solicitation may be a turnoff for healthcare consumers, but if these opportunities are approached in the right way, they can be perceived as valuable. If a patient registers for an educational program (and gives consent for subsequent contact), this may be perceived as having value by the patient. Ideally, though, cross-selling, follow-up sales, and the like should focus on the organization's core products and services rather than overextending to include a lot of products with which it normally would not deal.

Many healthcare organizations promote secondary products (e.g., pediatric services to obstetrics patients), and patient data provide the basis for the bundling of various services to the benefit of the patient. The main concern for many is observance of privacy laws, but this should not be a problem for anyone who really understands the issues. The retail angle really involves more product-oriented activities, whereas database marketing has its real appeal in increasing the use of services.

The degree of acceptance of more aggressive database marketing will be a function of how it is implemented. Clearly, the pharmaceutical companies have issued a call to action through their DTC marketing that has been well received by patients (if not by physicians). If the database marketing initiative encourages or facilitates the customer obtaining more information, that will be seen as a positive factor. Still, dangers of a backlash exist, in some cases as simple as someone repeatedly asking to be taken off the solicitation list and getting no response or as complex as the implications of dealing with patients with sensitive medical conditions.

Customer Relationship Management

Healthcare marketers are always searching for ways to have more impact and demonstrate real value within their organization. CRM strategies may prove to be the next hot area in healthcare marketing, and for good reason. Well-thought-out and executed CRM programs are generating substantial returns for many businesses, and new technologies only add to the possibilities. Healthcare organizations are beginning to recognize the benefits of CRM, and increased spending on CRM activities is predicted.

At the same time, however, CRM is largely misunderstood by many health professionals, and the industry will likely be slow to implement a lot of customer-driven business strategies. Despite the hype and media attention surrounding new customer service strategies, healthcare organizations need to make significant changes in how they do business to realize the true benefits of CRM.

The most common problem with implementing successful CRM programs is the fact that many organizations confuse a CRM strategy with a technology implementation. While technology is a great enabler and health-care systems should be leveraging technology to do more with their customer-driven initiatives, implementing technology is not the same thing as having a CRM program. The most important aspects of a true CRM initiative lie in how the organization as a whole defines its customers, identifies and segments their needs, and organizes around serving them in the most efficient and effective manner possible. Healthcare organizations need to balance the value they provide to customers with the value they generate for the organization itself.

Marketers should first identify the goals most important to the organization; these should lead the internal planning and implementation efforts. Some of the more common goals and objectives for developing and implementing technology-driven customer relationship programs include the following:

- Improving customer service and satisfaction
- Increasing profitability
- Reducing the number of negative customer experiences
- Allocating resources more efficiently
- Reducing the cost of customer interaction
- Attracting and retaining customers and prospects
- Staying in front of customers, and building stronger relationships over time
- Improving clinical outcomes

The majority of healthcare organizations use customer satisfaction as the key metric for defining CRM success. Given that most hospitals already use patient satisfaction as a key performance indicator, it should not be a big leap for management to see the value of CRM strategies that enhance customer satisfaction in all areas of the system. Marketers can then introduce more aggressive objectives aimed at increasing patient volume, revenue, and profitability.

Existing businesses often have difficulty changing the institutional mind-set from being sales or operations driven to being customer driven. Healthcare in particular seems to have a difficult time making the leap from being inside-out driven to being outside-in driven. A few healthcare organizations, like Kaiser Permanente, HealthSouth, Celebration Health, and the Mayo Clinic, have made significant strides in becoming more customer driven, but they tend to be the exception rather than the rule.

For that reason most healthcare marketers will not be able to integrate every aspect of their organizations into a CRM program, and they probably should not try. The success of these programs is not in how comprehensive or complex they are but in how well coordinated and orchestrated they are to the end customer.

Some areas that have potential for the application of CRM strategies (see Case Study 12.2) include the following:

- A disease management program for a chronically ill group of patients
- An employee assistance program
- A physician-to-physician marketing initiative
- A community health screening or prevention program
- Specific product lines like cardiology, women's health, and sports medicine
- An urgent care clinic
- A web site or online community
- A call center or customer service function
- The top ten referring physicians
- The top ten accounts or clients
- A "frequent customer" program or other affinity club

Internet Marketing

Although healthcare organizations were slow to jump on the Internet marketing bandwagon, recent years have seen a surge of interest in the use of the Internet for a wide range of marketing activities. Most hospitals now have web sites, and some healthcare organizations have actually led the way with regard to certain aspects of online marketing.

Significant growth has occurred in the number of consumers who search for healthcare information online. Whether for patients or caregivers, the Internet is used as a resource both before and after visiting the doctor. Because these consumers are information seekers, they are receptive to information provided by healthcare organizations. Some of the aura surrounding the Internet has been diminished because of the bad experience with dot-coms. Yet, there continues to be growth in the public interest in online healthcare information and evidence that increasing numbers of healthcare consumers are logging on.

Observers of the evolution of the Internet have noted the progression of healthcare organizations through the various stages of Internet marketing. The first stage involves simply a "brochure" site, indicating who the organization is and what it does. Most healthcare organizations have passed through this stage, but beyond that they are all over the board in terms of moving to stages of information provision, interactivity, and relationship building. A variety of factors determine the degree of sophistication to which various healthcare organizations have carried their online marketing efforts.

Healthcare web sites generally have moved beyond static marketing information and corporate descriptions, introducing a deeper level of service line and health content, more interactive features, and dynamic applications. Most web sites are still far from being truly integrated with their organization's marketing efforts or other information technology applications. A smaller number of health systems push customized health information and medical records out to consumers, allowing e-mail communication with physicians and performing some level of actual disease management online.

Today, many healthcare organizations are doing unique and sophisticated things online. The "Most Wired Survey" conducted by the American Hospital Association is a useful indicator of what health systems are doing with Internet technology. Some early pioneers in this arena were Columbia/HCA, Kaiser Permanente, United Healthcare, and many academic hospitals like the University of Alabama at Birmingham and the University of Iowa.

Today, most healthcare organizations have web sites and marketing budgets for promoting their brands online. They have moved beyond the brochure stage and now provide valuable information online. Many are now trying to figure out how to determine the return on investment as it relates to driving more patient visits, prescriptions, coupon redemptions, and, when possible, product sales. For most organizations, answering the return-on-investment question will put Internet marketing on equal footing with offline marketing.

The Internet has become a major channel in the whole DTC movement as pharmaceutical companies use the Internet to better communicate with patients. Sites include Sepsis.com, Schering-Plough's Claritin.com, and Novo Nordisk's Diabetes for Patients.com. The National Headache Foundation and Astra Zeneca recently teamed up to create a Migraine Mentors at Work program. The site is an online extension of a workplace-based education and disease management program giving users information on how to manage their illness. Pharmaceutical companies do their marketing not by pounding consumers over the head but by providing information, education, advice, summaries of scientific studies, tools, and shared experiences.

Healthcare marketers are successfully using offline techniques to draw consumers into their web sites to search for information or respond to specific offers such as finding a physician, viewing an infant photo, or signing up for a health screening. Once consumers are online, healthcare organizations are converting these browsers into prospects by capturing personal information in a customer database and having consumers sign up for interactive health news and medical reminders. This allows the hospital to continue to market to these consumers in a more personal way than just advertising on television or through the mail. (The various mistakes healthcare organizations can make in developing web sites are described in Box 12.1; Case Study 12.3 describes a successful healthcare Internet marketing initiative.)

Among the developments anticipated with regard to healthcare Internet marketing are the following:

- Better integration between the Internet and new and existing marketing program.
- Leveraging targeted marketing campaigns to bolster service lines
- Focusing on online CRM strategies
- Increased DTC online marketing
- Increased multicultural-marketing understanding of the specific healthcare needs of ethnic populations
- More integration with the entire media mix

Limitations to Contemporary Marketing Techniques

The various contemporary approaches to marketing presented here clearly have useful applications to healthcare. Indeed, healthcare may need many of these methods more so than other industries. However, some barriers exist to the incorporation of some of the more innovative and technology-based techniques into healthcare.

Some of these barriers reflect the practicality of adopting these techniques to healthcare. Often, healthcare organizations do not have the personnel or technical resources to implement such methods. They may lack the information technology infrastructure and often cannot access data in the manner necessary to support some of these techniques. Healthcare organizations are not likely to have the know-how to implement database marketing or CRM without bringing in outside consultants.

Not only are the necessary data often lacking, but concerns about the confidentiality of the patient data used for some of these techniques always exist. The enactment of HIPAA legislation has made many healthcare organizations gun-shy even when it comes to legitimate uses of personal health data. These concerns are reinforced by questions raised about the appropriateness of using patient data in this manner. The conservative nature of health professionals presents a barrier to uses of data that individuals in other industries would take for granted.

Such techniques will likely be slowly but surely incorporated into healthcare, particularly into those components such as pharmaceutical dis-

Box 12.1: Common Web Marketing Mistakes

Healthcare organizations have limited experience with marketing; this lack of experience is often reflected in their attempts to implement innovative marketing initiatives such as web sites. These mistakes can be grouped into several different categories.

Failure to Adequately Plan for the Project

The most common mistakes made by healthcare organizations are not having specific objectives or goals from the start and not having a formal plan or strategy.

Making Faulty Assumptions About Customer Wants and Needs

Healthcare organizations often make assumptions about what site visitors want without really understanding their needs and motivations, often because of a lack of front-end research. This approach often leads to a "build it and they will come" attitude that almost ensures failure. Each customer has unique needs, and the Internet allows for personalization at a low cost.

Entrusting the Process to Inappropriate Parties

Healthcare organizations may assign web site development to inappropriate parties, such as individuals from the marketing or information systems departments or an enthusiastic employee who is really into the Internet. This also may mean choosing a web developer based on price and failing to effectively negotiate with vendors.

Failure to Carefully Plan Content

Many organizations are careless about the choice of content and their content provider. The level of content quality and depth is critical, as site visitors are generally looking for in-depth information and will go to another site if they do not find it.

Lack of Integration with Other Marketing Activities

Many healthcare organizations fail to fully integrate their online marketing with other marketing activities and their strategic plan. Web sites are treated as stand-alone information and as promotional vehicles that are not well integrated into the other marketing efforts of the organization.

Assuming that the Project Is Finished

At some point healthcare organizations assume that "it's done." However, the process is never over when it comes to web sites; the Internet is dynamic and involves an evolving process.

Failure to Make a Long-Term Commitment

When revenue or volume improves, healthcare organizations often decide to slash marketing budgets. When the organization faces a crisis or downturn, marketing people often get the boot despite their pivotal roles in business development, cost cutting, and revenue-enhancement strategies. The organization must be prepared to support online marketing efforts with ongoing management resources and regular maintenance.

tribution where there are fewer qualms about use of data. The demands of a competitive and consumer-driven system will ask for this change, and contemporary consumers themselves are likely to insist on ever more interactive access to healthcare providers.

Summary

The 1990s witnessed the adoption of techniques from other industries and the development of new healthcare-specific approaches. These approaches generally emphasize organizational changes or the application of technology to marketing challenges. Both of these types of approaches place emphasis on relationship marketing.

Among the emerging techniques that take a different approach to the organization are direct-to-consumer marketing, business-to-business marketing, internal marketing, and concierge services as a marketing strategy. Emerging technology-based techniques include database marketing, customer relationship management, and Internet marketing. Techniques that involve information technology and intensive use of data have tremendous potential for healthcare but remain controversial in many ways. The enactment of HIPAA legislation has made many healthcare organizations gun-shy even when it comes to legitimate uses of personal health data.

The Internet is changing the face of healthcare marketing, just as it has affected numerous other industries. While healthcare is behind the curve when it comes to the establishment of effective Internet sites, most healthcare organizations are becoming increasingly "wired." In the future, the Internet is expected to facilitate the use of various other technology-based marketing techniques.

Discussion Questions

- What factors within marketing and/or healthcare are encouraging the adoption of more sophisticated marketing techniques?
- How has the discovery of the consumer by healthcare organizations influenced their approach to marketing?
- Why does direct-to-consumer marketing represent a radical departure from traditional approaches to marketing on the part of the pharmaceutical industry?
- What developments in healthcare have encouraged the growth of business-to-business marketing?
- In what ways can a customer database be used once it has been established by a healthcare organization?

- What factors have influenced the trend toward establishing and exploiting relationships rather than trying to get the immediate sale from the healthcare consumer?
- What characteristics of healthcare call for a cautious approach to the application of technology-based marketing techniques?
- Describe the progression that Internet marketing has gone through as this approach to marketing by healthcare organizations has matured.

Note

1. Much of the material in this chapter was drawn from the work of Daniel Fell, originally published by HealthLeaders.com.

Additional Resources

Barr, J., S. Lautenberg, and B. Stieckman. 1998. "Creating a Vision for Your Call Center." *Healthcare Information Management* 27 (1): 73.

Kleinke, J. D. 1998. *The Bleeding Edge: The Business of Healthcare in the New Century.* Gaithersburg, MD: Aspen.

Maidu, G. M., A. Parvatiyar, J. N. Sheth, and L. Westgate. 1999. "Does Relationship Marketing Pay? Marketing Practices in Hospitals." *Journal of Business Research* 43 (3): 207–18.

Shankland, S. 2003. "To DTC or Not to DTC." *Marketing Health Services* 23 (4): 44.

Soloman, S. 2001. "E-Marketing on a Shoestring." *Marketing Health Services* 21 (1): 35.

A CONCIERGE PLAN

The demands baby boomers have made on the healthcare system have driven a number of the changes that have occurred, and boomers appear to be a force behind the concierge practice movement. At least one hospital has seen the boomer surge as an opportunity and developed a hospital-sponsored concierge practice to cater to the needs of this population. Virginia Mason Medical Center in Seattle, Washington, is an integrated healthcare delivery system. Virginia Mason has been tracking the trends of baby boomers for some time and has identified the boomer as one of its primary targets in terms of program development.

Virginia Mason planners noted that consumers had become more educated. They were visiting their doctors armed with health-related articles from the Internet. They also saw a shift in patient perceptions of physicians. Whereas past generations placed physicians on a pedestal, today's healthcare consumers see the physician as only one point of reference for their healthcare needs. Virginia Mason staff concluded that today's patient wants to remain healthy, continue looking and feeling young, and have immediate and convenient access to personalized care. Furthermore, they are willing to pay for all of this.

Virginia Mason has responded to these demands through several channels, including expansion of its Cosmetic Services Group to include facial and body surgery, postsurgical reconstructive surgery, skin rejuvenation, hair replacement, laser vision correction, and massage therapy. It is also in the process of implementing an e-health strategy that will meet the growing online demands for consumer access and customization on the Internet. In addition, Virginia Mason has recently launched its first online store, featuring skin care products and gift certificates for skin care and massage services.

Probably the most innovative program developed by Virginia Mason is the Lewis and John Dare Center, which opened its doors in 2000 and is the only service-amenities program of its kind that operates as part of a major medical center. (Virginia Mason prefers *service amenities* to *concierge*.)

Answering the call for immediate access and personalized service, the Dare Center provides patients with around-the-clock access to their physicians via cell phone, pager, and e-mail. Office or home visits are common, and same-day appointments are the norm. Dare Center physicians coordinate specialist care within Virginia Mason and are directly involved in all aspects of their patients' care, including emergency room visits and hospital admissions. The center's objective is to provide individualized care that accommodates the needs, concerns, schedule, and lifestyle of each patient.

Dare Center physicians can guarantee this extended level of service because their patient panels have been drastically reduced from those of standard primary care practices. Each Dare Center physician is limited to 300 patients. This allows Dare Center family practitioners and internists time to get to know their patients and proactively help them generate a personalized health plan based on their unique healthcare needs. Dare Center physicians have even been known to visit a busy patient's office and administer treatment while the patient continues with his or her work schedule.

Patients who enroll in the Dare Center program receive the following:

- Direct and immediate access to their Dare Center physician by phone, 24 hours a day, seven days a week
- Unhurried appointments scheduled at their convenience
- Consultation in their home or office as needed
- Unlimited e-mail, fax, and phone consultations with their Dare Center physician
- Coordination of specialist referrals as needed
- Direct involvement of their Dare Center physician in any emergency care or hospitalization
- Friendly staff who know and understand their unique healthcare needs
- Free parking at each location
- Three convenient primary care locations

This service-amenities program, however, is not only reserved for boomers. Many members are boomer parents whose children have purchased a membership for them. Dare Center staff believe that being a member of such a program generates a feeling of security for all family members and that knowing their parents are taken care of is an indirect benefit for boomers, who are increasingly taking on the added burden of trying to navigate the healthcare system for their parents. Patients who participate in the Dare Center pay an annual fee, in addition to their regular insurance, of $3,000 per individual, $5,000 per couple, or $6,000 and up for a family.

Now in its second year of operation, Dare Center has a patient load of 900 and a retention rate of 96 percent. It also recently expanded to include five physicians and three locations. One of the benefits of a hospital-sponsored concierge practice is access to the extensive resources of the health system. With the availability of more than 45 medical specialties, patients know they are linked to one of the most comprehensive and advanced medical systems in the region.

Realizing the demand for such a program, Virginia Mason has consulted with several medical systems throughout the United States to provide insight into creating a service-amenities program in other regions.

12.2

PROMOTING HEART HEALTH USING CUSTOMER RELATIONSHIP MANAGEMENT

Health systems are increasingly turning to customer relationship management (CRM) for purposes of predictive segmentation. The application of this technique to the cardiology market has been pioneered by Customer Potential Management (CPM) Marketing Group. CPM developed a program for three hospitals in the eastern United States that are part of a national healthcare system with more than 100 acute care hospitals and related businesses in 17 states. The participating hospitals ranged in size from a small local hospital to a large regional medical center and are referred to here as Hospital A, Hospital B, and Hospital C.

The overall objective of this program was to educate consumers on the early warning signs of a heart attack and encourage them to take a proactive role by determining their heart health. The program also was designed to build awareness of the healthcare system's local cardiology services and to drive early intervention and service utilization.

This campaign used the Consumer Healthcare Utilization Index (CHUI), a predictive index developed by CPM, to select the top individuals in each market area most likely to benefit from the campaign information. Targeted individuals were referred for a Heart Health Exam, the fee for which ranged from $25 to $39, depending on the provider. The campaign also included a control group with the same characteristics.

Area-referring physicians and providers were briefed on the campaign and encouraged to participate in screening patient results and referrals. This effort was designed to include physicians in the campaign, promote hospital cardiology services, and extend information to more patients.

The following objectives were identified for the project:

- Identify individuals at risk for a heart attack and provide early intervention (promotion of low-cost Heart Health Exam)
- Provide consumers with beneficial education (heart attack signs and symptoms)

- Strengthen positioning with primary care physicians and cardiologists
- Increase total charges attributed to cardiac-related services

The approach involved delivering segmented messages to male and female prospects drawn from the databases of the three facilities. The solicitations were limited to one per household and targeted to individuals 35 and older living in households reporting at least $30,000 annual income.

The package for the promotion consisted of a 7.5-inch by 5-inch four-color, self-mail piece with two executions segmented by gender. The primary offer was the Heart Health Exam, which included an EKG screen with a free EKG wallet card, body mass index measurement, lipid screen, and a cardiac education booklet. The secondary offer was a free take-home health-risk assessment.

The cost per package, including materials, lettershop services, and postage, differed for each hospital based on how many pieces were printed and how many were actually mailed and ranged from $0.71 to $1.39 per package. Package prices for Hospitals B and C were higher because they printed large quantities for future mailings.

Active responses were identified as those who scheduled Heart Health Exam appointments and were tracked through the appointments. A complete record of the organization-initiated communications—outbound dialogs with customers and prospective customers through direct mail—was maintained. These communication records were matched against individuals and households within the database to assess activities, behaviors, and service utilization within the product line promoted.

A 5 percent sample of the system's CRM database was flagged as a static market control group for each hospital. The control group was selected using the same criteria as the organization-initiated communications group that received the mailing. The control group did not receive the mailing but was tracked and matched against individuals and households within the database to assess activities, behaviors, and service utilization compared with those who did receive the mailing.

Hospitals A and B showed significant positive results on the basis of their list selection of individuals with high predictive index scores. While Hospital C reported positive results as well, fewer data were available for this site. At Hospital A nearly half of those who signed up for the Heart Health Exam had abnormal EKG readings. When combined with individuals who had minor abnormal EKG readings, the percentage of those with some sort of abnormal reading rose to 54 percent. At Hospital B the EKGs of those who signed up for the Heart Health Exam revealed abnormal EKG readings for well more than half (61 percent) of the participants. EKG scan results were not available for Hospital C.

The real measurement of success for a marketing campaign is the revenue received for marketing dollars spent. An accurate calculation of return on investment must also be done, by examining the control group, to account for utilization that might have occurred without the campaign.

The use of CHUI methodology for targeting potential cardiology patients generated positive benefits to the participating hospitals. The combined response results for the first six months of this campaign indicated the following:

- Patient response rate of 5.36 percent (control group response rate of 1.61 percent)
- Marketing response increase of 333 percent
- Net profit of $1,868,711
- Marketing lift (after factoring-out control group) of $1,684,643
- Return on investment of $44.78 for every $1.00 spent in marketing costs

The campaign results for the first six months demonstrated that this health system was successful both in identifying the most appropriate individuals for cardiology services and in generating a reasonable return on investment. The significance of these numbers illustrates that CHUI allows organizations to target at-risk individuals for intervention with appropriate education, health maintenance, and wellness programs.

12.3

EFFECTIVE WEB INTEGRATION: A HOSPITAL CASE STUDY

Most hospitals today have established an Internet presence. Yet, despite a strong consumer interest in performing transactions online, a relatively small percentage of hospital and health system e-health sites have progressed much beyond electronic brochures and relatively limited interactivity. Research shows that more than 40 percent of e-health sites operated by hospitals and health systems offer little or no consumer-focused health information. Many hospital and health system e-health initiatives remain the purview of the marketing or information systems departments and do not yet demonstrate ownership by, and interconnectivity with, clinical departments.

Mercy Health Partners (MHP) in Toledo, Ohio, is a six-hospital region of Catholic Healthcare Partners, a large multihospital health system operating in five midwestern states. MHP is one of the two large health systems that dominate the Toledo market; it offers a complete spectrum of health services, including primary, secondary, and tertiary programs and a significant medical education function. Within its six hospitals more than 40,000 annual inpatient admissions are generated by more than 1,600 medical staff members.

MHP previously operated nine largely independent and unconnected web sites covering a variety of entities and programs. In October 2000 the organization launched its completely redesigned web site, MercyWeb.org, in an effort to consolidate the many earlier web sites into a single, branded Internet presence for the entire organization. MercyWeb.org is intended as the primary portal to a number of MHP e-health initiatives.

After only a few months of operation, MercyWeb.org had grown to an average of approximately 2,500 unique monthly visitors, with more than 13,000 visitor sessions per month. Yet, with only a few months' experience in optimizing the MercyWeb.org site, MHP decided to begin work to accelerate the evolution of the site and its functionality. MHP marketing and business development staff embarked on an effort to transfer ownership of the organization's e-health initiatives to the clinical operating divisions in a well-organized approach to ensure optimal integration of e-health into the operating processes of the health system.

Although MercyWeb.org was widely viewed as a successful e-health initiative, those primarily responsible for MercyWeb.org understood that it was not embraced as a tool by clinical staff throughout the organization; many, if not most, had not visited the site themselves. The site was largely perceived by staff as a marketing tool under the auspices of the marketing and business development group. MercyWeb.org had not yet been fully integrated into the operating practices of the organization. The MHP marketing and business development team identified four keys to ensuring the optimal success of the organization's e-health initiatives:

- *Clear strategic fit:* The e-health initiatives must be clearly connected to the overall strategy and positioning of the organization, and they must have a measurable objective.
- *Beyond electronic brochures:* The web portal must go beyond electronic brochures to include enhanced functionality, interactivity, personalization, and patient-hospital transactions.
- *Integration with operating practices:* Web site functionality must be integrated with existing and future offline databases and other applications used as part of the care delivery and supporting processes, to effectively blur any distinction between online and offline patient interactions.
- *E-cultural transformation:* The organization must engage in an e-cultural transformation to ensure that staff and physicians understand the potential of information technologies, feel comfortable in their use, and are encouraged to identify new ways to use them to further the organization's objectives.

With these four broad objectives in mind, the marketing and business development leadership decided to focus further e-health initiatives on individual centers of excellence, beginning with The Heart Center, Mercy Children's Hospital, and Mercy Occupational Health. A complete online extension of each clinical area was to be developed and launched within several months under the direction and control of the clinical leadership for each center of excellence.

The first of the three targeted online centers of excellence was MHP's cardiovascular disease program, The Heart Center. This center of excellence transcends the organization's three acute care hospitals in the Toledo area and represents a "product line management" focus of the organization. The project to establish The Heart Center Online began with the appointment of a steering committee composed of the director of The Heart Center, the senior vice president for marketing and business development, three physicians, seven MHP managers/supervisors, and four representatives of the consulting group. Two representatives of the MHP information systems department provided staff support.

Five work teams—content, marketing and research, return on investment, technology, and training—were established from the members of the steering committee and other staff who were enlisted to develop The Heart Center Online. Combined, the five work teams made up the implementation team. The steering committee met prior to the launch of the project and then, along with the implementation team, met monthly for four months. Each of the five work teams also met as needed, ranging from weekly to monthly during the four-month development process.

After three months of development the collective effort of the teams had produced a beta version of The Heart Center Online that would be tested, redesigned, and refined over the following month. Four months from the first implementation team meeting the group celebrated the completion of The Heart Center Online, which included more than 300 pages of online content, features, and functionality devoted to cardiovascular diseases and conditions. When the site was first shown in its completed form to the implementation team, the pride within the room was nearly palpable. In addition to creating a robust, vibrant online presence, the group had accomplished its task within only four months, moving from the initial blank slate to the "brain map" and finally to The Heart Center Online.

The cost of the project was approximately $100,000, amortized over two years, but because MHP participated in a beta project development with the consulting group, the actual cost was approximately one-half the normal cost, or about $50,000 over two years. Although considerable enhancements to the site will occur in the future to add increased value and payoff for MHP, results of The Heart Center Online are already beginning to appear.

Source: Campbell, G. S., D. Sherry, and D. J. Sternberg. 2002. "Effective Web Integration: A Hospital Case Study." *Marketing Health Services* 22 (2): 40–42.

IV

MANAGING AND SUPPORTING THE MARKETING EFFORT

I t is one thing to come up with a marketing idea, but it is quite another to coordinate a marketing campaign or implement a marketing plan. These activities require an understanding of the process and the skills to manage the process. This section addresses the nuts and bolts involved in organizing, developing, and implementing marketing initiatives. The end-to-end marketing process is described, and techniques for evaluating the effectiveness of marketing initiatives are discussed. The various support activities that make effective marketing possible, such as marketing planning and marketing research, are explained.

Chapter 13 outlines the steps in the marketing process, from concept to marketing plan to project implementation. It provides basic information on the activities necessary for bringing a marketing project to fruition. It discusses the role of outside agencies of various types and explains the budgetary process for marketing activities. Techniques for assessing the effectiveness of a marketing initiative are described.

Chapter 14 presents an overview of the marketing research function as applied to healthcare. The importance of research in the marketing process is emphasized and the types of research are outlined. The various techniques for researching the market, products and services, locations, and pricing are described.

Chapter 15 introduces the reader to marketing planning and the role it plays in healthcare. Although presented late in the book, planning activities should occur early in the marketing process and guide the marketing initiative. The steps in the planning process are outlined with special consideration to the healthcare environment. The importance of plan implementation is discussed.

Chapter 16 describes sources of data to support the marketing process. Marketing is a data-driven endeavor, and healthcare, unlike other industries, has not developed a clearinghouse of marketing data. Thus, the healthcare marketer must develop inordinate skills at identifying and accessing the data needed for marketing research and marketing planning. This chapter describes methods for identifying, accessing, interpreting, and applying health-related data in the marketing process.

13

MANAGING AND EVALUATING THE MARKETING PROCESS

The marketing process entails the full range of activities involved in developing a marketing plan or implementing a marketing campaign. It begins with the decision to carry out a marketing effort and ends with the evaluation of that effort.

This chapter describes the steps in the organization, implementation, management, and evaluation of a marketing initiative and the unique nature of this process as applied to healthcare. This chapter emphasizes the manner in which the many components of the marketing process come together to create a marketing campaign.

From Marketing Plan to Marketing Campaign

Marketing is not an act but a process. As such, certain steps must be followed in implementing a marketing project. While circumstances vary from situation to situation, certain commonalities are involved in all marketing campaigns. The importance of these steps for both plan development and campaign implementation cannot be overemphasized. This process assumes that certain conditions are in place (e.g., the organization is promoting well-defined products that lend themselves to marketing, an overarching strategic plan within which this initiative fits is in place, adequate information is available on the various potential target audiences, and an adequate understanding of consumer behavior exists).

The extent to which the staff of the healthcare organization is involved in the process will be a function of the extent to which the marketing is internalized within the organization. The nature of the organization's marketing arrangement will influence the manner in which the process is carried out. A number of options are available to a healthcare organization in terms of marketing arrangements, and each has different implications for the organization.

One option is for the healthcare organization to fully outsource its marketing function. This is typical of many organizations in the early years of healthcare marketing and still common among smaller organizations, such as physician offices, that cannot support an in-house marketing function. In this case all of the activities related to the marketing process are handled by an entity or entities outside the organization. The process can never be fully outsourced, of course, as the client organization must provide information on the product to be marketed, provide feedback on marketing strategies, and approve the materials developed.

Another option may be for the healthcare organization to mostly outsource the marketing function while carrying out some of the activities in-house. This would typically happen in cases in which an organization has a marketing professional on staff but none of the other capabilities required. In this case the marketing "director" would coordinate the process but leave most of the actual tasks to agencies with which it contracts outside the organization. In other cases a large organization, like a hospital, may have some of the capabilities required for marketing in-house but no formal marketing function. It may have copywriters, graphic artists, printing facilities, web site developers, and other personnel or capabilities that would contribute to the marketing function.

A third option involves the in-house administration of most aspects of the marketing process, essentially establishing an in-house agency. Even here, healthcare organizations that have an internal marketing function are likely to continue to outsource some aspects of the process. The organization may not have certain specialized skills or the ability to handle certain activities. Even a well-developed marketing department within a healthcare organization is not likely to have the contacts and skills for negotiating media purchases or implementing a direct-mail campaign.

A few healthcare organizations are able to support virtually all of the functions required for marketing. Most multifacility health systems, for example, are likely to have a centralized marketing department. This department coordinates the marketing activities for the system and ensures that a consistent message is conveyed by all corporate entities. Even here, however, the organization may still have to rely on outside parties for at least some functions.

Obviously, the extent to which the process is incorporated into the operations of the hospital will determine the amount of control, and responsibility, the healthcare organization has for the marketing function. Even with "totally" outsourced marketing functions, time, energy, and money are required of the client organization. If key staff have to spend two person days, for example, explaining a complicated service to the marketers, this involves considerable direct and indirect costs. Diverting resources from other functions to the marketing campaign may involve unanticipated opportunity costs.

Organizing the Project

The first step in any marketing process involves getting organized for the effort, or planning for planning. Certain groundwork has to be laid before the campaign can be implemented. Part of this organizational process involves the identification of someone to champion the effort, whether it is a broad-scale planning initiative or a short-term promotional campaign. The champion is someone who believes in the value of the idea or approach and supports it in the face of numerous possible obstacles and even opposition within the organization.

The planning phase provides the foundation on which the rest of the process is built. To create an effective marketing program, the problem being addressed, audiences being targeted, and environment in which the program will operate must be understood. Market research is used to analyze these factors and develop a workable strategy for effecting behavioral change. As noted above, it is assumed that a body of relevant knowledge on the service area and its population already exists.

Defining the Target Audience

As above, the content of this step will depend on whether a marketing plan or specific marketing campaign is being pursued. The target audience should be defined through market research and market segmentation analysis. A marketing program has as its core the wants and needs of its consumers, determined through the market research methods that identify the target audience and how it thinks, feels, and behaves in relation to the issue the program addresses. These methods include quantitative research that generates objective data on the target population and qualitative research that provides insight into why people think or do what they do.

Determining the Marketing Objectives

The marketing objectives should be determined within the broad context of the organization's strategic plan if a marketing plan is under consideration. If the focus is on a specific marketing initiative, the objectives should be in keeping with those of the overall marketing plan. Here, as elsewhere, the objectives established should be specific, include quantifiable concepts, and be time limited. The marketing objectives should be based on where the consumers are located on the *hierarchy of effects,* the stages through which a buyer moves from first seeing an advertisement to buying the product or using the service.

Determining the Resources Required

A well-thought-out marketing budget is critical. The *marketing budget* is the section of the overall marketing plan or project plan that indicates projected costs. The expense component of the budget may be based on one of several methods: percentage of sales, competitive parity, "all you can afford," or an objective-and-task approach. A percentage-of-sales approach is commonly used in other industries but has limited application in healthcare.

The resources required for marketing include not only the direct costs (e.g., creative development, media time) involved but also the costs for the personnel, production facilities, and other resources required for carrying out the project. For initiatives built around advertising, media costs are likely to be the major expense. These expenses include the cost of advertising through various channels of communication such as print, electronic, outdoor, and direct mail.

The marketing budget for a specific initiative should consider such direct costs as personnel expenses, market research costs, creative costs, production costs, media expenses, and a variety of other resource requirements. Indirect costs must also be considered. Even if the campaign is essentially outsourced, there will be staff time required by the marketing agency as well as some overhead costs. (See below for more detail on budgetary issues.)

Developing the Message

This phase of the marketing program involves the development of the marketing message and the promotional materials for delivering it. Based on the results of the research conducted in the planning stages of the program, concepts and materials are typically created and pretested with members of the target audience. The message involves the combination of symbols and words the sender wishes to transmit to the receiver and indicates the content the sender wants to convey. The message embodies the campaign theme, primary topic, subject, motif, or idea around which an advertising campaign is organized as well as the campaign slogan that comes to be identified with the product or service.

Testing the marketing concept with a group of target consumers is common to learn whether the concepts have the appropriate consumer appeal. The pretesting phase involves using various methods to test messages, materials, and proposed tactics with the target audience to determine what works best to accomplish the program's objectives. It may be necessary to go back and forth several times between development and pretesting to make the necessary changes in the messages, materials, or overall strategy.

Positioning concepts must be developed and evaluated by members of the target audience. *Positioning* refers to the way the product is perceived by the target audience relative to other similar products. Generally, positioning is based on the key selling point of the product. Selecting the best positioning statement is often based on the result of concept testing through focus groups or in-depth interviews.

Using the information obtained from concept testing, materials are created and then tested using prefinished executions that may include theme lines, posters, news clips, videotapes, brochures, public service announcements, or product packaging. These materials should be evaluated in terms of memorability, impact, communication, comprehension, believability, acceptability, image, persuasion, and other key attributes.

With printed materials, the readability of the text is crucial, particularly for audience from lower socioeconomic status. The readability of printed text may be assessed by checking sentence length and number of polysyllabic words. Readability testing is generally recommended for materials with a lot of text, such as longer print ads, brochures, or information kits. It is often helpful to have health communication peers and representatives of intermediary organizations review such materials as well.

When the process reaches a certain point, it is customary to develop a *marketing brief* that presents the specifics of the campaign (see Box 13.1). This is essential if the organization is going to "shop" the project to various marketing agencies. The production of a brief is important, even if virtually every aspect of the project is being handled in-house, to have a thumbnail sketch of the marketing project and its objectives.

Having compiled the appropriate information necessary on the product, market, and various promotional options, the subsequent steps in the campaign can be implemented.

Specifying the Media Plan

Projects will differ in the extent to which they emphasize the use of media. Few projects, however, will have no media component. Even those that involve no advertising are likely to distribute press releases or other communiqués that end up in the media. The *media plan* outlines the objectives of the advertising campaign, the target audience, and the specific media vehicles that will be used to reach that audience. This step applies more directly to the marketing campaign than to overall plan development. The media plan involves the determination of the medium, vehicle, and scheduling of the

Box 13.1:
Developing
the
Marketing
Brief

In dealing with marketing agencies the client commonly presents a brief as a starting point for the planning of the project. (If the healthcare organization is in the process of selecting an agency, the brief will be what prospective agencies react to in making their presentations.) The brief contains the specifics of the proposed campaign to the extent they are known at the time. The degree of marketing sophistication of the healthcare organization will no doubt determine the extent of the brief, but it is important that any agency involved be given something to which to respond.

The brief typically includes the following components:

- Description of the good or service to be marketed
- Situational information on the company and product
- Objectives of the marketing campaign
- Proposed strategy
- Anticipated budget
- Timelines
- In-house personnel and their potential contributions
- Means of evaluating the campaign's effectiveness

The marketing agency or agencies will respond to the brief, addressing each issue presented. They will offer their interpretation of the marketing challenge, suggest a creative and media strategy, and indicate the control mechanism to be used and the allocation of agency responsibilities. The agency will also present relevant terms and conditions for performing the project.

message. If the marketer is thinking "advertising," she needs to consider whether it will be print or electronic. If electronic, will it be radio, television, or the Internet? If she chooses television, will it be network or cable? If cable, what channel, time slot, and frequency are appropriate?

In addition, the media plan must consider the reach, frequency, and waste involved, all of which must be balanced when developing an ad campaign. The *reach* is the number of people exposed to an ad; the *frequency* is the number of times the same person sees the ad within a defined time period; and the *waste* is the number of people reached who were not intended to be reached. This last issue is particularly important in healthcare marketing, given that the patronage of some categories of patients (based on payer class) would *not* be encouraged by the healthcare organization.

The steps involved in media planning include the following:

- Defining the objectives
- Identifying the audience
- Establishing a media budget
- Evaluating media options
- Selecting the type of medium
- Determining the specific form of that medium
- Negotiating media relationships
- Developing the media schedule
- Implementing the plan
- Evaluating the plan

Implementing the Marketing Campaign

Marketing implementation turns marketing strategies and plans into marketing actions to accomplish the specified marketing objectives. During the implementation phase the program is introduced to the target audience. Preparation is essential for success, and implementation must be monitored to ensure that every element proceeds as planned. The process shifts at this point from the planning function to the implementation function and from the concept people to the operational staff. Marketing planning has the advantage over other types of planning in that the same people are likely to be involved in both planning and implementation.

To approach plan implementation systematically it is important to develop both a detailed marketing project plan and an implementation matrix. The *project plan* systematically depicts the various steps in the planning process and specifies the sequence they should follow. The project plan also indicates the relationships that exist between the various tasks and, importantly, the extent to which the completion of some tasks is a prerequisite for the accomplishment of others.

The *implementation matrix* should list every action called for by the plan, breaking each action down into tasks if appropriate. For each action or task the responsible party should be identified, along with any secondary parties who should be involved in this activity. The matrix should indicate resource requirements (in terms of staff time, money, and other requirements). The start and end dates for this activity should be identified. Any prerequisites for accomplishing this task should be identified at the outset (and factored into the project plan).

The resource requirements from the implementation matrix should be combined to determine total project resource requirements. This information feeds back into the fourth step, the point where required resources are estimated. Once the requirements are identified, project activities may have to be addressed in relation to available funds and any other fiscal constraints. (See Chapter 15 for an additional discussion of marketing plan implementation.)

Evaluating the Campaign

The evaluation of the marketing initiative should be top of mind from the outset of the process and, in fact, should be built into the process itself. It should involve ongoing monitoring of the process, including benchmarks and milestones for assessment along the way. While the evaluation process is important for all types of planning processes, it is particularly important in marketing planning. Because the objectives of the marketing process are usually highly focused, measures of marketing effectiveness are essential.

Evaluation techniques are of two types: process (or formative) analysis and outcome (or summative) analysis. Both have a role to play in the project, although outcome evaluation is particularly important for the marketing process. Process evaluation assesses the efficiency of the marketing effort, whereas outcome evaluation addresses its effectiveness. Campaign effectiveness can be measured in a variety of ways, and any project will likely involve more than one means of evaluation. This is particularly the case in healthcare, where the intangible benefits of a marketing initiative are often as important as the tangible ones.

When marketing programs seek mass-media coverage for their promotional activities they need to be able to evaluate the success of these activities. An effective way of determining media "hits" is to subscribe to a clipping service that tracks the publication of print items. The frequency of play for the program's broadcast public service announcements can also be tracked through the use of a media monitoring service such as Arbitron.

While the marketing program is in effect, process evaluation should take place intermittently in each part of the program. As detailed in the implementation phase, this step includes media monitoring and analysis as well as evaluation of program activities. The key measurement areas to track include awareness of the product, advertising awareness and recall, knowledge level, attitudes and perceptions, images of product and users, experience with the product, and behaviors (trial and repeat). At this stage the target audience should be asked questions that are specific to the particular product or campaign, in addition to the earlier, general questions about attitudes and behaviors regarding the topic.

Impact evaluation is an aspect of outcome evaluation that assesses whether the marketing campaign actually induced the desired change (e.g., an increase in consumer approval, greater patient volume). The actual impact of the marketing program is often difficult to assess accurately. Can one public service announcement produced by the health department through its social marketing initiative, for example, cause a drop in morbidity and mortality from heart disease? Probably not, but many such efforts may combine synergistically and become a contributing factor in health status improvement. Because marketing campaigns are relatively short lived, the effect of a particular spot on overall trends may be impossible to determine. However, we can at least compare mortality and morbidity rates before and after implementation of the program as one form of measurement.

The most effective way of establishing a cause-and-effect relationship between healthcare marketing efforts and changes in behavior and health outcomes is to conduct an intervention study in one or more communities, with matched communities as controls. Assuming no significant differences between the intervention and control communities, marketing activities may be linked to changes in the communities with precision and reliability.

The Players in the Marketing Process

The marketing process can involve a variety of personnel and departments or organizations, depending on the extent of outsourcing involved. If marketing is fully internalized within the healthcare organization, virtually all of these components will be found in-house. If the process is partially outsourced, some will be found in-house and others will be contracted out. Of course, if the process is essentially outsourced, virtually all of these components will exist external to the organization. Following are some of the entities that may be involved in the marketing process.

Agencies

The term *agency* covers many different entities in the marketing industry. It could refer to full-service marketing agency, creative shop, media independent, a la carte operation, or other entity. The term could even be applied to an in-house entity that carries out agency functions. Although these may be referred to informally as *advertising agencies,* many provide a wide range of services beyond advertising support. A *full-service agency* is an organization that can offer start-to-finish services to its clients. An *a la carte agency* is a specialist shop that offers uniquely tailored services. A la carte is the approach to the advertising function whereby the various services a client requires, such as creative work and media buying, are handled by separate specialized agencies.

The main functions of agencies include the following:

- Planning campaigns
- Designing creative components
- Scheduling and buying media
- Buying and integrating other promotional materials
- Administration and accountancy for the process
- Implementing campaigns
- Monitoring and evaluating results

For healthcare organizations that intend to outsource some or all of their marketing functions choosing an appropriate agency is an important step. This is not a decision to be taken lightly, and it requires some meaningful research into the options available (see Box 13.2).

Clients

The healthcare organization is typically the client in the marketing process, and the other entities strive to serve the needs of the client. If the marketing function is internalized, the client will typically be another department within the organization. The client should not be considered a passive customer in the marketing process but should play an important role that includes the following:

- Providing the rationale for the marketing campaign
- Selecting and briefing the marketing agency
- Providing input into and approving campaign plans
- Integrating promotional planning into marketing planning
- Evaluating and controlling the campaign
- Financing the process

Media Suppliers

Media suppliers include the commercial television companies, commercial radio companies, newspaper and magazine owners, poster companies, and a variety of other organizations that make media available to the campaign. Various entities, depending on the nature of the campaign, must be factored into the process.

Promotional-Material Suppliers

A variety of other specialist suppliers exists, from printers to producers of promotional gifts to exhibition organizers to organizers of corporate hospitality. These specialist services are bought directly by client companies or managed through advertising agencies.

Any healthcare organization involved in marketing will have to deal with an agency at one time or another. If the organization has professional marketing staff in-house, this process is facilitated. Many organizations, however, have limited experience dealing with marketing agencies, and the individuals involved in the search for an agency may be relatively unfamiliar with the whole process.

As in selecting any type of consultant, the client organization should have its requirements well defined before any discussions with prospective agencies. Some health professionals may argue that they know little about marketing and are really relying on the agency to provide guidance. Even so, a well-developed description of the service to be marketed, ultimate goal of the campaign, and potential interfaces with other organizational components should be available for presentation to prospective agencies.

With requirements in hand, the organization should develop a list of potential agencies. It should be emphasized that in only very unusual circumstances should an agency that does not have experience in healthcare marketing be considered. Healthcare is different, and so is healthcare marketing. Not only is there the danger of a highly visible gaffe of some sort if the agency does not know healthcare, but the issue of the time required to explain basic aspects of the organization and its services to an uninformed marketing person must also be considered.

Given the fact that relatively few marketing agencies have experience in the healthcare industry and even fewer *specialize* in healthcare, this list is likely to be relatively short. Healthcare organizations are followers for the most part, and in this situation it may be beneficial to be a follower rather than a leader. Ideas should be solicited from other healthcare organizations concerning the available agencies and their capabilities. A positive experience on the part of another healthcare organization is probably the best recommendation that can be provided.

The agencies that appear to be qualified in healthcare marketing or are recommended by colleagues should be asked to present their credentials for review. This would include examples of current or past work, staff capabilities, and the company's history. A brief that contains the specifics of the proposed campaign should be presented to the agencies; this includes situational details, objectives, proposed strategy and tactics, target-market data, budget and time scales, performance evaluation information. The degree of marketing sophistication of the healthcare organization will no doubt determine the extent of the brief, but it is critical that the prospective agency be given something to which to respond.

In many industries it is standard operating procedure to make several agencies jump through major hoops before a decision is made. The intent, of course, is to select the best possible agency for the particular campaign. Given the nature of healthcare and the services being marketed, this seems like an extravagant waste of time. Nine times out of ten the healthcare organization does not need the very best agency; it needs a good one that can meet its needs. Here again, recommendations from other healthcare organizations may play a role.

While it is important that the agency chosen has the requisite capabilities, the agency also must be easy to work with. *Easy* in this case means an agency with staff who understand healthcare and the constraints healthcare organizations face in marketing, who know the time demands made on health professionals, and who have an appreciation for the mission of the client organization. Because marketing resources will likely be limited, the sooner the topic of costs can be broached, the better.

Some considerations in healthcare may be less important in other industries. Concern always exists over the extent to which the agency's culture and management style fit with that of the healthcare client. Another issue is potential conflict with existing business handled within the agency network. A healthcare organization that incurs significant costs as a result of treating smoking-induced health problems may not find a comfortable fit with an agency that maintains cigarette firms among its major accounts.

Once an agency has been selected, the organization must negotiate contractual terms. A variety of factors must be considered in developing the project budget, and this net should be widely cast. The healthcare organization needs to be aware of any hidden costs, particularly if it is a neophyte in the marketing arena. Agencies may assume that everyone knows that certain expenses will be incurred, but an organization without experience in marketing may not be aware of them. The contract should cover not only the amount of remuneration but the terms and timing of payments, issues of nonperformance and termination, and ultimate decision-making authority. In most cases some type of confidentiality agreement will be required as part of the contract as well.

Marketing Consulting Firms

Marketing consulting firms vary with regard to the services they offer; they range from those that offer specialized services (e.g., market research, media planning, evaluation) to those that offer a full array of services. Their input may be broad (e.g., determination of the overall strategic plan) or narrow (e.g., provision of a targeted mailing list).

Components of a Marketing Department

Should a healthcare organization endeavor to establish in-house marketing capabilities, several components to the internal agency need to be considered. These reflect the range of activities involved in the marketing process. Even if the organization retains external marketing resources, it must know about the various elements involved.

The components that would typically be established in a marketing department include those described below.

Creative Department

The creative department typically houses the "ideas people" and, in basic terms, deals with words and pictures. This department typically handles the copy, graphics, and art direction. The visual and audio portions of posters, billboards, brochures, television or radio spots, and web-based promotions are typically created by this department.

Media-Planning and -Buying Department

Determining media needs and negotiating for the placement of advertisements is an industry in its own right. This area is fairly specialized and may be difficult to totally bring in-house. Media-buying experts presumably know the most suitable type of medium, best time slots, and best prices. The more central media is to the campaign, the more important this function becomes.

Production Department

The production department is ultimately responsible for producing the promotional material, whatever form it may take. This may be as simple as translating art from the creative department into printed materials or as complicated as producing a video spot for television. As with media buying, this function is difficult to fully bring in-house because of the specialized equipment and expertise that may be required.

Account Management Department

The account management department represents the primary ongoing interface with clients. In an external agency an account manager will be assigned to handle the healthcare client. While this same terminology may not be used with an in-house department, different individuals may be assigned to work with different internal clients. Either way, account manager responsibilities include (1) attending client meetings, (2) writing reports, (3) coordinating activities, (4) presenting agency findings, and (5) feeding back client comments. The account manager has ultimate responsibility for the client's satisfaction.

Traffic Department

The traffic department has the responsibility for getting the artwork or film to the magazine or television station on time. When the promotional campaign involves a number of different media, this process becomes complicated and accurate timing becomes crucial.

The Marketing Budget

The marketing budget as a component of the marketing process requires special discussion. Budgeting is an essential financial discipline that represents a particularly tricky problem in marketing given the difficulty in determining both likely demand for a product and likely cost of achieving a given sales target. For healthcare organizations unused to marketing this becomes an important consideration, whether an in-house department is being planned or an external agency is being used. In fact, the budget issue may be considered at two different levels. On the one hand, the annual budget will require figures on the expected expenditures for marketing in the coming fiscal year. On the other hand, each marketing campaign requires a budget to address its specific needs. Presumably, the cumulative campaign budgets for the year will approximate the annual budget that has been established.

While most people may feel they know what a budget is, the marketing budget serves a number of purposes above and beyond accounting. The marketing budget serves to do the following:

- Set targets to be achieved
- Establish financial and time frameworks for all components of the project
- Control these activities to ensure they remain within budget
- Motivate staff to maintain control of their own budgets
- Assign responsibility, and allow managers to take responsibility for their actions
- Communicate project objectives
- Motivate and stimulate the staff
- Increase coordination between all business units, all departments, and all staff

The factors that make up the marketing budget are numerous and varied. Many are obvious, but others are not and may be overlooked by those unfamiliar with marketing planning. In addition to direct costs incurred for marketing, indirect costs will likely be incurred as well. In an industry like healthcare opportunity costs will also likely come into play. The expenses that must be budgeted for include the following:

- Direct personnel costs of marketing personnel
- Market research costs
- Creative costs

- Production costs
- Printing costs (if applicable)
- Postage (if applicable)
- Promotional items (if applicable)
- Media costs
- Evaluation costs

Expenses indirectly attributable to the marketing campaign may include the following:

- Administrative expenses or the cost of management, secretarial, accounting, and other administrative services, which include

  — Salaries of directors, management, and office staff
  — Rent and rates
  — Insurance
  — Telephone and postage
  — Printing and stationery
  — Heating and lighting

- Distribution and selling expenses, which include

  — Salaries of marketing and sales directors and management
  — Salaries and commissions of sales staff
  — Travel and entertainment expenses of salespeople

As noted elsewhere, a considerable amount of time will likely be required of nonmarketing staff as they work with marketing personnel in the development of the marketing plan or marketing campaign. This not only involves the direct cost of staff time but, in healthcare in particular, may also involve considerable disruption in the operation of the organization.

The factors that ultimately affect the size of the promotional budget include the following:

- Geographic market to be covered
- Type of product (industrial, consumer durable, or consumer convenience items)
- Distribution of consumers
- External factors (e.g., competitors' promotional budgets)
- Other salient factors

Marketing Management

Marketing management is an art and science in its own right and is particularly challenging in healthcare. *Marketing management* can be defined as the analysis, planning, implementation, and control of programs designed to create, build, and maintain beneficial exchanges with target buyers for the purpose of achieving organizational objectives. Ultimately, this involves the oversight necessary for managing the start-to-finish marketing process. The marketing control process includes, among other things, measuring and evaluating the results of marketing strategies and plans.

Strong marketing management is particularly important in the healthcare industry. Healthcare organizations have had limited experience with marketing in most cases, and it remains a new and different experience for many. Healthcare organizations often have diffuse objectives and a range of customers. They also may have a variety of stakeholders with competing agendas. In any case considerable skepticism with regard to the efficacy of marketing is likely, so strong controls are required.

Many in healthcare express concern over the potential negative fallout from marketing. Healthcare organizations must be careful not to convey the wrong image or appear to recklessly expend resources on marketing. The damage done by a poorly conceived, targeted, or implemented campaign may be difficult to rectify.

Management has two distinct aspects: (1) managing the process (i.e., forecasting, planning, monitoring, and controlling) and (2) managing the people, within the organization and outside it, who are involved in the process. The first aspect emphasizes the existence of structures and resources that support the various functions involved in the process. The second aspect involves the direct management of the personnel who perform these functions. These types of resources are not readily available in most healthcare organizations, but they are necessary for marketing to be integrated into the corporate structure.

Summary

The marketing process entails the full range of activities involved in developing a marketing plan or implementing a marketing campaign. It begins with the decision to carry out a marketing effort and ends with the evaluation of that effort. The extent to which the staff of the healthcare organization is involved in the process will be a function of the extent to which the marketing is internalized within the organization.

A number of options are available to a healthcare organization in terms of marketing arrangements, and each has different implications for the organization. These range from virtually total outsourcing of the marketing function to developing the full range of marketing capabilities in-house. The circumstances of the organization at that point in time will determine the extent to which these tasks are internalized. The extent to which the process is incorporated into the operations of the hospital will determine the amount of control, and responsibility, the healthcare organization has for the marketing function. Even with an essentially outsourced marketing function, staff can be expected to spend substantial time interacting with marketing consultants.

The management of the marketing process requires the coordination from a number of different activities more or less carried out in a specified sequence. This includes establishing a planning team (and possibly identifying a champion), defining the product, identifying the target audience, specifying marketing objectives, and developing a marketing strategy. The next steps include developing the message and identifying the mechanism for delivering it. The marketing concept will be pretested and modified as appropriate prior to implementation of the marketing campaign.

The evaluation of the marketing initiative should be top of mind from the outset of the process and, in fact, should be built into the process itself. Evaluation techniques are of two types: process (or formative) analysis and outcome (or summative) analysis. Both have a role to play in the project, although outcome evaluation is particularly important for the marketing process.

Campaign effectiveness can be measured in a variety of ways, and any project will likely involve more than one means of evaluation. This is particularly the case in healthcare, where the intangible benefits of a marketing initiative are often as important as the tangible ones. Impact evaluation is an aspect of outcome evaluation that assesses whether the marketing campaign actually induced the desired change.

The planning process can involve a variety of personnel and departments, depending on the extent of outsourcing involved. Health professionals should become familiar with the agencies, marketing consulting firms, media suppliers, and the variety of other players in the marketing arena. Every marketing initiative will require interaction with at least some of these entities. If the healthcare organization seeks to internalize the marketing function, the functions performed by each of the parties must be considered.

The marketing budget is used to both set annual goals for marketing activities and guide the implementation of specific marketing initiatives. The budget should consider both direct and indirect costs as well as any hidden costs that the health professional may not anticipate. In health-care, the indirect costs could become significant, if personnel are pulled away from their core functions and the operation of the healthcare organization is disrupted.

Discussion Questions

*   Why is the careful planning of a marketing campaign considered so important?
*   What role may the marketing agency play in the development and implementation of the marketing plan?
*   In what ways should the client for a marketing campaign play an active role in the process?
*   What is a marketing *brief*, and why is it so important to the marketing process?
*   What are the component units usually found within a marketing department, and what functions do they serve?
*   What are the indirect costs that a marketing budget must take into consideration?
*   Why is strong marketing management probably more important in healthcare than in other industries?
*   Why is evaluation in healthcare somewhat different from that process in other industries?
*   Why is it important for marketers to use different types of evaluation in the assessment of a marketing project?
*   Why may different approaches to evaluation be used for different marketing techniques?
*   Why is measuring the return on investment from marketing more of a challenge in healthcare than it is in other industries?

Additional Resources

Kotler, P. 1999. *Marketing Management: Analysis, Planning, Implementation and Control.* Englewood Cliffs, NJ: Prentice Hall.

Kotler, P., E. L. Roberto, and N. Roberto. 1989. *Social Marketing: Strategies for Changing Public Behavior.* New York: The Free Press.

Weinreich, N. K. 2003. "Research in the Social Marketing Process." 2003. [Online article; retrieved 11/13/03.] http://www.social-marketing.com/process.html.

14

MARKETING RESEARCH IN HEALTHCARE

Virtually any marketing initiative will involve some marketing research. *Marketing research*, often used interchangeably with *market research*, encompasses market research, product research, pricing research, promotional research, and distribution research (Chartered Institute for Marketing 2001). The marketing-research process serves to identify the nature of the good or service, characteristics of consumers, size of the potential market, nature of competitors, and any number of other essential pieces to the marketing puzzle. While this chapter is not intended to enable the reader to become an accomplished marketing researcher, it should instill an understanding of the marketing-research process and an appreciation of the role of marketing research in healthcare.

The Scope of Marketing Research

The scope of healthcare marketing research today is extremely broad. Those who remember the fledgling attempts to introduce marketing research into healthcare two decades ago would be impressed with the breadth of activities now subjected to marketing research. Indeed, at one time an accomplished marketing researcher in healthcare only had to have some familiarity with demographic data and be able to conduct a patient satisfaction survey. Now, marketing researchers are confronted with an extensive array of tools and techniques for carrying out this process.

The scope of marketing research in healthcare understandably reflects the scope of marketing in the industry (Rynne 1995). As perceptions of marketing on the part of health professionals have expanded from the narrow (and rather naive) notion of advertising as marketing, the accepted scope of marketing research has expanded. Researchers are now asked to address issues considered beyond both their expertise and purview in the past (Gaus and Fraser 1996). Technologically driven innovations such as database marketing and the Internet have further expanded the options available to marketing researchers.

To provide a perspective for the scope of marketing research it may be noted that the content of marketing research may range from something as focused as, "How will consumers react if we raise our monthly fitness program fee from $25 to $40?" to such a diffuse question as, "What effect will the integrated delivery system planned by a competitor have on our market share?" Marketing research is expected to contribute to functions as broad as corporate-strategy development on one end of the spectrum and to functions as narrow as the measurement of patient satisfaction on the other. Some recent examples of marketing research drawn from the author's experience include the following:

- Determining the appropriate location for an urgent care center
- Identifying employer needs in the area of occupational medicine
- Determining if a particular market could support an oncology service
- Determining the level of demand among surgeons for robotic surgery equipment
- Measuring enrollee satisfaction with a managed care plan
- Identifying appropriate market niches for a small hospital in a highly competitive market
- Measuring the potential business for a national managed care corporation in a state
- Determining the types of services desired in a planned community-based clinic

This list provides some indication of the scope of marketing research now being undertaken in healthcare. There are few aspects of healthcare today, it seems, that cannot benefit from the application of marketing-research techniques. (Box 14.1 provides vignettes on healthcare marketing research initiatives.)

Healthcare marketing research also has been expanding in terms of its set of users. *Users* here refers to both the types of organizations conducting marketing research and the types of professionals within healthcare organizations using the results of marketing research. Marketing research has historically been limited to large hospitals, national health systems, and some for-profit healthcare entities (e.g., pharmaceutical companies). Only recently have organizations providing direct patient care become heavily involved in marketing research. Today, organizations from the home health agency to the urgent care center network to the national managed care organization require input from marketing research.

The following vignettes provide a sample of the types of marketing research activities undertaken in today's healthcare environment.

Identifying Unmet Healthcare Needs

A market researcher was engaged by a local health agency to help identify segments of the population that were affected by untreated health problems. The agency required this information for the development of its strategic plan. The market researcher collected census data and health-related statistics on the service area to identify potentially high-risk populations. Once target populations were identified, a consumer survey was conducted with households sampled from the target areas. The level of health problems among the sample was determined, along with the extent to which these problems were being treated. This information served as a basis for determining the existing level of unmet needs and an indication of the types of services that needed to be provided.

Evaluating a New Service

A hospital's behavioral health department wanted to explore the possibility of establishing an outpatient eating-disorders program. The market research department was asked to explore the market potential for such a program, as well as its feasibility in the target community. The market researchers identified the characteristics of individuals who were most likely to be affected by eating disorders and developed an estimate of the number of potential cases in the community. Because insurance coverage was lacking in many cases for this condition, the potential market's ability to pay had to be determined. Furthermore, the market penetration of existing competing programs had to be determined. The information on effective market potential and strength of competitors allowed a rational decision to be made on this new program.

Monitoring Changing Market Characteristics

A group of internal medicine specialists had developed a large Medicare practice. Over time, they noticed a trend toward a lower level of visits and the failure of some regular patients to return for care. A market researcher was engaged to assess the situation and found that, because of changing community characteristics, the elderly population was slowly but steadily relocating to a quieter, safer neighborhood some distance from the clinic. As the practice was still strong, there was no need to panic. The market researcher set up a mechanism for monitoring changes in the composition of the market area served by the practice. The researcher was able to keep the practice apprised of resident turnover and indicate, if appropriate, that the time had come to consider another practice location.

Conducting a Physician Supply-Demand Analysis

Hospital administrators were attracted to a growing suburb some distance from the hospital's downtown location. Although some physicians had located in the area to take advantage of the new market emerging, it was felt that adequate opportunity existed for the placement of a multispecialty clinic in the community. The market research department was asked to conduct a physician supply-demand analysis for the target area to determine what specialties should be included. The researchers began by developing an inventory of existing private practitioners in the target area, as well as any urgent care centers or other facilities that might be a factor in the competition for patients. The next step was to evaluate the resident population in terms of its need for physicians. Using a computer model for projecting demand for various services the researchers were able to determine the numbers and types of physicians this population required. The level of need was compared to the existing physician inventory to indicate the types of physicians that were overly abundant or in short supply. The results indicated the types of specialists likely to be the most successful at that location.

Predicting the Changing Demand for Inpatient Care

Hospital administrators were concerned about the shift away from inpatient care that was occurring in the community. The patient census had been steadily declining, and some nursing units had already been closed. While there definitely appeared to be a downward trend in admissions, the administrators wondered if this trend was short term or likely to continue into the future. The market research department first reviewed past utilization patterns to determine if the trend was a general one or if certain services or patient groups were more affected. Having found that the decline was across the board, the researchers conducted a demographic analysis of the hospital's historical market area. This analysis determined the size and characteristics of the future population in the service area. Given the stable population and the changing age structure of the market area, the researchers concluded that this decline was a long-term trend and that nothing in the analysis suggested optimism for future increases in inpatient admissions. With this knowledge, the hospital was able to shift gears and begin positioning itself to capture the outpatient care that was bound to increase in volume.

Source: Adapted from Berkowitz, E. N., L. G. Pol, and R. K. Thomas. 1997. *Health Care Market Research.* Burr Ridge, IL: Irwin Professional Publishing.

The variety of users of market data within healthcare organizations has expanded as well. The demand for market data has soared, and the requests are coming from all directions. Human resources departments need information on the future labor pool. Finance professionals need demand projections to forecast future revenue. The managed care department requires detailed data for negotiating contracts with employers. Each of the departments providing patient care needs to anticipate future volumes for planning purposes. The facilities planning staff need to know how to allocate floor space commensurate with future demand. The physician-relations staff need information for medical staff development purposes, and so on.

The scope of healthcare marketing research has also expanded in terms of its degree of involvement in the strategic issues facing the organization. Gone are the days when marketing research focused primarily on the measurement of corporate image or response to advertising campaigns. As the level of input of marketing has increased, so has the salience of marketing research (see, for example, Seltman 1994). Issues now under consideration at any major healthcare system may include human resources analyses, managed care assessments, evaluation of facilities for acquisition, assessment of the impact of competitor activities, or justification of the organization's tax-exempt status. The potential involvement of the organization's marketing researchers appears to be limited only by the sphere of involvement of the organization.

The scope of marketing research has also broadened in terms of the target for the research. At one time marketing researchers' primary targets were patients and perhaps the general public. The focal point for marketing research today has expanded from patients to consumers to employees to medical staff to employers, and so on. It seems few populations do not have some relevance for marketing research.

Marketing research in healthcare has also expanded in terms of the techniques used. The reader will recognize some of the standard marketing research techniques used in other industries, although they have likely been tailored for use in healthcare. After all, healthcare is different, and the field requires a unique set of marketing research skills. New research techniques are continuously being developed, and old techniques are being adapted for new circumstances. Existing tools like desktop marketing systems are being enhanced in keeping with changing demands and new technology. The simple mapping of health-related phenomena has become transformed into sophisticated spatial-analysis techniques through the availability of advanced geographic information systems. The research capabilities offered by the Internet have further expanded the resources available to the market researcher.

Marketing research in healthcare has also expanded in terms of its participants. Perhaps more so than other industries, healthcare is demanding a multidisciplinary approach to market analysis. While most market analysts have an understanding of survey research, the qualitative techniques gaining popularity often require skills that are less common. As marketing research broadens its scope, need will increase for individuals with training in sociology, anthropology, demography, epidemiology, organizational development, and other disciplines.

Marketing Research and Healthcare Decision Making

Perhaps the most important development related to marketing research in healthcare has been the increasing contribution of research to the decision-making process. Healthcare has become increasingly market driven, and data generated through market research drive marketing. The days when the characteristics of the market could be ignored are long gone in healthcare. Increasingly, healthcare goods and services are offered in direct response to the identified needs of the market.

The nature of today's healthcare environment calls for a more aggressive approach when it comes to market research. The marketer must be constantly alert to the emergence of a new market opportunity or threat *before* it has been officially recognized as a problem. In addition, the analyst must have monitoring capabilities in place that will flag any out-of-range statistic and alert him or her to a possible market opportunity or threat. For example, if a marketing researcher maintains a database on physicians within the market area, he should be one of the firsts to spot an area in which a shortage of certain types of physician manpower has occurred. Such market audits have become essential to decision makers.

Marketing research is becoming increasingly important also because U.S. consumers—including healthcare consumers—have become increasingly diverse. Once the consumer came to be recognized as a key player, the diverse nature of consumers had to be examined. Despite past predictions of growing homogeneity, Americans have become more racially and ethnically diverse, maintained and enhanced regional differences, and adopted such a variety of lifestyles as to daunt any marketer (Pol and Thomas 2001). This growing diversity has served to change the characteristics of the U.S. healthcare consumer and resulted in a loss of the predictability that characterized much health behavior of the past.

In many segments of healthcare today the market pie is no longer growing. A good example is the slumping demand for inpatient care. Success, therefore, will rely less on new customers than on existing ones. This situation means that healthcare organizations making decisions about the market will have to know more about their existing customers than ever before.

Other factors also make market data an essential fixture in healthcare decision making. A poorly sited facility, mistimed marketing initiative, overlooked key niche market, or misdirected product development can all incur tremendous costs. The costs involved in building and outfitting a clinic, mounting a marketing campaign, and developing a product are growing, and losses associated with one bad decision may require ten good decisions to offset.

Perhaps more important in an environment of increasingly scarce resources are the opportunity costs of a wrong decision. Siting a clinic in one place means other, potentially more favorable sites were not selected. Money spent on one promotion cannot be spent on another, perhaps more appropriate one. Product development resources spent on one service could have been spent on one with more potential. Overlooking a critical niche may mean that a competitor has outpositioned the organization in the market.

Decision making in healthcare must increasingly rely on accurate, timely, detailed, and complete data. Market data must supplement the knowledge base of the decision maker, which is acquired through experience and intuition. Marketing research should be a complement to rather than a substitute for a manager's direct contact with the marketplace. Increasingly, market analysts are working closely with the decision maker in the generation of the appropriate knowledge base for the process.

Finally, marketing research should drive marketing strategy. As discussed in Chapter 11, marketing initiatives should not exist in a vacuum, but should support an overarching marketing strategy that in turn supports the organization's long-range plans. This strategy should be driven by the marketing research the organization has undertaken. If, for example, research indicates that the organization is actually a niche player (and furthermore, the public sees the organization in this light), the marketing strategy should capitalize on this positioning.

Steps in the Marketing-Research Process

Marketing research can take a variety of forms and is not always a formal, expensive process. Any type of information gathering on the marketplace constitutes marketing research. Although the focus here is on the formal aspects of market research, more less-formal approaches, such as observation and mystery shoppers, have a role in healthcare marketing research (see Box 14.4).

Much of the time and effort involved in marketing can be attributed to the research activities that lead up to and support the marketing function. The type and amount of research undertaken during the marketing process are dictated by a number of factors, including the kind of marketing initiative being formulated, the nature of the organization, the available resources, and the intended use of the findings. A critical skill for the marketer is the ability to determine the type and scope of research appropriate for a particular marketing initiative.

In an ideal world, the research necessary to support marketing would be an ongoing function within the organization. It is not practical to initiate discrete research projects from scratch to support every marketing initiative. By the time most organizations can mount a data-collection process, the marketing campaign period is likely to be over. With ongoing monitoring systems in place it is possible to track changes in physician referral patterns, trends in admissions, or emerging market niches, for example. Because of the various aspects of marketing that could come into play, this chapter can only serve as an introduction to the research activities that support marketing.

The marketing-research process can be conceptualized as a multistage endeavor. The exact number of stages varies from marketing analyst to marketing analyst and from problem to problem, but all research designs include certain basic elements. The process leads from the initial inquiry (e.g., Is the management of eating disorders a service worth pursuing?) to the ultimate decision made by the organization (e.g., A pilot eating-disorders program should be initiated). No two experts agree completely on the steps involved in the research process, and research that supports health services marketing has unique characteristics that distinguish it from the process in other industries. The steps below represent the general order of activities in the research plan, although there is nothing sacred about the order in which they occur. The steps in the design process sometimes interact and often occur simultaneously. These steps should be modified as appropriate to suit the particular marketing exercise.

Identifying Issues

Issue definition is an important step in the marketing-research process. Unless the issues are properly defined, the information produced by the research process is unlikely to have much value. In marketing research the "problem" is likely to be defined in terms of a process or the specific issues related to a process. The scope of the research could be broad or narrow, depending on the issues that require research.

In marketing research the first step typically involves developing a generalized understanding of the community or organization for which marketing is occurring. A reasonable knowledge of the nature of the organization needs to be developed as well. For any marketing initiative, information on the product or service is required, as well as information on the market area.

A review of the existing literature is an obvious place to start the research process. *Literature* is used here in a broad sense. In traditional research, literature typically refers to the professional journals in which the field's conventional wisdom is codified. Unfortunately, health services marketing has yet to develop a body of professional-journal resources comparable to that of other fields. The literature for health services marketing will include not only standard journals but also newsletters, government reports, technical papers, professional meeting presentations, annual reports, and the publications of professional associations. (The American Marketing Association, for example, sponsors an online special interest group devoted to healthcare marketing.)

Today, marketers can gain access to the Internet for literature reviews and other sources of relevant information. Most bibliographical databases can be accessed through the Internet, and any number of other sources—some quite serendipitous—can be uncovered by accessing the World Wide Web. Another type of electronic literature review involves the growing volume of e-mail exchanges among the informal network of health professionals. An increasing amount of health-related data are becoming available via the World Wide Web, which is becoming a standard research tool.

Marketing initiatives are typically triggered by some event or situation, and isolating the relevant issues becomes an important early task in the research process. Triggering events could include the introduction of a new service, a move on the part of a competitor, or the identification of a new market for an existing service. A more precise statement of the issues may imply a very different research problem from the concern that originally initiated the process.

During this step the researcher will probably want to state some assumptions that will drive the marketing-research process. Do any audiences have priority? Are any issues or questions off limits? What time constraints are involved? Assumptions should be stated early in the process so that researchers will have guidance in research design.

Research Objectives

Once the problems have been identified, the research objectives should be determined. The type of objectives will then determine the research design. This phase specifies what the researcher ultimately wants to get out of the process. What questions do we want answered? What body of knowledge do we want to establish through this process?

The approach used to address the research objectives is determined by the type of organization and marketing envisioned. In formulating the research design to support the marketing effort four general categories of research—exploratory, descriptive, causal, and predictive—should be considered based on the type of information required

The goal of *exploratory research* is discerning the general nature of the problem or opportunity under study along with the associated factors of importance. Exploratory research is characterized by a high degree of flexibility and usually relies heavily on literature reviews, small-scale surveys, informal interviews and discussions, and a subjective evaluation of the data. Exploratory designs are typically used for initial information gathering at the outset of a marketing initiative. The objective here is to gain insights into the marketing context and to gather information, even if anecdotal, that may inform further marketing research.

Descriptive research involves the development of a factual portrait of the various components of the community or organization being examined. Market profiles, community assessments, and resource inventories are examples of the products of descriptive research. Any source of information can be used in a descriptive study, although most studies of this nature rely heavily on secondary data sources and survey research. Carefully designed descriptive studies are the bread and butter of marketing research, and they provide the basis for any subsequent research. The bulk of the effort in marketing-oriented data collection is geared toward descriptive studies, with no pretense of explaining the "why" of any of the observed findings.

Causal (or inferential) research attempts to specify the nature of the functional relationship between two or more variables in the situation under study. For example, a study of the relationship between place of medical training and physician referral patterns would probably involve an analysis of cause-and-effect relationships. A study on the market response to a promotional campaign would seek to isolate and identify the ways in which increased advertising, for example, fostered an increase in outpatient visits. Causal-research designs typically infer relationships, as a direct causal relationship usually cannot be conclusively demonstrated.

Little of the marketing-oriented research conducted in healthcare in the past could be characterized as causal. Although causal research has contributed to an understanding of the motivation for consumer behavior in other industries, health services marketing has a long way to go to arrive at this level of sophistication.

Predictive research uses the findings of earlier types of research as a basis for forecasting future events and conditions. Predictive modeling has only recently been adopted by healthcare organizations. Health plans and managed care organizations, for example, can benefit immeasurably from being able to identify at-risk enrollees and predict (and hopefully influence) their future utilization of services.

Developing the Research Plan

As in any research process, a carefully thought-out research plan must be developed. The initial information-gathering stage should provide a guide to the types of data that will be required. The nature of the marketing initiative will dictate certain research requirements as well as the objectives of the research plan, and various action steps will specify the effort required. The categories of data to be considered, the means of collecting the relevant data, the indicators to be used, and the analytical techniques to be employed, among other attributes, are included in the research plan. The research plan specifies the sequence in which various research efforts are to be carried out, responsible party or (parties), resources required, and time frames involved. The plan should also specify the products expected from the research effort.

Because most marketing research is essentially descriptive, the analytical methods used may be fairly straightforward. Data analysis involves converting a series of observations, however obtained, into descriptive statements or conclusions about relationships of the phenomenon under study. The types of analyses that can be conducted depend on the nature of the sampling process, the measurement instrument, and the data-collection method. A variety of analytical approaches can be used for converting raw data into information that supports the marketing process. The healthcare marketer should probably be familiar with the techniques used in demographic analyses, methods developed by epidemiologists, and approaches to evaluation analysis.

Once the research plan has been developed, the marketer must estimate resource requirements, which involve time, money, and personnel. If the research is to be conducted in-house, resources can be broken down into direct expenses (e.g., to hire additional interviewers) and in-kind contributions such as staff time, office space, and supplies. Time refers to both the time needed to complete the project and the time commitment required of personnel. The financial requirement is the monetary representation of the personnel time, computer resources, and materials needed. In addition, the opportunity costs incurred by those participating in marketing-oriented research must be calculated to the extent possible. If an outside consultant or resource is to implement the process, the determination of costs must be calculated differently.

Project management tools like the *program evaluation review technique* (PERT) and the *critical path method* offer useful aids for estimating the resources needed for a project and for clarifying the marketing-and-control process. PERT involves dividing the total research project into its smallest component activities, determining the sequence in which these activities must be performed, giving a time estimate for each activity, and presenting a flowchart that allows a visual inspection of the overall process. The time estimates allow marketers to determine the critical path through the chart.

Data Collection

Data collection involves the actual process of acquiring the raw data that will be converted into the information needed for the marketing analysis. In considering the alternatives available for any project each approach must be evaluated in terms of its unique advantages and disadvantages. In using any approach the researcher must address and be cognizant of special concerns to ensure that the data collected will be reliable and valid.

The data-collection process can take a variety of forms, but it will typically involve both primary data collection and the use of secondary data. Secondary data are virtually always collected first because they are likely to be readily available without much additional expense. Primary research is likely to be used when certain types of data cannot be acquired through secondary research. For example, in collecting data to support marketing for a new health service, an analyst may (1) examine hospital records for information relating to past introductions of similar services (secondary data), (2) conduct a set of interviews to determine current consumer attitudes about the service (primary survey data), or (3) conduct a pilot study that measures consumer reception of the proposed service (primary experimental data).

Because an unlimited amount of data on an infinite number of topics can be collected, the marketer must ensure that any data collected are relevant to the issues at hand. In particular, care must be taken to ensure that the data collected are actionable. Some things may be interesting to know, but if they do not contribute to the process, they may not be necessary. Specifically, the marketer should list the questions that need to be answered by the end of the study and should structure the data-collection process accordingly. Furthermore, the potential use for any information to be collected should be determined in advance. (The use of secondary data in marketing research is discussed in Chapter 16.)

Analysis and Conclusions

The main objective in analyzing the data that have been collected is the generation of conclusions related to the marketing issues. The conclusions drawn will rely heavily on the analysis outlined in the research design. Properly chosen analytical techniques should generate useful findings and conclusions related to market share, utilization trends, or changing market characteristics. These conclusions should provide the basis for subsequent marketing activities. Some of them, in fact, become a part of the assumptions that have been stated and restated throughout this process.

The formulation of recommendations is a relatively new role for the researcher but one likely to grow in significance. Historically, marketing research was seen as a technical support function. The researcher's role was to turn over numbers to administrators, who would make the appropriate decision. As marketing issues have become more complex and research methods more sophisticated, marketers are increasingly asked to offer recommendations. Rather than providing the decision maker with three objectively compared options for review, the analyst is likely to be asked to indicate the best choice among the three given the results of the various analyses.

Presenting Marketing-Research Results

Marketing-research findings are virtually useless unless they can be presented in a fashion that allows decision makers to understand them and to take appropriate action. If the intended audience cannot benefit from the research findings, the effort has been wasted. Regardless of the quality of the research process and the accuracy and usefulness of the resulting data, the findings will not be used if they are not communicated effectively to the appropriate decision makers. Furthermore, many executives cannot easily ascertain the quality of a research design, questionnaire, or experiment. They can, however, easily recognize the quality of a report. Therefore, the report is often used as an indicator of the quality of the research itself. (Box 14.2 describes the use of geographic information systems in the presentation of marketing-research findings.)

Effectively communicating research findings to healthcare professionals is a particular challenge for healthcare market researchers. Written or oral reports may be presented to hospital administrators, physicians, financial analysts, venture capitalists, and a range of other professionals. These individuals and groups typically will be well-educated, highly positioned executives at the height of their careers and the top of their fields. Even if the audience is composed of only department heads, they will have a certain level of technical or managerial skill. On the other hand, few will have the technical background to understand some of the more arcane aspects of research methodology and statistical analysis. Each of these audiences holds different perspectives and biases.

Primary Data-Collection Methods

Virtually every marketing study requires the collection of primary data. There will always be situations in which the desired information is simply not available, particularly in an industry undergoing the rapid and dramatic changes that characterize healthcare today.

The major advantage of primary data is that the information is collected for the particular problem or issue under investigation, making the

<table>
<tr><td>

Box 14.2:
Using
Geographic
Information
Systems in
Analyzing and
Presenting
Marketing
Research

</td><td>

The use of geographic information systems (GIS) in marketing research has long been common in other industries. Few marketing studies in other industries would be complete without maps illustrating the distribution of markets, consumer segments, usage rates, and other essential data. Furthermore, the use of spatial-analysis techniques for developing sales territories and decision making is not uncommon in other industries.

</td></tr>
</table>

While mapping applications have been available to healthcare organizations for more than 20 years, most organizations have failed to incorporate mapping and spatial analysis into their operations to the extent found in other industries. Given the importance of the spatial dimension of many aspects of healthcare, the status of GIS in healthcare is surprising; the lack of buy in on the part of healthcare organizations is perhaps attributable to the recent development of marketing and planning functions and to the slow adoption of computer technology in healthcare overall.

Unlimited opportunities for the use of GIS exist in healthcare. In its most basic form, maps can be used to illustrate any number of health-related phenomena. Maps can be used to illustrate the distribution of resources (e.g., hospitals, physicians, urgent care centers), patterns of patient flow, demand for health services, market shares, and so forth. From a marketing perspective nothing depicts concentrations of potential customers better than a map.

Beyond mapping are unlimited opportunities for the application of spatial-analysis techniques by healthcare organizations involved in marketing research. GIS systems can be used to track trends in population growth and compositional change, determine drive time to various healthcare facilities, compare potential facility sites on several variables simultaneously, and monitor the progression of disease through the service area. Specialized applications like the accessibility analysis for managed care plans can also provide information for marketers.

As GIS software becomes more sophisticated but less expensive and easier to use, it is anticipated that healthcare marketers will begin to use mapping and spatial-analysis capabilities to a greater extent.

data more directly relevant and current than most secondary data. Another major advantage is that primary data collection allows the organization to maintain the proprietary nature of the information collected. Conducting primary research also gives the planner control over the types of information elicited, rather than having to rely on questions asked by another party with perhaps quite different intentions.

Primary data collection, however, has some disadvantages. The collection of primary data can entail significant costs and require an extended period to complete. The administration of primary research also requires some fairly sophisticated skills that may not be available within the organization.

When initiating primary research activities, the means of data collection must be determined. The "right" data-collection method depends on a number of factors, and there are many alternatives from which to choose (Creswell 1994). Several commonly used methods for collecting primary data are described below. (Box 14.3 compares quantitative and qualitative approaches to research.)

Observation

Observational research involves techniques in which the actions or attributes of those being studied are observed either by another individual or through a mechanical recording device such as a video camera. Information is not so much elicited from the subjects as it is observed. Data collection by means of observation is performed according to specified rules based on stated objectives.

Before observation can be used in marketing research three minimum conditions must be met. First, the data must be accessible via observation. Motivations, attitudes, opinions, and other internal conditions cannot be readily observed. On the other hand, behavior in a waiting room, for example, can be observed and recorded. Second, the behavior must be repetitive, frequent, or otherwise predictable. Third, an event must be of relatively short duration. Thus, we are usually restricted to observing activities that can be completed in a relatively short time span, such as clinic visits or segments of activities with a longer time span.

Observational methods are typically used in marketing research when data cannot be obtained through interviews or from secondary sources. This approach is particularly useful when a process is being analyzed. For example, a hospital may place a trained observer in its waiting area to observe the admitting process. Observers may track individual emergency patients from their initial encounter in the admitting area through their examination in the emergency room. Some organizations use a mystery shopper program (see Box 14.4) to improve the organization's ability to perform this type of observational research. By actually going through the admissions process, for example, these simulated patients may obtain more information about the process than any other method would yield.

Observational techniques are characterized as either participatory or nonparticipatory. In participatory observation the researcher becomes part of the group or activity being observed. Participant observation allows the observer to analyze the group, situation, or process as an insider. Also, because the observer becomes part of the group, the impact of the observation process on behavior hopefully is minimized. However, the partici-

For a number of years the importance in healthcare of quantitative data has eclipsed that of qualitative data. Researchers and managers became enamored with surveys in particular and the ability to apply statistical analyses. Because there was a substantial body of knowledge regarding survey research, it was relatively easy to conduct virtually any kind of study that involved interviewing patients, their families and friends, healthcare professionals, and physicians as well as other players in the healthcare arena. Some even argued against the use of qualitative data, claiming that such information was neither scientific nor rigorous.

Certainly, quantitative methods have their advantages. Survey data lend themselves to a wide range of statistical analysis, and the findings from quantitative analyses can be generalized to other populations. The presumed objectivity of survey research and the ease with which quantitative data can be collected and analyzed make this approach popular with marketing researchers. The process generates definitive results (at least within a known range of error) that can be used with confidence in decision making.

Recent years have seen something of a reaction against quantitative methods, and qualitative approaches have made a comeback. Some, particularly in marketing research, contend that survey research generates misleading results more often than not (Beckwith 2000). It has become common for healthcare providers to conduct focus groups and naturally occurring group interviews on a regular basis. In addition, observation techniques

pant observer typically cannot take notes or otherwise record the observations being made. Thus, the observer must rely on memory for the recording of observations at a later date. The greatest concern, of course, relates to the possibility of the observer's mere presence altering the behavior of those being observed.

Nonparticipant observation involves a situation in which the researcher is detached from the individuals, situations, or processes being observed. In some cases the observer may view the subjects from afar or, in more controlled environments, through the one-way mirror of an observation booth. The advantage of this approach is that the process typically does not affect the phenomena being observed, as the subjects do not know they are being observed.

Although observational data are useful in observing what people do, they cannot address *why* people behave the way they do. Thus, observational research must often be supplemented with personal interviews or some other form of data collection to determine the motivations underlying the observed behavior.

and content analyses are being used to supplement the quantitative approach. New software designed for the analysis of qualitative data has furthered these efforts.

The benefits of qualitative data are coming to be appreciated, and methodologies have been devised to facilitate the analysis and interpretation of qualitative data. Data collected through focus groups, in-depth interviews, and observation provide a richness of detail and a perspective that may not be generated through quantitative analysis. In situations where opinions, choices, and perceptions are involved qualitative data are de rigueur.

Admittedly, qualitative data have their limitations. They cannot be easily subjected to statistical analysis, nor can they be generalized to other populations. Their use is limited to the generation of general conclusions and as a basis for hypothesis development. In this sense they provide guidance for the development of quantitative-research initiatives.

Contemporary researchers recognize the value of both types of data, in particular focusing on situations in which the two should be collected simultaneously. Surveys are no longer just a set of closed-ended questions with boxes to check. Open-ended questions are used, and the answers are actually being analyzed. Even when qualitative and quantitative data are not gathered simultaneously, the value of one type over the other in answering important questions is being emphasized.

Reference: Beckwith, H. 2000. *The Invisible Touch.* New York: Warner Books.

In-Depth Interviews

In-depth (or one-on-one) interviews typically involve one respondent and one interviewer. The in-depth interview is of value when the respondent must be probed regarding his or her answers. Complicated questions, or those that do not lend themselves to simple dichotomous responses, often require personal interviews. The interview does not necessarily follow a defined set of questions asked in a predetermined order but probes and questions as necessary to elicit the required information.

In-depth interviews are sometimes referred to as *key informant interviews.* They typically last 30 to 45 minutes but can take several hours. The interviewer has latitude to ask ad hoc questions, follow up on responses that appear worthy of further exploration, and generally elicit the best information possible within this research framework.

In-depth interviews appear to be the most useful in situations in which more superficial data-collection techniques will not work, including those in which extensive probing is required; the subject matter is com-

<table>
<tr>
<td>

**Box 14.4:
Mystery
Shoppers in
Healthcare**

</td>
<td>

Other industries more accustomed to heated competition have long used *mystery shoppers* to collect market intelligence. Until recently the healthcare industry had limited interest in marketing in general and resisted aggressive methods of competitive analysis. However, as competition has become more acute in healthcare and the industry has become more consumer driven, methods like the mystery shopper have

</td>
</tr>
</table>

been adopted from other industries. While there is still resistance to blatant efforts at acquiring intelligence on competitors, aggressive approaches like the mystery shopper are being applied in a variety of ways.

The mystery shopper can take a variety of forms and can be used for collecting information on one's own organization as well as on competing organizations. In the case of healthcare the term *shopper* is probably not appropriate, and the shopper may take many forms. As a better understanding of an organization's processes and level of service has become mandatory, healthcare organizations have begun to use this approach by admitting pseudopatients to hospitals or mental institutions, sending would-be patients to the emergency room to observe operations, or arranging for potential "patients" to call a number advertised for the organization to monitor the type of responses telephone callers experience. These shoppers could be employees of the organization or, better, outside data collectors who have limited prior knowledge of the target organization.

plicated, confidential, or sensitive; or group influence (e.g., as in a focus group setting) may be a distraction.

Ostensibly, in-depth interviews can be conducted with anyone presumed to have knowledge of a particular topic. However, in healthcare in-depth interviews are usually carried out with key informants who possess a particular set of knowledge (e.g., technical innovators), have a broad perspective for the issues (e.g., hospital administrators), are in a position to be familiar with the perspectives of a large number of people (e.g., human resources managers), or are likely to hold influential opinions (e.g., hospital medical staff members).

It is difficult to imagine undertaking any marketing initiative within a healthcare organization without including in-depth interviews with key informants. One initial task is to identify the problems or opportunities being faced by an organization; in-depth interviews provide an excellent setting for this. In fact, such interviews are typically used as a basis for constructing the survey forms used in subsequent quantitative research.

Personal interviews have some limitations. This method requires skilled interviewers, and even then potential for bias on the part of inter-

Using this approach, healthcare organizations can develop an unprecedented level of appreciation for their own operations, the knowledge of their personnel, and the level of customer service provided. Data collected in this manner can be used to revise procedures, institute training programs, introduce policies and procedures, and even institute personnel changes.

More aggressive organizations may use mystery shoppers to collect information on their competitors. The same methods may be used to study the operations of a competitor, determine the volume of services being performed, or identify the sources of patients patronizing a competitor. This could involve a process as simple as walking the halls of a competing hospital on the pretense of visiting a patient, calling a competitor to quiz them on their services, or sitting in on patient education sessions offered by a competitor. It could involve masquerading as a couple investigating nursing home or assisted-living facilities for an aged parent.

This form of qualitative data collection is not likely to provide all of the hard data necessary for a thorough market analysis unless a systematic data-collection approach is undertaken. More often, mystery shoppers provide information that can serve as the basis for more formal data-collection activities in the future. While the use of mystery shoppers is not widespread among healthcare organizations, this method of data collection will likely become common as healthcare organizations become increasingly market driven.

viewers or misrepresentation on the part of respondents exists. There is also the danger of experts going off on a tangent; a physician respondent on a soapbox, for example, may be difficult to rein in.

Group Interviews

In recent years one of the most popular qualitative-research techniques in healthcare has been the group interview. Group interviews can be fairly structured, as in the case of focus groups, or more informal, as in the case of naturally occurring groups. *Focus groups* consist of a group of people assembled to discuss a particular topic of interest under the direction of a professional moderator. The objective is to have people express their feelings or views on a range of interests. *Naturally occurring groups* in healthcare may include all persons working the same shift in a particular department or the families and friends of patients admitted to a hospital.

Focus groups can be used for several purposes. For example, information from focus groups may be used in the construction of a survey instrument. A second frequent use of the focus group is in needs assessment. For example, a hospital may want to better understand the type of programs or services it could provide that would be valuable to referring physicians.

Focus groups are often used to test ideas for new programs or services. For example, an orthopedic medicine group may conduct focus groups among parents of youth between the ages of 6 and 18 to assess the feasibility of establishing a pediatric sports-medicine program.

Another valuable use of focus groups is in examining the underlying meaning of survey results. Often, in conducting a quantitative survey the organization examines the response and finds, for example, that 50 percent of the emergency room patients thought the service was unsatisfactory. A focus group among emergency room users may help reveal the reasons behind the quantitative findings.

The focus group method should never be used as the primary tool for marketing research. It does serve, however, to provide useful insights that can contribute to the formulation of issues and the development of subsequent research activities. As such, focus groups are a useful supplement to the other types of research employed.

Survey Research

Many, if not most, marketing projects will involve some survey research. Survey research takes three common forms: mail-out surveys, personal interviews, and telephone interviews. Computerized interviews and fax-based surveys are also becoming common.

While many healthcare organizations conduct survey research themselves, others may contract with an outside consultant. Survey data may also be obtained through participation in a syndicated survey or an omnibus survey. With the syndicated survey, a number of organizations share the cost of the research. While participants may have the option of supplying a few custom questions, for the most part all participating organizations will receive the same information. Omnibus surveys are ongoing (often panel) surveys the organization can buy into. The survey firm regularly asks questions of a panel of several thousand respondents, and the healthcare organization can submit questions to be asked of the pool of respondents. Each of the forms of survey research that an organization may undertake is described below.

Mail Surveys

Mail surveys are a common method of administering sample surveys. Mail surveys involve the development of a survey instrument, identification of an appropriate sample of respondents, and mailing of survey forms to the sample. Returned survey forms are analyzed according to predetermined analytical techniques.

Mail surveys have the advantage of being a relatively inexpensive way to collect data. Typically, costs involve the reproduction of the survey form and postage to send and return it. Mail surveys also provide anonymity to the respondent and eliminate potential interviewer bias. Mail is also an efficient way to contact individuals dispersed over a large geographic area. For this reason mail surveys are often used in healthcare to collect patient satisfaction data.

This data-collection method does have several disadvantages. Response rates to mail-out surveys are often low. The instruments are self-administered, leaving the items open to interpretation on the part of the respondent. Turnaround time may be lengthy, and the short time frames characterizing much healthcare marketing, for example, may preclude the use of this method.

Personal Interviews

A second method of surveying individuals involves personal (or face-to-face) interviews. An individual interview is a valuable way to collect data when the respondent must be probed regarding his or her answers. Complicated questions, or those that require explication on the part of the interviewer, can best be handled in a face-to-face situation. In contrast to the in-depth interview, these interviews are relatively short, involve a larger number of respondents, and require that those interviewed are representative of the population being studied. Personal interviews also require a lower level of interviewing skill and less substantive knowledge of the topic than in-depth interviews.

In marketing research the focus is often on specific audiences. For this reason on-site interviews are often conducted. The waiting rooms of clinics, emergency departments, and other healthcare facilities offer such an opportunity. This survey approach has become popular in recent years because it has the advantage of face-to-face interviewing without the expense of the door-to-door canvassing involved in community surveys.

Community surveys were once routinely conducted, but they are much less common today. With the community survey, a sample of households is selected, and an interviewer or a team of interviewers contacts individuals in their homes for the interviews. Today, the costs involved in community surveys have become nearly prohibitive. Furthermore, the perceived danger involved in sending interviewers into various neighborhoods has made many research organizations reluctant to use this approach. At the same time it is difficult to find respondents at home during much of the day, and potential respondents are increasingly reluctant to open their doors to strangers.

Another drawback is the potential for interviewer bias. Untrained interviewers may condition responses by their reactions to answers or by their mannerisms, or they may fail to accurately follow the wording of a survey. In terms of cost the personal interview is the most expensive survey approach. Trained interviewers are required, and all travel costs for interviewers must be considered in the budget.

Telephone Interviews

The third common survey technique involves the telephone interview. While there have been increasing complaints from consumers about the intrusive nature of telephone surveys, this methodology still offers many advantages. Telephone interviews represent a quick way to acquire information. Using multiple interviewers in a telephone interview bank, considerable data can be acquired in a short time frame. If the interviewers have some "hook," a high response rate can generally be obtained. Telephone interviewing allows for a reasonable degree of probing by the interviewer. On the other hand, while it is often difficult for a respondent to terminate a personal interview, terminating a telephone interview is easy.

Telephone interviews have an inherent sampling bias in that they require the respondent to have a telephone. While telephone ownership is high in the United States, certain areas or populations may have significantly lower telephone ownership than the national average. Low-income populations and racial and ethnic minority groups, in particular, have lower-than-average levels of telephone installation. Furthermore, cellular phones have replaced landline phones for many segments of the population.

Increasingly, people are requesting unlisted telephone numbers, making the phone directory, always a questionable sampling frame, even less useful. One method to address this problem uses computerized programs to perform a random-digit-dialing sequence, working from the prefixes used in an area and generating the last four digits randomly. Still another approach involves randomly selecting numbers listed in the phone directory or other directories and systematically adding or subtracting one from the last digit. (See Dillman 1978 for the definitive reference on the effective administration of mail and telephone surveys.)

Computer-assisted telephone interviewing has become increasingly common among survey researchers, and inexpensive software has made this technology available to most interviewers. A computer-assisted telephone interviewing system involves a survey workstation in which the telephone interviewer enters answers to survey items directly into the questionnaire programmed into the system. The responses are automatically entered into the computer and typically directly into the database to be used for analysis. The intelligence built into the software application can flag out-of-range answers, adjust subsequent questions based on earlier answers, and automatically lead the interviewer through a series of branching questions.

Computerized Interviews

Computer-based interviews have become increasingly popular as software has become more user friendly and the general public has become more comfortable with computers. In computerized interviewing the computer presents the survey items to the respondent on the screen in much the same form as it would take on a printed interview questionnaire.

Onsite computerized interviewing is being used in more and more healthcare settings. The most frequent use to date is for collecting patient satisfaction data. After a clinic visit, for example, a respondent may be asked to sit down at a computer station and fill out the questionnaire shown on the screen. The more user-friendly systems allow the user to touch the appropriate response on the screen. Others may instruct the interviewee to strike certain keys on a keyboard.

This onsite approach to data collection has the advantage of capturing the information when it is top of mind. It allows researchers to obtain responses from virtually every patient rather than relying on a sample. The provision of information is easy for the respondent, and the computer-assisted system often has the ability to modify itself during the course of the interview, edit the responses, and even perform analysis. Computerized interviewing saves time and resources and eliminates much of the paper involved in survey research. The results of the surveys can typically be obtained in hours, if not minutes.

The disadvantages of this approach are that the survey must be relatively short, survey items must be simple and completely clear, and patients must be willing to cooperate, especially if they suffer from computer phobia. There is always the fear that patients may resent being asked to go to this extra trouble, especially if they are not feeling well or have just paid a large fee. In addition, some analysts feel that patient satisfaction responses are not valid unless they have had some time to age; they would contend, for example, that surveys conducted two weeks after the visit are more valid than those conducted at the time of the visit.

It has become increasingly common to administer surveys through the use of facsimile machines. While this is not a particularly useful data-collection approach, it is proving to be a reasonably efficacious method for conducting surveys with certain target audiences. A faxed questionnaire seems to carry more significance with certain hard-to-reach groups of respondents than a mailed one. It is more likely to reach the respondent than a mail questionnaire or even a telephone call. Returning responses is also easier via fax than through the mail. Hard-to-reach respondent groups, such as physicians or employee benefits managers, seem to be particularly appropriate for this approach. Recent legal rulings may make the use of fax surveys less feasible.

Some researchers have begun to administer surveys via the Internet, and the growing level of Internet penetration among the general public has made this medium increasingly popular. Assuming that the target population is "wired," data collection via the Internet is convenient and inexpensive. To date, this approach has worked best in the case of an existing network of customers, an advisory board, or other groupings that may already be linked by e-mail rather than for general consumers. As penetration rates increase and consumers become more familiar with this data-collection approach, the use of the Internet for survey research will undoubtedly increase.

Summary

Marketing research encompasses market research, product research, pricing research, promotional research, and distribution research. As perceptions of marketing on the part of health professionals have expanded, the accepted scope of marketing research has expanded. The demand for market data has soared, and the requests are coming from an ever-growing variety of data users and, in an environment of increasingly scarce resources, so are the opportunity costs of a wrong decision.

Marketing research can take a variety of forms and is not always a formal, expensive process. Any type of information gathering on the marketplace constitutes marketing research. Research can be conceptualized as a multistage process. The exact number of stages varies from marketing analyst to marketing analyst and from problem to problem. The process leads from the initial concept to the ultimate decision made by the organization. The steps in the marketing-research process are similar to those in other industries, although certain modifications may be required for healthcare. The nature of the research plan will be a function of the research questions that have been formulated.

Most marketing research projects will require some primary research, and a number of techniques, each with its own advantages and disadvantages, can be used. Qualitative techniques include observation, interviews, and focus groups. Quantitative techniques emphasize mail surveys, with personal and telephone surveys being options. Computerized surveys are becoming increasingly common with improved technology and a more Internet-oriented population.

Discussion Questions

- What developments have made marketing research increasingly important in healthcare?
- In what ways has the scope of marketing research in healthcare broadened in recent years, and what accounts for the expanded scope?
- How can we explain the growing influence of marketing research on the decision-making process for health professionals?
- What are the relative advantages and disadvantages of primary research and secondary research?
- Why has most research in healthcare to date been descriptive in nature rather than causal or predictive?
- What are the relative merits of quantitative and qualitative research, and why are both important to marketing researchers in healthcare?
- How has contemporary technology served to improve the effectiveness of marketing research in healthcare?
- Why is it important to "triangulate" research findings when conducting marketing research in healthcare?
- What potential does the Internet carry as a research tool?

References

Chartered Institute for Marketing. 2001. Ilia Afanasieff's Marketing Encyclopedia. [Online material. Creation 06/11/01; retrieved 05/30/03.] http://www.nets.kz/ilia.nets.kz/marketing.html.

Creswell, J. W. 1994. *Research Design: Qualitative and Quantitative Approaches.* Thousand Oaks, CA: Sage.

Dillman, D. A. 1978. *Mail and Telephone Surveys: The Total Design.* New York: John Wiley & Sons.

Gaus, C. R., and I. Fraser. 1996. "Shifting Paradigms and the Role of Research." *Health Affairs* 15 (2): 234–42.

Pol, L. G., and R. K. Thomas. 2001. *The Demography of Health and Healthcare.* New York: Wolters Kluwer.

Rynne, T. 1995. *Healthcare Marketing in Transition.* Burr Ridge, IL: Irwin Professional Publishing.

Seltman, K. D. 1994. "Wanted: A Little Marketing." *Journal of Healthcare Marketing* 14 (2): 40–43.

Additional Resources

Aday, L. A. 1989. *Designing and Conducting Health Surveys*. San Francisco: Jossey-Bass.

Berkowitz, E. N., L. G. Pol, and R. K. Thomas. 1997. *Health Care Market Research*. Burr Ridge, IL: Irwin Professional Publishing.

MARKETING PLANNING

While marketing planning is well-established in other industries, it is a relatively new function in healthcare. Until the 1980s healthcare providers typically did not engage in formal marketing activities, thereby obviating the need for marketing plans. While some sectors of the industry, such as insurance, pharmaceuticals, and medical supplies, have a long history of marketing planning, organizations involved in patient care have only recently established marketing-planning functions. Growing numbers of hospitals, physician groups, and other organizations involved in direct patient care are now trying to develop marketing expertise. While most healthcare organizations have some level of marketing expertise today, marketing activity does not automatically translate into skills in marketing planning.

Marketing planning may be defined simply as the development of a systematic process for promoting an organization, product, or service. This straightforward definition masks the wide variety of activities and potential complexity that characterize marketing planning. Marketing planning can be limited to a short-term promotional project or comprise a component of a long-term strategic plan. It can focus alternatively on a product, service, program, or organization.

A marketing plan should be in place prior to any marketing effort—large or small—and the systematic implementation of a marketing initiative is not possible without benefit of a marketing plan. While this chapter will not turn the reader into a marketing planner, it should instill an appreciation of the importance of the marketing-planning process and the role of planning in the marketing endeavor. (For additional information on marketing plans see Hillestad and Berkowitz 1991 and Thomas 2003.)

The Nature of Marketing Planning

Purpose

Of the various types of planning that could be carried out by a healthcare organization, marketing planning is the most directly related to the customer. Marketing plans are, by definition, the most market driven and are single minded in their focus on the customer. The emphasis on promotion in the definition above assumes that the organization or service is being promoted to someone. Whether the targeted customer is the patient, referring physician, employer, health plan, or any number of other possibilities, the marketing plan is built around someone's needs. Although a consideration of internal factors is often pertinent (and internal marketing may be a component of many marketing plans), the marketing plan focuses on the characteristics of the external market with the objective of influencing change in one or more of these characteristics.

Relative to many other types of planning, marketing planning is narrow in focus and short term in duration. Although marketing plans geared toward changing the image of an organization are understandably broad, many marketing initiatives focus on a particular good or service. The intent of most marketing plans is to effect change in consumer knowledge and behavior. Thus, marketing effectiveness is measured in terms of changes in consumer awareness and attitudes or, more concretely, on the basis of changes in volume, sales, revenue, or market share.

While all planning activities should be time delimited, marketing plans are often obsessive in this regard. Clear target dates are virtually always included, as the content of marketing campaigns is often time sensitive. A marketing plan that calls for the establishment of consumer awareness prior to the opening of a new clinic does not allow much margin for error.

The approach to marketing planning varies depending on the focus of the project. A lot depends on whether the plan is generated for a new organization or service or for an existing one. In the former case the intent of the marketing plan would be to create awareness, generate initial business, and establish a customer base. These approaches to acquiring customers will be different from those used at a later stage to retain existing customers.

For an existing organization or service the intent may be to enhance or improve the organization's image. The objectives may include changing existing customer behavior, such as convincing customers to switch from a competitor or encouraging the customer to consume more services. Because information on existing customers is available, the approach here focuses on capitalizing on this knowledge to derive as much business as possible from existing clients. This knowledge can also be used to expand the customer base to new clients.

Although marketing planning is often seen as a stand-alone activity, it should fit within the context of the organization's overall strategic initiatives. Thus, the objectives of the marketing plan should correspond with those outlined in the strategic plan. A marketing plan should be an inherent component of any formal business plan as well. Even if established relationships exist with customers for an existing product, a marketing plan is required; a plan is even more important if new customers are being sought or new services are being introduced. Potential investors reviewing a business plan are not likely to give much credence to the business proposition in the absence of a marketing plan.

Levels of Planning

Marketing planning can take place at a variety of levels. At the "highest" level a plan could be developed for a facility or health system. Thus, a hospital attempting to brand itself may develop a master marketing plan to encompass virtually all aspects of the organization's marketing effort. Such a plan would be comprehensive in approach and broad in scope. Its time horizon may be relatively long in marketing terms (i.e., strategic), involving, say, a two- to five-year planning period. The objectives of this plan are likely to be both broad and specific, with efforts to make the brand a household term accompanied by such mundane tasks as reprinting the organization's letterhead.

Most marketing plans, however, are geared toward a "lower" level of operation. The typical marketing plan focuses on a particular service, program, or even event. A marketing plan developed to roll out a new service, office site, piece of equipment, or a promotional plan for a series of patient education seminars would be fairly narrow in scope and short term in duration (i.e., tactical). Similarly, a plan aimed at increasing patient volume or market share would have relatively narrow goals. The objectives would be more restrictive than those for a facilitywide plan and be measured in terms of consumer awareness of the new service, attendance at the patient education sessions, or increases in patient volume.

While the planning process is similar for both of these levels of planning, and those in between, the respective approaches have differences, which are noted as appropriate in the sections that follow.

The Marketing-Planning Process

Planning for Planning

A great deal of preparation is involved in the planning process; thus, planning for planning consumes much of the early effort. The first step in any planning process involves identifying the mandate under which the planners are to operate. A marketing campaign may be initiated for any number of reasons. It may be driven by the actions of competitors, some political motivation, some immediate financial consideration, or other factors. The "why" of the marketing initiative will likely color all subsequent activities and should be addressed early in the process.

Much early marketing-planning activity is organizational in nature and involves identifying the key stakeholders, decision makers, and resource persons who must be taken into consideration. If the organization has an established marketing department, much of the initial work (e.g., background research) may have already been completed and the key players may be in place. However, in the case of a newly established marketing function or the marketing of an unfamiliar service, additional organizational effort will likely be required.

While there is no foolproof combination of team members that ensures success, certain categories of participants should be involved, including those who have familiarity with the service or product, the market, and the organization's distribution channels. During the research phase representatives of the target audience should be involved, whether these be patients, physicians, or employers.

The internal participants in the planning process should be drawn from a wide range of functional areas, starting with management. Certainly, the staff of the marketing department should play a key role and, if a research department exists, the efforts of the two should be combined. Depending on the issues, the finance; human resources; or other key departments, including clinical departments, may play a role. Furthermore, it is difficult to imagine an efficient planning process being carried out today without the full cooperation of the information systems department.

During this early stage the planning process that will be observed needs to be specified. The format for the process, objectives of the process (not the plan at this point), and such practical issues as frequency of planning team meetings should be considered. Importantly, the purpose of these meetings (e.g., work session, progress reporting, decision making) must be specified.

Stating Assumptions

There is often a tendency to rush into the development of a marketing plan without carefully considering the assumptions under which one is operating. However, the stating of assumptions at the outset and throughout the planning process is critical. An example involves assumptions about the type of image the organization wants to convey. There is a big difference between presenting the image of an aggressive, profit-seeking enterprise driven by hard-bitten business principles and the image of a humble, community-based organization intent on serving the needs of the population.

Assumptions should be stated with regard to the potential consequences of the marketing initiative. In today's reimbursement environment, for example, a healthcare provider does not want to attract all potential consumers for a good or service. The organization wants to attract those who can be reasonably expected to pay. At the same time it should not appear that the provider is deliberately excluding certain classes of patients.

The nature of the assumptions made at the outset reflect the extent to which a product or service is already in the market and has some level of awareness and utilization. In addition, the extent to which marketing activities are already underway will affect the assumptions under which the planner operates. Other assumptions may relate to the type of approach or appeal to be considered.

Initial Information Gathering

To the extent that a healthcare organization already has a marketing function in place it may be unnecessary to perform many of the tasks associated with initial information gathering. The marketing staff will typically have already examined most aspects of the environment as part of their ongoing market-research activities, and at most some updating of information on certain aspects of the environment will be necessary. In the case of a newly formed marketing department or the introduction of outside marketing resources a wide range of data-collection activities may be necessary.

The data-collection process begins by gathering general background information on the organization through a review of any materials that have been prepared on the organization and the particular good or service to be marketed. In addition to determining the attributes of the organization or its services that may not be adequate for marketing planning, the planner needs to determine the degree to which the organization or service is different from others and the extent of these differences.

In a large organization such as a hospital the marketing staff are not likely to be familiar with all services, especially those that have not been heavily marketed in the past. New services are frequently added by a hospital, and some existing services may be marketed for the first time. These situations will likely call for additional background-information gathering.

This initial information-gathering process should also reveal something about the history of the organization, service, or product being marketed. While planning is futuristic in outlook, the organization's future is likely to be inextricably intertwined with its past. Current relationships take the form they do because of historical developments, and past experiences and relationships will color any future developments. The organization's life history will be instructive in developing a plan for its future, and the corporate culture will exert a strong influence on the marketing mind-set.

An early step typically involves inventorying marketing resources and determining the extent to which current marketing activities relate to the proposed project. Ongoing marketing activities are easily overlooked (especially if they are not labeled as such), but duplication of effort should be minimized. At the same time the possibility of marketing activities operating at cross purposes needs to be avoided.

As part of this process, potential barriers to the marketing initiative should be noted. Immutable patterns of behavior should be identified, particularly if internal marketing is to be involved. Supporters of services within the organization that may be considered in competition could become an issue. For example, the director of the emergency department may not react favorably to a marketing campaign meant to direct patients away from the emergency room to urgent care centers affiliated with the hospital. While some barriers can be surmounted, others may not be. These understandings become a part of the assumptions that drive the process.

It may be beneficial to obtain information on similar marketing initiatives in other markets, especially if the initiative involves a product, market, or approach with which the marketer has limited familiarity. The planner should be able to incorporate information about marketing approaches that have and have not worked when similar organizations or services were being marketed in other contexts.

As the planning process moves forward more formal data collection will likely be required. The extent of this data-collection effort will depend on the nature of the organization and type of marketing initiative. A national organization courting a mass market (e.g., a pharmaceutical company promoting an over-the-counter product) will probably perform an analysis involving substantial detail at the national level. On the other hand, a home health agency licensed to practice in a single county is not likely to need much detail with regard to national trends to develop a marketing plan. Depending on the nature of the initiative, the marketer is likely to review broad social trends, lifestyle trends, changes in consumer attitudes, health industry trends, and industry or product life-cycle information. The marketer may also consider regulatory, political, and legal developments along with technological developments. Regardless of the type of organization the question should be, "What environmental constraints are likely to affect this organization, and what can be found out about them?"

The Market Audit

Because of the nature of marketing planning, the planner must have an adequate understanding of many aspects of the organization. The development of a marketing plan requires an in-depth understanding of the organization's products and services and the manner in which customers are processed.

Detailed information on existing marketing activities is needed. Similar information will typically be required on competitors in the market area.

As a result the marketing-planning process will typically involve an audit of both internal and external factors. In performing the internal audit some or all of the following aspects of the organization would be of interest:

- *Services/products.* What are the services provided or products produced? What are the characteristics of these services and products?
- *Customer characteristics.* How many customers does the organization have, and what are their characteristics? What are the most pertinent demographic characteristics? Where do patients reside, and what is the "reach" of the organization? What is the case mix of current customers? What are the financial categories of the patient base?
- *Utilization patterns.* What volume of services and products is consumed by the organization's customers? How does this volume break down by service line or procedure?
- *Pricing structure.* How is pricing determined for the organization's services and products? How does this price structure compare with that of competitors and the industry average? How price sensitive are the goods and services offered?
- *Marketing arrangements.* What marketing programs are currently in place, and how is marketing structured? What type and level of resources are available for marketing? Are processes in place for internal marketing?
- *Locations.* To what extent are operations centralized or decentralized? How many satellite locations are operated, and how were these locations chosen? Are there markets not being served by existing outlets?
- *Referral relationships.* How are customers referred to the organization? To what extent are there formal referral relationships? How dependent is the organization on referrals?

Determining Strategies

The *strategy* refers to the generalized approach to be taken to the challenges of the market. Strategies set the tone for subsequent planning activities and in effect set the parameters within which the planner must operate. Ideally, the strategy employed for a marketing initiative will support the organization's mission statement and reflect the strategies embodied in the organization's strategic plan. Thus, if the organization's strategy involves positioning itself as the "caring" organization, marketing initiatives should support this approach.

The marketing-planning process should be guided by strategic considerations. Organizational strategies set the tone for marketing activities and set the parameters within which the marketer must operate. The strategy could, for example, be framed in terms of an educational initiative, a public relations rather than an advertising approach, a soft-sell versus a hard-sell approach, and so forth. It should reflect strategies established for the organization. Of course, on some occasions a particular marketing situation may call for a departure from the established approach.

Setting Goals

A *goal* represents the generalized accomplishments the organization would like to achieve through the marketing plan. The goal or goals established for the marketing plan should reflect the information generated by means of the background research and be in keeping with the organization's mission statement. The goal of the marketing plan will be broad in scope and limited in detail. It should be stated in a form such as, "To establish Hospital X as the top-of-mind facility in this market area." Alternatively, for a service-oriented initiative the marketing plan's goal may read, "To dominate the market niche for occupational medicine in this market area."

Marketers entering healthcare from other industries will likely be surprised with the diffuse nature of goals in healthcare (see Box 15.1). For many marketers the only possible goal is improvement in the bottom line; they cannot fathom that any initiative would not have this goal as its primary aim. This is clearly not the situation for many healthcare marketing initiatives.

Setting Objectives

Having established a goal for the marketing initiative, the next step involves the formulation of objectives to support the attainment of that goal. *Objectives* refers to the specific mechanisms for accomplishing marketing goals. While goals are general statements, objectives are specific. Objectives should be clearly and concisely stated. Any concepts must be operationalizable and measurable. Objectives must also be time bound, with clear deadlines established for their accomplishment. Furthermore, objectives must be amenable to evaluation, a particularly critical consideration because the success of the marketing plan will typically be measured in terms of the extent to which objectives have been achieved.

For every goal a number of objectives may be specified, as action will likely be required on a number of different fronts to reach the specified goal. Marketing objectives are stated in such terms as, "The proportion of the general population for whom Hospital X is top of mind will be increased from 10 percent to 25 percent within six months" (in support of the stated goal of making Hospital X top of mind in the community).

**Box 15.1:
The Diffuse
Goals of
Healthcare
Marketing**

We are constantly reminded that healthcare is different from other industries, particularly when marketing is considered. The mission of the healthcare organization is likely to be quite different from that of organizations in other industries undertaking marketing-planning activities. The mission may emphasize the charity or service orientation of the organization rather than a bottom-line concern with profits. The mission will also likely be more diffuse than that for organizations in other industries. A mission of "improving the health status of the community" is a lot different than the bottom-line-oriented missions of most corporations in other industries.

The objectives of the healthcare organization are also likely to be much more diverse that those of its counterparts in other industries. The hospital, with its myriad functions and interests, is the epitome of the multipurpose organization. A marketing plan for an organization this complex must be able to consider a wide range of perspectives, especially when few of these components were established with an eye to the bottom line.

The constituencies of healthcare organizations are typically quite different from those of other industries. Although a growing number of healthcare organizations must be accountable to stockholders, most are more directly accountable to other types of constituencies. A public hospital may have to cater to politicians, consumer interest groups, vested interests in the medical community, and other entities. A church-affiliated hospital not only has a board of directors to which it reports, but it may also be accountable to the denomination's leadership as well.

Healthcare organizations are also different in the sense that they are required in one way or another to provide comprehensive services. In other industries an unprofitable product line can simply be eliminated. Hospitals and some other healthcare organizations, however, may feel they cannot compete on equal terms unless their service offerings are comprehensive. A hospital's decision to drop an unprofitable obstetrics operation may have negative implications for other aspects of the organization. Indeed, state regulations may mandate the existence of the unit, and eliminating it may not be an option.

Any barriers to accomplishing the stated objectives of the organization should be identified and assessed at this point. Barriers to marketing objectives could arise for a variety of reasons, some of which (e.g., lack of resources or talent) may be common for any type of plan. Ethical or legal considerations may be associated with some types of marketing, including situations in which advertising may be prohibited for certain health professionals. Issues of appropriateness and taste may also be a consideration. It may be found, for example, that the educational level of the target audience is a barrier to introducing a new high-tech procedure or that a new

The healthcare industry is still primarily not for profit in orientation. The main objective is to provide a service needed by the community or fill a gap in the organization's complement of services. If the marketing effort contributes to profitability, that is a plus. However, in no other industry would an organization knowingly enter into a business venture that has no prospect of being profitable.

This situation reflects, among other things, the intangible aspects in the provision of health services. In many cases the intent is not to make a profit on the specific business but to use a service line to support other aspects of the operation. Perhaps the best example involves the establishment of a network of urgent care clinics that will be marginally profitable at best, with the notion that 20 percent of the patients will be referred to the organization's specialists and 20 percent of these will end up being admitted to the organization's inpatient facility. The indirect benefits in this case are considered more important than any profits that would derive directly from the operation of the urgent care centers.

Healthcare marketers must appreciate this characteristic of the industry and adapt their marketing-planning approaches to the realities of the healthcare field. The notion of "bottom line" is simply different in healthcare than in other industries.

procedure is considered experimental by the public, thereby making potential patients apprehensive.

Prioritizing Objectives

The objectives specified to support the marketing goal are likely to address different dimensions of the initiative. While all of the objectives may be considered important or even essential, it may not be feasible to pursue all of them, or at least not all at the same time. Indeed, some objectives may potentially operate at cross purposes.

An example of a potential dilemma is a situation in which the project has multiple objectives in support of the establishment of a facility as the dominant provider in a specified market area. One objective may involve increasing top-of-mind awareness of the facility, whereas another may focus on increasing patient volume. While some overlap in the efforts directed at these two objectives will likely occur, the approach to making the facility a household word is likely to be different from one that emphasizes incentives for patients to try this new facility. If the resources are not available to pursue these two objectives simultaneously, it may be necessary to prioritize marketing efforts.

One approach that may be used for prioritizing the objectives of a marketing plan involves the traditional four Ps of marketing: product, price, place, and promotion (see Box 4.3 in Chapter 4). The decision could be made, for example, to focus on the product in the marketing initiative at the expense of price, place, and promotion. Thus, the objectives most directly related to promoting the characteristics of the product would be emphasized. Alternatively, it may be appropriate to capitalize on the price advantage of the product, thereby encouraging an emphasis on objectives focused on the pricing dimension.

One other consideration at this point is the possibility of unanticipated consequences resulting from the meeting of any of the objectives. Although it may appear tedious, specifying the likely consequences of carrying out each objective is important. This should involve a determination of both intended and unintended consequences. Too often, the positive aspects of the situation are examined in isolation from the negative consequences that result from the pursuit of the objective. These issues should be considered in the formulation of assumptions.

Specifying Actions

The next step in the marketing-planning process is the specification of the actions to be carried out. It is one thing to indicate what should be done; it is another to specify how it should be operationalized. For each of the objectives identified a set of actions must be specified. These actions take a wide range of forms, from ensuring that postage is available to support a direct-mail initiative to enlisting a celebrity spokesperson as a means of reaching an objective.

If the objective of a specialty practice is to raise the awareness of its new sports-medicine program, for example, a number of actions must be carried out, possibly including selecting an advertising agency, allocating funds for marketing, packaging the program, and aligning promotional referrers. Many of these actions imply a certain sequence, and at this point the original project plan may be further refined to specify the sequencing of the action steps.

The action steps developed for a marketing plan may be relatively standardized. Marketing initiatives are likely already underway, and this activity may be frequently carried out by the organization. A reasonable understanding of marketing resource requirements is likely to have been previously established, and parties may already have responsibilities that would be directed toward the planning initiative. Case Study 15.1 presents examples of goals, objectives, and activities.

Implementing the Marketing Plan

Planning is ultimately only an exercise, albeit a meaningful one. The payoff comes in the implementation of the plan. The planning process creates a road map that the marketer must use to get where he or she wants to go.

To a certain extent planning is talk, but implementation is action. Marketing planners have an advantage in that the handoff from planning to implementation is likely to be smoother than for other types of planning; indeed, the same parties will likely be involved in both functions.

To approach plan implementation systematically it is important to develop both a detailed marketing project plan and an implementation matrix. The *project plan* systematically depicts the various steps in the planning process and specifies the sequence they should follow. The project plan also indicates the relationships that exist between the various tasks and, importantly, the extent to which the completion of some tasks is a prerequisite for the accomplishment of others.

Project planning tools like Gantt charts help create a framework within which planners can work. Project management tools such as the program evaluation review technique (PERT) and the critical path method (mentioned in Chapter 14) are useful aids for estimating the resources needed for the project and clarifying the planning-and-control process. PERT involves dividing the total research project into its smallest component activities, identifying the sequence in which these activities must be done, assigning a time estimate for each activity, and presenting the activities on a flowchart to allow a visual inspection of the entire process. The time estimates allow marketers to determine the critical path through the chart. These tools can be readily accessed today using computer software packages.

The implementation matrix should list every action called for by the plan, breaking each action down into tasks if appropriate. For each action or task the responsible party should be identified, along with any secondary parties who should be involved. The matrix should indicate resource requirements (in terms of staff time, money, and other requirements). The start and end dates for this activity should be identified. Any prerequisites for accomplishing this task should be identified at the outset and factored into the project plan. Finally, some benchmark that allows the planning team to determine when the activity has been completed should probably be stated.

The resource requirements from the implementation matrix should be combined to determine total project resource requirements. Once identified, the extent of the requirements may have to be addressed in relation to available funds and any other fiscal constraints.

There are well-established techniques for implementing a marketing plan. The implementation plan can focus on a traditional media campaign with heavy advertising, or it may emphasize direct marketing. Perhaps internal marketing is the most efficacious approach to take, or the situation may call for business-to-business marketing. If a media approach is chosen, the type of media to be used becomes an issue for the implementation plan. The techniques used will be dictated by the nature of the marketing initiative.

The Evaluation Plan

As stated in Chapter 13, the evaluation of the marketing initiative should be considered on the first day of the process and built into the process. Evaluation should involve ongoing monitoring of the process, including noting benchmarks or milestones along the way. Evaluation is particularly important in marketing planning because the objectives of the marketing process are usually highly focused.

Process (or formative) analysis and outcome (or summative) analysis are two types of evaluation techniques. Both types have a role in the project, although outcome evaluation is particularly important for the marketing-planning process. Process evaluation should assess the efficiency of the marketing effort. For the outcome evaluation, changes in image or sales volume must be measured, with the success of the project calculated in relatively precise terms.

Increasingly, marketers are being asked to justify a marketing initiative in terms of return on investment. Not only does this require a carefully constructed marketing plan, but it also demands detailed record keeping with regard to both the expenditures and revenues associated with the marketing initiative. Some type of cost-benefit analysis should be conducted prior to the initiation of the project, and every effort should be made to track the benefits that accrue to the organization (in terms of visibility, perception, market share, volume, and revenue) as a result of the marketing effort. Case Study 15.2 presents a sample marketing plan that includes the above elements.

Summary

While marketing planning is well established in other industries, it is a relatively new function in healthcare. Most healthcare organizations have some level of marketing expertise today, but marketing activity does not automatically translate into skills in marketing planning. A marketing plan should be in place prior to any marketing effort large or small, and the systematic implementation of a marketing initiative is not possible without benefit of a marketing plan.

Relative to many other types of planning, marketing planning is narrow in focus and short term in duration. Although marketing plans geared toward changing the image of an organization are understandably broad, many marketing initiatives focus on a particular good or service. Marketing planning can take place at a variety of levels. At the "highest" level a plan can be developed for a facility or health system. The objectives of this plan are likely to be both broad and specific, with efforts to make the brand a household term accompanied by such mundane tasks as reprinting the organization's letterhead.

Most marketing plans, however, are geared toward a "lower" level of operation. The typical marketing plan focuses on a particular service, program, or even event. A marketing plan developed to roll out a new service, office site, or piece of equipment, or a promotional plan for a series of patient education seminars, is fairly narrow in scope and short term in duration (i.e., tactical).

The marketing-planning process involves certain steps that carry the planner from the initial framing of the issues to the ultimate implementation plan. The organization must establish goals and objectives and a strategy for accomplishing these ends. Objectives must be prioritized and the unintended consequences of meeting an objective must be considered. The action steps subsequent to formulating objectives should be laid out in an implementation plan. Project planning tools are often used. An evaluation plan should be built into the overall marketing plan.

Discussion Questions

- In what ways does marketing planning differ from other types of planning in which a healthcare organization may be involved?
- What determines the level within the organization at which planning should occur?
- Why is it important to lay out the assumptions underlying the plan on the front end?
- What are some of the types of data that are generated through the internal audit?
- Within the planning context, how does one distinguish between goals, objectives, and activities?
- Given that it may not be possible to pursue all possible objectives, what are some of the criteria that may be used to prioritize objectives?

References

Hillestad, S. G., and E. N. Berkowitz. 1991. *Health Care Marketing Plans.* Gaithersburg, MD: Aspen.

Thomas, R. K. 2003. *Health Services Planning, 2nd ed.* New York: Wolters Kluwer.

Additional Resources

Bashe, G., and N. Hicks. 2000. *Branding Health Services.* Gaithersburg, MD: Aspen.

Berkowitz, E. N. 1996. *Essentials of Health Care Marketing.* Gaithersburg, MD: Aspen.

Berkowitz, E. N., L. G. Pol, and R. K. Thomas. 1997. *Health Care Market Research.* Burr Ridge, IL: Irwin Professional Publishing.

Kotler, P., and G. Armstrong. 2000. *Marketing: An Introduction.* Englewood Cliffs, NJ: Prentice Hall.

Rogers, S. C., and R. H. Thompson, Jr. 1992. *The Medical Marketing Plan.* Burr Ridge, IL: Irwin Professional Publishing.

Rynne, T. J. 1995. *Healthcare Marketing in Transition.* Burr Ridge, IL: Irwin Professional Publishing.

Siegel, M., and M. Doner. 1998. *Marketing Public Health.* Gaithersburg, MD: Aspen.

Wayne, J. A. 1998. *Strategic Marketing of Your Long-Term Care Facility: A How-to Approach.* Springfield, IL: Charles C. Thomas Publishers.

SAMPLE GOALS, OBJECTIVES, AND ACTIVITIES

Southern Neuroscience Center (SNC) had completed a strategic planning process and set the goal of becoming recognized as the premier neurological specialty group in its region. A marketing plan was developed to support that goal. Sample components from the marketing plan follow.

Marketing Goal

The marketing goal was stated as, "To establish SNC as the premier neurological specialty center in the minds of consumers in its market area."

Marketing Objectives

1. Increase top-of-mind awareness of SNC from 40 percent of consumers to 60 percent of consumers within 12 months.
2. Improve patient satisfaction ratings for SNC patients from 80 percent excellent ratings to 90 percent excellent ratings within 12 months.
3. Increase the number of physicians regularly referring to SNC by 25 percent over the next 12 months.

Marketing Actions

For Objective 1:

- Develop an advertising campaign for local television.
- Increase SNC event sponsorship from two events per year to four events during the next 12 months.

- Distribute an SNC newsletter to all relevant members of the medical community.
- Establish an interactive web site featuring consumer-oriented information on neurology and neurosurgery.

MARKETING PLANNING FOR A NEW PROGRAM

S outhCoast Institute, a rehabilitation hospital with a historical focus on inpatient services, perceived an opportunity to expand its outpatient capabilities in response to various developments in its market. A shift toward outpatient services would require considerable reorientation on the part of the staff—away from an inpatient mind-set—along with the planning and implementation of a number of new services.

Among the options for new services was the development of an aquatherapy program to supplement the services SouthCoast was already providing to rehabilitation patients. An aquatherapy program would expand the capabilities of the existing program and make physical therapy available for a wider range of patients than had historically been served by the inpatient program. Given that Medicare and most commercial health plans provide reimbursement for aquatherapy services, the program was seen as a potential source of additional revenue for SouthCoast. An aquatherapy program would further serve to differentiate the organization from other providers of rehabilitation services. While aquatherapy services could be utilized by SouthCoast's hospitalized rehabilitation patients, the intent was to bolster the fledgling outpatient program and attract other clients who were not involved with the hospital's inpatient program.

Planning for Planning

The decision to explore the development of an aquatherapy program was one result of a major strategic planning initiative being carried out by SouthCoast. Many of the organizational issues had been addressed within the context of the ongoing strategic plan. A planning team was already in place, and a planning framework had been established. The aquatherapy initiative was incorporated as a component of the overall implementation plan. It remained for the rehabilitation staff to develop and implement a marketing plan to support the development of this new program.

Initial Information Gathering

The initial steps in the information-gathering process involved collecting background data on existing aquatherapy programs in other markets. Data were compiled on the types of procedures and services offered by most programs, types of patients typically served, reimbursement prospects, and so forth. A general notion of what was involved in operating an aquatherapy program was developed.

At the same time a preliminary internal information-gathering process was implemented. This focused on the potential for developing the program within the confines of the existing rehabilitation-therapy framework. The analysis examined the availability of personnel to provide aquatherapy services, the potential for training additional staff, existing equipment and additional equipment needs, and, perhaps most important, the attitude of the medical staff with regard to this proposed service.

The internal information-gathering process uncovered a certified aquatherapist on staff who could serve as the service line champion. In addition, a pair of physical therapy aides could support the aquatherapy program with minimal additional training. Although the hospital did not have an existing therapy pool, renovation plans for the rehabilitation facility included the construction of a therapy pool and a regulation-size exercise pool. Furthermore, the medical staff primarily involved in referring patients to SouthCoast were generally supportive, and in some cases enthusiastic, about the prospects of aquatherapy.

Baseline Data Collection

These positive initial findings set in motion the formal data-collection process. Data were collected on the market potential for this service within SouthCoast's market area. The number of potential customers turned out to be much greater than anticipated. Potential sources of referral were identified and subsequently interviewed concerning their interest. Local health plans were contacted to determine their willingness to reimburse for this service, and aquatherapy programs in other markets were contacted to obtain their input.

Several secondary target audiences were identified that, while contributing no major revenue streams, would increase utilization of the pools and perhaps contribute to some fixed costs. These secondary audiences included community groups, swim teams, social service programs, and even a commercial audience of water aerobics customers willing to pay out of pocket. SouthCoast employees were found to have an interest in using the pools as part of their employee fitness program.

A competitive analysis was conducted and determined that no medically supported aquatherapy program was being offered within the community. Options for interim use of existing area pools were explored, and a suitable temporary site was identified for piloting the program. Preliminary financial statements were prepared to provide an estimate of the potential profitability of the service.

When the potential barriers were evaluated, few if any were found to exist. The only barrier identified was a lack of knowledge about aquatherapy in the community (even among medical practitioners). No inherent resistance was identified from any segment of the community.

Developing the Plan

With these background data indicating significant potential for a successful and profitable service, the planning team set a goal of establishing SouthCoast's program as the premier aquatherapy program in the region. In terms of strategy the team decided that an approach that emphasized education and relationship building was appropriate; the intent was to stay away from aggressive advertising and flashy promotions.

In support of this goal the following objectives were established:

- Create and implement a comprehensive internal marketing program for aquatherapy within six months
- Directly contact all potential referrers outside the institute and its affiliates within six months
- Recruit and train a marketing/liaison person to work with the aquatherapy program on a full-time basis within six months
- Identify and contact within six months all community groups that might potentially benefit from the recreational pool or the aquatherapy pool
- Integrate aquatherapy services into the institute's sports medicine and occupational medicine programs within one year

With these objectives in mind a number of action steps were identified:

- Create promotional material for distribution to potential referral agents
- Set up meetings with relevant internal parties (including medical staff) to explain the program
- Identify an appropriate person to train for liaison with the community
- Identify any appropriate external targets for promotional and educational activities

The fact that the program was new and unique in the area guided the development of the marketing plan. The appropriate message to be delivered was formulated, and the means of spreading it were determined.

In keeping with the educational/relationship-building approach the marketing mix focused on low-key promotional activities and avoided high-profile media advertising. For internal marketing the plan included a newsletter, articles in other internal publications, flyers in SouthCoast employee-pay envelopes, posters, special information sessions for staff and referring physicians, and a videotape to explain the purpose of the program. For external audiences the plan called for a newsletter, press releases (and other media coverage as appropriate), print advertising (probably limited to the yellow pages), limited electronic media (for the grand opening), videotape, exhibits (e.g., at schools, health fairs), and public presentations (e.g., at support groups, medical societies, voluntary health associations).

An implementation plan was developed as part of the marketing plan to identify the resources needed, required financial commitment, responsible parties for the various tasks, and timelines for all activities. The SouthCoast program director was given primary responsibility for implementing the plan. The physical therapist with aquatherapy certification would assist the program director.

An evaluation procedure was put into place to assess the progress of the program. Because it was a start-up operation, it would be easy to track the volume of services used. The plan also called for a pretest and posttest to be administered to referral agents to determine the extent to which they were made aware of the program. Satisfaction surveys were to be developed for administration to patients and referrers. The extent to which the program generated secondary benefits in the community (e.g., with community groups, schools, swim clubs) would be tracked and periodically reported.

SOURCES OF MARKETING DATA

Healthcare marketers require a wide variety of data made for planning and implementing marketing activities. They may be called on to determine market shares, profile potential markets, or initiate direct-to-consumer campaigns, all of which require extensive experience and knowledge of various data sources. This chapter examines the sources of data available to healthcare marketers and describes means of accessing, interpreting, and applying these data. The growing importance of the Internet as a source of marketing information is also explored.

The Data Challenge

The healthcare marketer seeking data to support the marketing process is presented with something of a paradox. The healthcare industry generates a wealth of data, but large portions of this bounty are inaccessible to marketers. Unlike other industries, healthcare has never developed national clearinghouses for bringing industry data into a central repository. When data are available, they often suffer from a variety of deficiencies. Because health-related information is often internally generated by a private healthcare organization, potentially useful health data sets may be unpublished, proprietary, or difficult to access. More recently the enactment of the Health Insurance Portability and Accountability Act (HIPAA) has erected additional barriers to access to health data by marketers (see Box 16.1).

Healthcare's increasingly market-driven approach has led to increased demand for market data. Despite this, the healthcare industry still lags behind other industries in the collection and dissemination of market-related data. The local orientation and autonomous nature of many healthcare organizations have impeded data sharing. Increasingly, the healthcare marketer's ability to access, manipulate, and interpret these data means the difference between the success and failure of a marketing initiative.

The primary purpose of this chapter is to outline the categories of data required for various marketing initiatives, describe the ways in which

When HIPAA of 1996 was enacted, it was intended to clarify issues related to personal health information. In reality, it has served to cloud the issue. Although the medical privacy section was accepted in December 2000 and finalized on April 14, 2001, the debate over the ultimate implications of HIPAA for healthcare marketing continues.

The good news is that the majority of marketing activities in which healthcare providers participate are still allowable under the HIPAA provisions. The concept relates to the promotion of products or services by a *covered entity*—an organization (healthcare or otherwise) covered by the privacy provisions.

Naturally, healthcare providers, many of whom have begun HIPAA implementation in earnest, have been scrambling to fully understand the proposed changes and where these fit into current HIPAA-related efforts. The most recent changes to HIPAA cut a broad path through the various sections under the medical privacy portion of the federal regulation. According to officials at the Department of Health and Human Services (HHS), the initial marketing regulations satisfied no one because they were too complicated and ambiguous for both industry and consumer groups.

Covered entities expressed confusion over the Privacy Rule's distinction between healthcare communications that are excepted from the definition of marketing and those that are considered marketing but are permitted subject to the special conditions in Section 164.514(e). Questions have been raised concerning disease management communications, refill reminders, and general health-related educational and wellness promotional activities. Every healthcare provider or entity that communicates with its patients must address the following two issues.

First, what is the definition of marketing, and what kinds of communication are allowed without authorization by patients? The initial definition of marketing has hospitals and healthcare providers worried that they can no longer use the information in their patient records, classified as protected health information (PHI), to inform their patients about healthcare services or programs that may directly affect their health. However, it

data are generated, and indicate sites where data may be accessed. In view of the growing number of types and sources of health-related data, this chapter cannot present an exhaustive discussion of this topic. It should, however, direct the reader to the most important sources of data for health services marketing. While many of the information sources discussed in this chapter have been introduced in specific contexts earlier in the book, important characteristics of these sources—such as frequency of release, geographic specificity, and methodological limitations—are presented here.

appears that most of the types of communication healthcare organizations conduct with their patients are allowable under the current marketing exclusions.

Second, the fact that the maintenance and improvement of health is one of the key tenets of a relationship, between caregiver and patient must be considered. Within this trust relationship, providers should be able to send information to their patients about recommended screenings and immunizations, new procedures, treatments, and health-related seminars.

HHS officials ultimately conceded that when hospitals, physicians, and other care providers offer information to their patients to help maintain their health, they further and advance the goal of improved health. Patients expect their physicians, hospitals, or other direct treatment providers to share medical information for core activities essential to the provision of healthcare. The changes enacted would permit doctors, hospitals, pharmacists, and health plans to communicate freely with patients about individual treatment options and other health-related information.

HHS ultimately conceded that it does not want the marketing provisions to interfere with the relationship and dialog between healthcare providers and their clients. The proposed revised definition of marketing is, "to make a communication about a product or service to encourage recipients of the communication to purchase or use the product or service."

For now the biggest concern healthcare providers have concerning HIPAA and marketing is how the regulations will affect their ability to communicate with patients about programs and services that could improve their health and in what situations the use of PHI is permissible. The majority of communication programs healthcare entities are conducting today are *not* prohibited by the proposed changes to the HIPAA Privacy Rule and do not require prior authorization.

Source: Paddison, N. V. 2002. "Where Do We Go From Here?" *Marketing Health Services* 22 (3): 14–18.

A number of the data sets described here are not what most users would consider health data. However, much of what affects the healthcare industry does not result directly from health-related events. Marketers have always used demographic data, and the 1990s saw an increase in the demand for data thought in the past to be unrelated to healthcare, including data on such topics as employment, housing, and crime. Therefore, this discussion has been expanded to include data sets that reflect the more general environment affecting healthcare marketing activities.

Data Dimensions

The data being considered for use in marketing activities can be categorized along a number of dimensions. By categorizing data along these dimensions some organization is introduced into the data-management process. Some of the most important dimensions are addressed in the sections below.

Community Versus Organizational Data

The compilation of health data can be approached on two levels: community and organizational. The former involves the analysis of community-wide data, whether the community is a nation, state, county, or market area. Community-level data focus on top-of-the-organization statistics, as opposed to detailed internal data for organizations. The emphasis is more likely to be on overall patterns of health service delivery and dominant practice patterns rather than on the details of the operation of specific organizations. Thus, community-level data provide the marketer information on such phenomena as patient flow into and out of the service area, levels of overcapacity or undercapacity affecting the area's health facilities, and adequacy of various types of biomedical equipment within the service area.

At the organizational level, data analysis focuses on the characteristics and concerns of specific corporate entities such as hospitals, physician groups, and health plans. The emphasis is likely to be on the details of the organization's operation vis-à-vis the activities of competitors. The overall pattern of system operation is of interest only to the extent that it affects the particular organization. The specialty physician practice, for example, is primarily interested in the details of competing specialty practices (e.g., patient volume, market share, procedures performed) rather than more general data on the health service area.

Internal Versus External Data

Marketers require data on both the internal and external environments. While healthcare organizations have naturally turned first to internal information sources, data on the external environment have become increasingly important. Data related to the external environment are sometimes difficult to locate and access, but relative to internal data they are more available to the public. The healthcare marketer's ability to access, manipulate, and interpret external data sets is increasingly the difference between success and failure.

Internally generated data represent a ready source of information for marketers. Healthcare organizations routinely generate a large volume of data as a byproduct of their normal operations, including data related to patient characteristics, utilization patterns, referral streams, financial transactions, personnel, and other types of information that almost always have a demographic dimension. To the extent that these data can be extracted from internal data-management systems, they serve as a rich source of information on the organization and its operation.

Data on the internal characteristics of the organization typically include information on patient characteristics, utilization trends, staffing levels, and financial trends, among others. Internal data are usually compiled through an *internal audit,* which typically includes analysis of the organization's structure, processes, customers, and resources. The internal audit may compile data generated through standard reports produced by the organization's data-management systems (e.g., patient-activity reports), but additional "runs" are often required of the data systems to obtain the necessary data. Few data-management systems within healthcare organizations were set up with the generation of data for marketing in mind, and many are too inflexible to produce custom data sets. In these cases the internal audit will likely require some primary research. Financial data are an increasingly important aspect of internal data with which marketers must be familiar. Marketers must be aware of the profitability of various services provided by the organization, the pricing process, and the cost-benefit situation with regard to various marketing approaches.

Most of the data-collection effort on the part of healthcare marketers will be directed toward external data. As healthcare providers have become more market driven and the emphasis has shifted to externally oriented marketing activities, the interest in external data of all types has grown. Marketing activities must address the external environment in which they operate. They need to take into consideration national, state, and local trends in healthcare delivery, financing, and regulation. Marketers need to be aware of developments in the local market that will affect their initiatives. They particularly need to have an understanding of the characteristics of other healthcare organizations within the market area, especially their competitors.

Primary Versus Secondary Data

Another useful distinction is made between primary and secondary data. Primary data-collection activities involve the use of surveys, focus groups, observational methods, and other techniques for the stated purpose of obtaining information on a specific topic. Secondary data are those gathered for some purpose besides marketing research but nevertheless have value to marketers. Indeed, most of the data used in marketing research come from secondary sources.

Primary research requires a much more detailed treatment than can be afforded in this framework and is better addressed in a research methodology context. Also, primary research activities are usually focused narrowly on specific issues facing an organization at a particular time under certain conditions. While the value of primary research has become well established within healthcare, as evidenced by the growing number of patient satisfaction surveys and focus groups being conducted, these activities usually generate proprietary data unlikely to be disseminated outside the sponsoring organization. (This chapter focuses on secondary sources of data, whereas primary research is addressed in Chapter 14).

Geographic Level

Another dimension of health data that should be noted is the geographic dimension. Data are made available for a variety of different geographic units and for various levels of geography. Data may be collected for *administrative units,* or "official" entities set up for administrative purposes, including states, counties, municipalities, school districts, and other units defined for operational purposes. Much of the data available to marketers are collected for such administrative units. *Statistical units* are established primarily for data-collection purposes. The primary examples of these are the units established by the federal government for purposes of data collection during the decennial census. Thus, census regions, metropolitan statistical areas, census tracts, and census blocks are designated for essentially no other reason than data-collection purposes. These units are the basis for the compilation of most demographic data.

Functional units are established for carrying out some practical function and may be unrelated to administrative or statistical units. The best-known example is the ZIP code areas designated by the U.S. Postal Service; their primary function is to support efficient mail delivery on the part of the Postal Service. However, because they have become such a common unit for analyzing the spatial distribution of various phenomena, ZIP codes are frequently used as a geographic unit for marketing research. Another example of a functional unit is the Area of Dominant Influence established by the media to indicate the sphere of influence of radio, television, or other forms of media.

Healthcare marketers are likely to operate at different levels of geography, depending on the product being marketed and the type of organization involved. The Centers for Disease Control and Prevention (CDC), for example, may think in terms of national-level data and examine morbidity trends for the entire U.S. population. Similarly, a pharmaceutical company with a national market may also examine data at that level. A large specialty group will likely draw patients from a wide geographic area covering several counties; in this case the county is probably the best unit for data collection. A family practitioner in a solo practice is likely to serve a fairly circumscribed service area within a particular county. In this case the ZIP code may be the level at which data should be collected and analyzed.

The choice of geographic unit for analysis is important not only because of its implications for the service area under study but also because different types of data are available for different geographies. For many types of information the county may offer the most extensive range of data; generally, the smaller the unit of geography, the less extensive the data available. While use of ZIP code or census tract as the unit of geography may allow for more precise delineation of the service area, access to certain types of data becomes more limited. Thus, a trade-off will likely be involved between level of geography and the type of data available.

Temporal Dimension

One other dimension of data that needs to be taken into consideration by the marketer is the temporal dimension. Health professionals typically think in terms of current data—that is, data that relate to the present time frame or at least to the immediate past (e.g., the last set of lab tests). The nature of healthcare focuses the practitioner on the present, which is the reason for the interest in information management systems that can provide real-time access to data.

From a marketing perspective, current data are important but in some ways less important than future and even historical data. The value of current data rests with the data's ability to provide a baseline against which past and future figures can be compared. Marketing is future oriented, and effective marketing requires insights into likely future conditions affecting the healthcare environment. Because actual future data do not exist, efforts must be made to generate projections of future conditions relevant to the community or healthcare organization. Increasing emphasis is being placed on the production of projections by synthetic means of the future size and characteristics of populations and trends in health service demand and utilization.

Data-Generation Methods

The methods for marketing data generation discussed in this chapter are divided into five general categories: censuses, registration systems, vital statistics, surveys, and synthetically produced data. Censuses, registries, and surveys are the more traditional methods of generating data supportive of health marketing activities, although synthetically produced statistics such as population estimates and projections have become standard tools for most marketing analyses.

Censuses

A census of the population involves a complete count of the persons residing in a specific place at a specific time. The U.S. Census Bureau (within the Department of Commerce) conducts an enumeration of population and housing every ten years (the decennial census), and the 2000 enumeration was the 22nd decennial census.

Although a census theoretically includes a complete count of the population, it is increasingly difficult to strictly apply this term to the decennial census conducted in the United States. While the U.S. census ostensibly counts every resident, it falls short of a true census in two aspects. First, every decade a certain segment of the population is missed in the enumeration, resulting in some level of undercounting. While the undercount is typically less than 3 percent, its mere existence creates myriad problems.

Second, a large portion of the data on population and housing characteristics is obtained from a sample of the nation's households. Only a portion of the population and housing questions are asked of all U.S. households; the remainder are asked of approximately one of every six households. While the use of sampling significantly reduces the cost of conducting the census, it generates figures that some may incorrectly assume to represent complete counts.

The infrequent administration of the census is another source of problems. In a society where rapid change is common, collecting data at ten-year intervals has shortcomings. As time elapses after the census year, the usefulness of the data is diminished. Marketers typically require the most current data possible; even at the time of their release, census data have exceeded their shelf life. (The Census Bureau has instituted the American Community Survey [ACS], a national survey that involves a large sample of U.S. populations. The ACS is expected to eventually replace the decennial census and is discussed under the heading "Surveys.")

The census collects data on the number of persons residing in each living unit (i.e., house, duplex, apartment, or dormitory) and the characteristics of those individuals. Information is gathered on such characteristics as age, race, ethnicity, marital status, income, occupation, education, employment status, and industry of employment. The census also asks questions about the dwelling unit in which the respondent lives, including information on the type of dwelling unit (e.g., apartment, duplex), ownership status, value of owned house, monthly rent, age of dwelling unit, and a number of other housing characteristics.

Health-related items are noticeably absent from the census, as few have been mandated for collection through legislative action. Other government agencies, as discussed later, have a much more significant role in the collection of health-related data than does the Census Bureau.

The value of the census to marketers clearly rests with its demographic data. These data have direct application to the performance of market analyses and indirect applications as input into models for generating prevalence and demand estimates. Although the census is only conducted every ten years, the Census Bureau maintains the capacity for generating population estimates and projections on an ongoing basis. These figures may not be as detailed as some commercially produced ones (e.g., they are only calculated down to the county level), but they are broken down in terms of age, race, income, and other important variables. Census data may be accessed through a variety of sources. Many libraries are designated as depositories of U.S. government publications and maintain among their holdings most or all of the census reports in print, microfiche, or CD format.

A lesser known enumeration of business units, an *economic census,* is conducted every five years. The modern economic census was initiated in 1954 and is currently conducted in years ending in 2 and 7. The census covers businesses engaged in retail trade, wholesale trade, service activities, mineral industries, transportation, construction, manufacturing, and agriculture as well as government services. The information collected through the economic census includes data on sales, employment, and payroll along with other, more specialized data. These data are available for a variety of geographic units, including states, metropolitan areas, counties, and places with 2,500 or more residents.

While these data may appear unrelated to healthcare marketing, the economic census actually compiles extensive data on healthcare businesses. All businesses are assigned a code using the North American Industry Classification System (NAICS). Aggregated data on businesses within the NAICS categories that involve health-related activities (e.g., physician practices, pharmacies, medical laboratories) are available from this source. No other all-inclusive source indicates the number of hospitals, pharmacists, and chiropractors, for example, located in a particular area. As it does with the population and housing data, the Census Bureau is increasingly distributing data from the economic census in electronic form.

Registration Systems

A second method of data generation is represented by registration systems. A registration system involves the systematic compilation, recording, and reporting of a broad range of events, institutions, and individuals. The implied characteristics of a registry include the regular and timely recording of the phenomenon in question. Most of the registration systems relevant to this discussion are sponsored by some branch of government, although other types of registration systems are discussed as well.

The best-known registration activities in the United States are those related to *vital events* (i.e., births and deaths). However, other registries can prove valuable, especially when examining changes in the level and types of health services required by a population. These include registration systems supported by the CDC, Social Security Administration, Medicare, and the Centers for Medicare and Medicaid Services (CMS), among others. Statistics from these agencies are generally available, and many agencies are making efforts to provide actual raw data from their files.

Various agencies of state government also maintain registries, reflecting the fact that many health-related activities are regulated at the state level. The health department in each state is likely to maintain registries of various health conditions (e.g., cancer deaths), noteworthy public health problems (e.g., hazardous waste sites), and program participation (e.g., family planning counseling). In addition, the state health department or some other designated agency is responsible for maintaining registries of physicians and other healthcare personnel, hospitals and other health facilities, and categories of health information.

Commercial data vendors also maintain registries of various types, including registries of health personnel (often extending beyond clinical personnel to purchasing agents, chief information officers, and so on) and health facilities, from urgent care centers to ambulatory care centers to hospitals. In some cases vendors serve to supplement registries maintained by government agencies or professional associations. In others they may be developed to fill a void in the market.

A variation on registries that is finding increasing use in health-related research is the *administrative record*. Administrative record systems are not necessarily intended to be registries of all enrollees or members of an organization or group but rather a record of transactions involving these individuals. Thus, the list of all Medicare enrollees would constitute a registry, but the data generated by virtue of Medicare enrollees' encounters with the healthcare system would be under the heading of administrative record (as not all Medicare enrollees would use services during a given period). Data sets on Medicare activity made available by the federal government involve administrative records that are useful for a number of purposes. Some examples of useful registries are described below.

Health departments at the county (or county equivalent) level are charged with filing certificates for births and deaths and thus become the initial repositories of vital statistics data. These data are forwarded to the vital statistics registry within the respective state governments. The appropriate state agency compiles the data for use by the state and transmits the files to the National Center for Health Statistics (NCHS). NCHS has the responsibility of compiling and publishing vital statistics for the nation and its various political subdivisions (see Box 16.2).

The CDC has been involved in disease-surveillance activities since the establishment of the Communicable Disease Center in 1946. Surveillance activities now include programs in human reproduction, environmental health, chronic disease, risk reduction, occupational safety and health, and infectious diseases. These data are compiled into registries that serve as a basis for much of our epidemiological information.

Data registries constitute the main source of data on many categories of health personnel. Most health professionals must be registered with the state in which they practice. In addition, most belong to professional associations whose rosters become de facto registries. Like other registries, the registration of healthcare personnel involves the regular and timely recording of persons entering a given profession. Registries of health personnel—either government or professional—require constant updating, making them more prone to error than certain other types of registries.

Commercial data vendors maintain databases of physicians and other personnel, some of which are comparable to the more traditional databases maintained by professional organizations and government agencies. Data vendors may identify emerging professions or "marginal" practitioners that do not have an association base or are not tracked by the government. Other vendors repackage data from government organizations or association sources and resell the data in modified form.

The federal government is the major source of nationwide data on health facilities. The National Master Facility Inventory (NMFI), maintained by NCHS, is a comprehensive file of inpatient facilities. The institutions included in this data-collection effort are hospitals, nursing homes and related facilities, and other custodial or remedial care facilities. The NMFI is kept current by periodic additions of names and addresses of newly established facilities licensed by state boards and other agencies. Annual surveys are used to update information concerning existing facilities.

Arguably, the nation's most complete hospital registry is maintained by the American Hospital Association (AHA). Data are compiled annually on the availability of services, utilization patterns, financial information, hospital management, and personnel (AHA 2003). The database is continuously updated through an ongoing survey of the nation's hospitals. Some of the information is reprinted in secondary sources such as the *County and City Data Book* and *Health, United States*. Certain commercial data vendors have also established hospital databases. Solucient, one of the nation's largest health data vendors, produces an annual profile of hospitals based on its database.

Box 16.2: The National Center for Health Statistics

The National Center for Health Statistics (NCHS) is considered by many to be the Census Bureau of healthcare. As a division of the Centers for Disease Control and Prevention (CDC), NCHS performs a number of invaluable functions related to health and healthcare. For almost 40 years NCHS has carried out the tasks of data collection and analysis, data dissemination, and development of methodologies for research on health issues. NCHS also coordinates the various state centers for health statistics.

Part of NCHS's responsibilities include the compilation, analysis, and publication of vital statistics for the United States and each relevant subarea. This is a massive task, but the results of this work provide the basis for the calculation of fertility and mortality rates. These statistics in turn provide the basis for various population estimates and projections made by other organizations. The compilation and analysis of data on morbidity is another important function, and NCHS has been responsible for the development of much of the epidemiological data available on chronic disease and AIDS, for example.

In addition to the data compiled from various registration sources, NCHS is the foremost administrator of healthcare surveys in the nation. Its sample surveys are generally large-scale endeavors that fall into two categories: community- and facility-based surveys. Perhaps NCHS's most important survey is the National Health Interview Survey (NHIS), in which data are collected annually from approximately 49,000 households. The NHIS is the nation's primary source of data on the incidence or prevalence of health conditions, health status, number of injuries and disabilities characterizing the population, health services utilization, and a variety of other health-related topics. Other surveys that involve a sample from the community include the Medical Expenditure Panel Survey, the National Health and Nutrition Examination Survey, and the National Survey

Because most health facilities are licensed by the state, information is usually available from the state agency charged with that responsibility. Increasingly, local organizations such as marketing and regulatory agencies and business coalitions maintain facilities databases. For facilities other than hospitals some private data vendors have begun collecting and disseminating data. Vendors now sell data on health maintenance organizations, urgent care centers, freestanding surgery centers, and a variety of other types of facilities.

Surveys

Sample surveys are frequently used to supplement data from other sources. A sample survey involves the administration of a survey form or questionnaire to a segment of a systematically selected target population. The sam-

of Family Growth. Another survey, the National Maternal and Infant Health Survey, involves a sampling of certificates of birth, fetal death, and infant death.

One of the newer surveys has become the most important source of information on the increasingly important topic of ambulatory care. The National Ambulatory Medical Care Survey samples the patient records of 2,500 office-based physicians to obtain data on diagnosis, treatment, and medications prescribed, along with information on the characteristics of both physicians and patients. Important facility-based surveys include the National Hospital Discharge Survey and the National Nursing Home Survey.

The data collected through NCHS studies are disseminated in a variety of ways. Much of the information is disseminated as printed material. NCHS's publications include the annual *Health, United States* (the official government compendium of statistics on the nation's health) and *Vital and Health Statistics*. Data from NCHS surveys are also available in tape, diskette, and CD formats. NCHS sponsors conferences and workshops offering not only the findings of NCHS research but also training in its research methodologies. NCHS-generated data sets are being made increasingly available via the Internet.

From the perspective of a health data user NCHS can offer other resources. By contacting the appropriate NCHS division one can obtain detailed statistics, many unpublished, on all of the topics for which NCHS compiles data. NCHS staff are also available to help with methodological issues and provide that "one number" the health data analyst may require. In short, NCHS is a service-oriented agency that performs a number of invaluable functions for those who require data on health and healthcare. Much of the information required for the U.S. system to adapt to the changing healthcare environment, in fact, will be generated by NCHS.

Source: Thomas, R. K. 2003. *Health Services Planning, 2nd ed.* New York: Wolters Kluwer.

ple is designed so that the respondents are representative of the population being examined, allowing conclusions concerning the total population to be drawn based on the data collected from the sample.

The federal government is the major source of survey research data related to healthcare. Primarily through NCHS, the federal government maintains a number of ongoing surveys that deal with hospital utilization, ambulatory care utilization, nursing home and home health utilization, medical care expenditures, and other relevant topics. The National Institutes of Health and the CDC also conduct surveys, although more episodically, that generate data of interest to health demographers (see Box 16.3).

Some surveys conducted by professional associations and voluntary organizations should be noted as well. The American Medical Association regularly surveys its members, as does the AHA. Voluntary health associ-

The combined agencies of the federal government represent the nation's largest data-collection force. Led by the National Center for Health Statistics (NCHS), federal agencies conduct a variety of surveys on health-related issues. The following sections describe a sample of these federal survey activities that have particular relevance for healthcare marketing.

The National Health Interview Survey (NHIS) is an ongoing survey of the non-institutionalized civilian population in the United States. Each year a multistage probability sample of 49,000 households is interviewed. The data gathered are quite detailed and include demographic information on age, race, sex, marital status, occupation, and income. Information is compiled on physician visits, hospital stays, restricted-activity days, long-term activity limitations, health status, and chronic conditions.

The National Health and Nutrition Examination Survey (NHANES) is conducted by NCHS and the Centers for Disease Control and Prevention (CDC). This survey has been designed to collect information about the health and diet of people in the United States. NHANES is unique in that it combines a home interview with health tests performed in a mobile examination center. Tens of thousands of interviews are conducted annually, and examinations are performed on some 5,000 of the interviewees during a 12-month period. NHANES collects information on physical health status, dental health, and nutrition.

The National Hospital Discharge Survey (NHDS) is a continuous nationwide survey of inpatient utilization of short-stay hospitals. All hospitals with six or more beds reporting an average length of stay of fewer than 30 days are included in the sampling frame. A multistage probability sampling frame is used to select hospitals from the National Master Facility Inventory and discharge records from each hospital; the resulting sample has ranged from 192,000 to 235,000 discharge records. Information is collected on the demographic, clinical, and financial characteristics of patients discharged from short-stay hospitals.

The National Ambulatory Medical Care Survey (NAMCS) is a nationwide survey designed to provide information about the provision and utilization of ambulatory health services. The sampling frame is office visits made by ambulatory patients to physicians engaged in office practice. A sample of the records of these physicians for a randomly assigned one-week period is then examined; recent samples contained about 35,000 records. Data regarding the age, race, and sex of the patient are gathered, along with the reason for the visit, expected source(s) of payment, principal diagnosis, diagnostic services provided, and disposition of visit.

The National Nursing Home Survey (NNHS) is a periodically conducted national survey of nursing and related care homes and their residents, discharges, and staffs. Last administered in 1999, data are collected using a two-stage probability design. Once facilities are selected, residents and employees of each facility are sampled. Six separate questionnaires were used to gather data in the most recent survey. The first stage addresses characteristics of the facility and involves an interview with the administrator or a designee. The second stage focuses on cost data and is completed by the facility's accountant or bookkeeper. Information on the current and discharged residents is obtained by interviewing the staff member most familiar with the medical records of the residents. Additional resident data are gathered using telephone surveys of the residents' families. Full- and part-time employees, including nurses, complete a nursing staff questionnaire. This data set includes approximately 1,400 facilities, 5,100 discharges, 3,000 residents, and 14,000 staff records.

The National Home and Hospice Care Survey (NHHCS), last conducted in 2000, involves the collection of data from a sample of 1,200 home health agencies and hospices. Patient questionnaires are administered for the various agencies, and information on the demographic and health characteristics of the patients served by these agencies is collected.

The National Survey of Family Growth (NSFG), last administered in 1995, involves a survey of approximately 10,000 women ages 15 to 44. NSFG collects data on factors affecting birth and pregnancy rates, adoption, and maternal and infant health. Specific characteristics examined include sexual activity, contraception and sterilization practices, infertility, pregnancy loss, low birth weight, and use of medical care for family planning and infertility.

The Medical Expenditure Panel Survey (MEPS) was initiated in 1996 as a replacement for previous surveys focusing on expenditures for health services. Cosponsored by the Agency for Healthcare Research and Quality and NCHS, MEPS is designed to generate data on the types of health services Americans use, the frequency with which they use them, how much is paid for these services, and who pays for them. In addition, MEPS provides information on health insurance coverage.

The Behavioral Risk Factor Surveillance System (BRFSS), sponsored by the CDC, was initiated in 1995 to collect information on the health behavior and lifestyles of the U.S. population. More than 90,000 persons respond to the survey annually. The BRFSS includes data collection on such timely items as smoking, alcohol and drug use, seat beat use, and obesity, as well as other factors that might contribute to one's health risk profile.

In the area of behavioral health the Center for Mental Health Services conducts an annual survey of mental health organizations and general hospitals that provide mental health services. These surveys collect data on the characteristics of all providers of behavioral health services and on the characteristics of the patients served. Other related surveys include samples of patients admitted to various treatment programs.

The Current Population Survey (CPS) is the Census Bureau's mechanism for gathering detailed demographic data between the decennial censuses. Since 1960 the sample size has ranged from 33,500 to 65,500 households per year. Data are collected on many of the items included in the census of population and housing (e.g., age, race, education). Questions are included on some health issues and on fertility issues that have implications for healthcare. Of particular interest to the healthcare industry are the data on health insurance coverage for the U.S. population. These data were the basis for recent estimates of the size of the population that lacks health insurance.

This sample does not exhaust the list of government sources of data relevant to health services marketing. Publications of the federal National Technical Information Service provide a good starting point for finding other relevant databases, and of course NCHS's web site provides links to most of these surveys.

Source: Thomas, R. K. 2003. *Health Services Planning, 2nd ed.* New York: Wolters Kluwer.

ations like the American Cancer Society and the American Heart Association may commission surveys of consumers, patients, or physicians. Foundations may fund projects that involve the collection of data through primary research.

A few surveys sponsored by commercial data vendors also contain data useful for health services marketing. These organizations sponsor nationwide surveys every year or two that may include as many as 100,000 households. These surveys collect data on health status, health behavior, and healthcare preferences. Certain market research firms collect health-related data as part of their consumer surveys, and public opinion pollsters may also collect data on health and healthcare. Some of the data collected in this manner are considered proprietary and are generally not available except to clients. Other vendors make data available for purchase to the general public.

Synthetic Data

Synthetic data refer to figures generated in the absence of actual data through the use of statistical models. Synthetic data are created by merging existing demographic data with assumptions about population change to produce estimates, projections, and forecasts. These data are particularly valuable given the restrictions on census and survey activities because of budgeting and time considerations. Because of the large and growing demand for information for years in between the administration of the census, the production of synthetic data has become a major business. As no actual data are available for future points in time, any such data must be produced through synthetic means.

The demand for synthetic data is being met by both government agencies and commercial data vendors. Within the federal government, population estimates for states, metropolitan statistical areas, and counties are prepared each year as a joint effort of the Census Bureau and the state agency designated under the Federal-State Program for Local Population Estimates. The purpose of the program is to standardize data and procedures so that the highest-quality estimates can be generated.

A number of commercial data vendors have emerged in recent years to supplement the efforts of government agencies. Data generated by these vendors have the advantage of being available down to small units of geography (e.g., census block group), and they are often provided in greater detail (e.g., age and gender breakdowns) than government-produced figures. Such vendors also offer the flexibility to generate estimates and projections for custom geographies (e.g., market area) for which government statistics are not available. The drawback, of course, is that some precision is lost as one develops calculations for lower levels of geography and for population subgroups. However, the ease of accessibility and timeliness of these vendor-generated figures have made them a mainstay of healthcare marketers.

A major category of synthetic data involves estimates and projections of health services demand. Because few sources of actual data on the use of health services exist and projections of future demand are often required, a variety of approaches have been developed for synthetically generating demand estimates and projections. The general approach involves applying known utilization rates to a current or projected population figure. To the extent possible these figures are adjusted for, at a minimum, the age and sex composition of the target population. Utilization rates generated by NCHS are the basis for most such calculations.

Commercial data vendors have led the way in the development of demand estimates and projections. Some vendors have developed calculations for the full range of inpatient and outpatient services, although these are often available only to established customers. Other vendors can provide selected data on, for example, the demand for a particular service line.

Sources of Data for Healthcare Marketing

A variety of sources of data for healthcare marketers are available today, and the number continues to grow. The following sections group these sources into four main categories: government agencies, professional associations, private organizations, and commercial data vendors. The products available from these sources fall into two categories: (1) reports that summarize the data and (2) the actual data sets themselves. Although the sources presented in each section refer to the agencies and publications responsible for the specific data set being discussed, numerous compendia exist that marketers may find useful (see Box 16.4).

Government Agencies

Governments at all levels are involved in the generation, compilation, manipulation, and dissemination of health-related data. The federal government, through the decennial census and related activities, is the world's largest processor of demographic data. Other federal agencies are major managers of data for the related topics of fertility, morbidity, and mortality statistics.

A large share of the nation's health data are generated through NCHS, the CDC, the National Institutes for Health, and other organizations. The Bureau of Health Resources (Department of Health and Human Services) maintains a master file of much of the health data compiled by the federal government entitled the *Area Resource File.* Other federal sources outside health-related agencies, such as the Bureau of Labor Statistics (e.g., health occupations) and the Department of Agriculture (e.g., nutritional data), create databases of supporting data. The number and variety of databases generated by federal agencies are impressive, but the variety of agencies involved means that databases vary in coverage, content, format, cost, frequency, and accessibility.

State and local governments are also major sources of health-related data. In fact, a survey of health data users indicated that various state agencies were their primary source of data for marketing research (Thomas 1996). State governments generate a certain amount of demographic data, with each state having a state data center for demographic projections; vital statistics data can often be obtained in the most timely fashion at the state level. University data centers may also be involved in the processing of demographic data. Local governments may generate demographic data for use in various marketing functions. City or county governments may produce population projections, while county health departments are responsible for the collection and dissemination of vital statistics data.

Professional Associations

Various associations within the health industry represent another source of health-related data. Chief among these are the American Medical Association (and related medical specialty organizations) and the AHA. Other organizations of personnel (e.g., American Dental Association) and organizations (e.g., National Association for Home Care) maintain databases on their members and activities related to the organization's membership. These databases are typically developed for internal use, but they are increasingly being made available to outside parties.

A number of organizations formed in recent years focus specifically on health data, whereas others have established formal sections that deal with health data within their broader contexts. The National Association

Currently, no national clearinghouse for data on health and healthcare in the United States exists, making identifying and acquiring needed data a challenge for healthcare marketers. There are, however, a few compendia of health data that may prove useful for many purposes. While no one of these publications provides all of the data a marketer is likely to need, they offer a reasonable starting point. Not only do they compile specific data on certain topics, but they can also often direct the reader to the origin of the data and other useful resources.

The best-known compendium of health-related data is *Health, United States.* This work is published annually by the National Center for Health Statistics (NCHS) and includes data gathered from NCHS and many other sources. The publication includes data on health status, health behavior, health services utilization, healthcare resources, healthcare expenditures, and insurance coverage. These data are available mostly at the national level, although some state and regional data are available.

A companion publication, *Mental Health, United States,* is published less frequently than *Health, United States* but represents a source of data on behavioral health and facilities for the treatment of mental disorders. The statistics are based on data collected by the Center for Mental Health Services.

Another more specialized compendium is also published by the Centers for Medicare and Medicaid Services (CMS). Simply referred to as *Data Compendium* (with the publication year presented as part of the title), this book brings together data on Medicare and Medicaid. The data are drawn primarily from Health Care Financing Administration files, although data from sources outside the agency are also included. The information compiled by CMS is presented only at the national level, with some data reported at the state level. No data are presented for substate levels of geography.

Because demographic data are so important to healthcare marketers, it is worthwhile to mention some compendia that focus on this type of data. The *County and City Data Book* is published every two years by the Census Bureau and includes more than 200 separate items for each county and 134 items for each city of 25,000 or more persons. Data of interest to healthcare analysts include population statistics; vital records; hospital, physician, and nursing home statistics; and certain insurance data.

The *State and Metropolitan Area Data Book* is published by the Census Bureau every four years and contains 128 data items for each state, 298 variables for each metropolitan statistical area, and 87 variables for each metropolitan statistical area's central city. *County Business Patterns,* also prepared by the Census Bureau, provides a comprehensive count of the various healthcare businesses operating in each U.S. county.

The *Statistical Abstract of the United States* is published every year by the Census Bureau. The abstract contains detailed data for the nation as a whole for 31 different subject categories (e.g., vital statistics, nutrition) as well as data for states and metropolitan areas. Most states publish a statistical abstract that includes comparable data for that state and its counties and cities.

of Health Data Organizations, for example, brings together disparate parties from the public and private sectors who have an interest in health data. The National Association of County and City Health Officers has become active in terms of access to health data for local marketing purposes. The Health Information and Management Systems Society is one of the largest organizations addressing this issue as a collateral consideration to data-management systems issues.

In recent years many professional associations have made an increasing amount of information on their members available to the research and business communities. Not only do such organizations have an interest in exchanging information with related groups, but they have also recognized the revenue-generation potential of such databases. Some of these databases include only basic information, whereas others offer a wealth of detail.

Private Organizations

Many private organizations (mostly not for profit) collect and disseminate health-related data. Voluntary healthcare associations often compile, repackage, and disseminate such data. The American Cancer Society, for example, distributes morbidity and mortality data as they relate to its areas of interest. Some of these organizations may commission special studies on fertility or related issues and subsequently publish this information.

Many organizations repackage data collected elsewhere (e.g., from the Census Bureau or NCHS) and present them within a specialized context. The Population Reference Bureau—a private, not-for-profit organization—distributes population statistics in various forms, for example. Some, like the American Association of Retired Persons, not only compile and disseminate secondary data but are also actively involved in primary data collection as well as the sponsorship of numerous studies that include some form of data collection.

Commercial Data Vendors

Commercial data vendors represent a fourth category of sources of health-related databases. These organizations have emerged to fill perceived gaps in the availability of various categories of health data and include commercial data vendors that establish and maintain their own proprietary databases, as well as those that reprocess or repackage existing data. For example, SMG Marketing maintains databases on nursing homes, urgent care centers, and other types of facilities and makes this information available in a variety of forms. Also included in this group are the major data vendors (e.g., ESRI Business Information, Claritas) that do not necessarily create health-related databases but incorporate health-specific databases into their business database systems.

Because of the demand for health-related data, several commercial data vendors have added health data to their inventories, and a few health-specific data vendors have emerged. These vendors not only repackage existing data into more palatable form, but some are also developing their own proprietary databases. At least three vendors are conducting major nationwide health-consumer surveys.

Because of the increasing demand for health-related data, improvement in the quality, coverage, timeliness, and availability of such data has become a priority for many organizations. The federal government has taken a lead in the public sector through its efforts to make its extensive health-related databases and registries available to the research and business communities. Through its various programs the federal government supports projects that involve the application of contemporary computer technology to the processing, manipulation, and dissemination of health-related data, an area in which healthcare lags far behind other industries. Commercial data vendors continue to develop proprietary databases and repackage and distribute databases produced by government or association sources.

The Internet is already becoming a force with regard to health data. Although the focus at the time of this writing has been on consumer-oriented health information on the World Wide Web, data for use by health professionals are not far behind. Bibliographical and text files are already becoming available, and some healthcare organizations are transferring patient data over the Internet. In the future there is every reason to believe that data for health services marketing and business development will be widely available on the World Wide Web.

Health Data and the Internet

As the world has discovered, the World Wide Web is becoming a global information depository that can be easily accessed via the Internet. At the time of this writing more health-related data were thought to be available via the Internet than on any other topic. Not only are there more sites dealing with more aspects of health, but some of the most extensive sites have been established by healthcare organizations.

Despite the spate of health-related data available via the Internet, until recently most of the data have been of limited usefulness to the health professional. The overwhelming majority of health sites offer data geared to healthcare consumers. The ready market has been for consumer data, and no shortage of consumer-oriented organizations eager to establish a presence on the web existed. Today, healthcare consumers can find a doctor, diagnose a condition, or order prescription drugs and nutritional supplements via the Internet.

By the mid-1990s the information needs of health professionals were beginning to be recognized. In response to this need various organizations responded by offering data via the Internet. This involved making data files available to be viewed, browsed, and downloaded. More advanced sites may actually allow the user to manipulate the data in some basic ways. Even commercial data vendors began searching for ways to make data more accessible via the Internet.

The federal government has led the charge to make raw data available on the Internet. Agencies such as the Census Bureau, CDC, NCHS, and CMS have expended significant effort toward posting their data files on the Internet. Not only do these data files represent improvements over the cumbersome output formats (e.g., print, magnetic tape) these agencies historically used, but web-based files can also be posted much more expeditiously than the data can be published in print form. Plus, many of these sites offer data for downloading at no charge, data that often had to be purchased from various agencies in the past. Some of these data sets would never be published in print form, making, for example, data available for levels of geography that would be much too cumbersome to publish in hard copy. As print versions of data reports are steadily eliminated by the federal government and other data generators, the importance of Internet distribution will increase.

The initial response of health data users has been enthusiastic. At last it has become possible to obtain data on a variety of topics from a single source. However, as one gets serious about using web-based data files from any of these sources, this enthusiasm can be quickly dampened because of the existing deficiencies in this approach.

The use of the Internet as a vehicle for making data files available for viewing and downloading represents a giant step forward in health data distribution. In fact, the Internet may truly come to be a single source for health-related data. Today, however, significant issues are associated with the data files being made available via this environment. Some barriers to efficient use will be obvious to users, but not-so-obvious ones could be disastrous. While hard-copy data files will continue to be useful, the presence of the Internet is likely to steadily expand the importance of electronic access to data files.

Summary

Healthcare marketers require a wide variety of data made for planning and implementing marketing activities, and healthcare is legendary for the massive amounts of data the industry generates. Marketers also use demographic data, and the 1990s saw an increase in the demand for data—including on such topics as employment, housing, and crime—that were thought in the past to be unrelated to healthcare.

Health-related data can be categorized along the dimensions of community versus organizational data, primary versus secondary data, or internal versus external data. These data sets can also be considered in terms of geographic level and time period (i.e., past, present, or future). Health-related data are generated through censuses, registries, and surveys. Increasingly, synthetic data are being used for estimates and projections. Each of the available sources of data has its advantages and disadvantages.

Healthcare marketers have a number of options for accessing health-related data. Government agencies at all levels are important sources, and the federal government is the major generator and disseminator of many of the types of data required by healthcare marketers. The Centers for Disease Control and Prevention, the National Center for Health Statistics, and the Agency for Healthcare Research and Quality are some of the federal agencies that make health-related data available to health professionals.

Professional associations, such as the American Medical Association and the American Hospital Association, compile data and make them available to the public. Not-for-profit associations, such as the American Cancer Society and the American Heart Association, assemble and distribute data to health professionals and the general public. Educational institutions and research organizations also provide a significant amount of data for health professionals. Increasingly, commercial data vendors have entered the field to supplement or, in some cases, supplant the data provided by other organizations.

The Internet has allowed health-related data to be distributed much more efficiently. The federal government has led the way in the posting of health data on the World Wide Web. Many state governments have extensive web sites devoted to health data, and private data vendors have established web sites for the distribution of health information on a fee basis. While the Internet allows the distribution of massive amounts of health-related data, there are numerous deficiencies that make the means of health-data dissemination problematic.

Discussion Questions

- Why has the healthcare industry failed to develop data clearinghouses and nationwide sources of market data like other industries have?
- Under what circumstances may it be necessary to collect primary data rather than use secondary data already available?

- What disadvantages of the decennial census as a data-collection method counter the fact that it involves complete coverage of the population?
- Why are registration systems and administrative records becoming increasingly important sources of data for healthcare marketing?
- What function does the National Center for Health Statistics serve, and why is this an important resource for healthcare marketers?
- Under what circumstances is it necessary to access synthetic data generated by government agencies or commercial data vendors?
- Why do healthcare marketers frequently use health-related data generated by agencies of state government?
- What are the advantages of accessing health-related data via the Internet, and what challenges does this source of data present?

References

American Hospital Association. 2003. *Hospital Statistics, 2003 ed*. Chicago: American Hospital Association.

Thomas, R. K. 1996. *Problems and Needs of Health Data Users*. Memphis, TN: Medical Services Research Group.

Additional Resources

American Hospital Association. 2003. *AHA Guide to the Healthcare Field, 2003 ed*. Chicago: American Hospital Association.

American Medical Association. 2002. *Socioeconomic Characteristics of Medical Practice, 2002*. Chicago: American Medical Association.

———. 2002. *Physician Characteristics and Distribution in the U.S., 2002*. Chicago: American Medical Association.

U.S. Bureau of Health Professions, Department of Health and Human Services. http://bhpr.hrsa.gov.

U.S. Bureau of Primary Healthcare, Department of Health and Human Services. http://bphc.hrsa.gov.

U.S. Census Bureau. http://www.census.gov. (See in particular "American Factfinder.")

———. Information on the North American Industry Code System. [Online information.] http://www.census.gov/epcd/www/naics.html.

———. 2002. *County Business Patterns, 2002*. Washington, DC: U.S. Government Printing Office.

U.S. Center for Mental Health Studies, Department of Health and Human Services. http://www.samhsa.gov/cmhs/htm.

U.S. Centers for Disease Control and Prevention, Department of Health and Human Services. http://www.cdc.gov.

————. *Morbidity and Mortality Weekly Review*. Atlanta, GA: Centers for Disease Control and Prevention.

U.S. Health Resources and Services Administration, Department of Health and Human Services. http://www.hrsa.dhhs.gov.

U.S. National Center for Health Statistics, Department of Health and Human Services. http://www.cdc.gov/nchs.

————. 2002. *Health, United States, 2002*. Washington, DC: U.S. Government Printing Office.

Wellner, A. S. 1998. *Best of Health: Demographics of Healthcare Consumers*. Ithaca, NY: New Strategist Publications.

THE FUTURE OF HEALTHCARE MARKETING

It may seem obvious that the "future" of healthcare marketing is ahead of it, but marketing is still relatively new in healthcare and most of what will ever happen in marketing is in the future. Virtually every development that affects healthcare—from emerging consumerism to the dominance of the baby boomers to the introduction of defined contributions—serves to increase the importance of marketing.

A future in which healthcare marketing takes on the sophistication and efficacy of marketing in other industries is foreseen, as healthcare becomes an increasingly market-driven endeavor. Chapter 17 summarizes the current state of healthcare marketing and where it is expected to go from here. The factors that will influence the future course of healthcare are discussed, along with some areas on which marketers may concentrate for the future.

17

HEALTHCARE MARKETING IN THE TWENTY-FIRST CENTURY

Although a book of this type is customarily concluded with a chapter that addresses the future of the particular field, this chapter takes on inordinate importance given the current state of healthcare. Because of the youth of the field, most of healthcare marketing's future is indeed in front of it. As the field matures and becomes increasingly tailored to the needs of healthcare, substantial changes can be anticipated. Furthermore, healthcare marketing is maturing in a highly volatile and unpredictable environment, and in no other industry is the ability to forecast its future direction so difficult yet so important. This chapter reviews the current status of healthcare marketing and attempts to specify, if not the future nature of the field, at least the factors that will influence its direction. A future in which healthcare marketing takes on the sophistication and efficacy of marketing in other industries is foreseen here, as healthcare becomes an increasingly market-driven endeavor.

Where Healthcare Marketing Is Today

It is difficult not to be optimistic about the future of marketing in healthcare. Much has been learned from past successes and failures. More effective techniques and better tools and sources of data are available to the healthcare marketer today. Marketers can measure patient satisfaction, they have access to much better consumer data, and new techniques like predictive modeling are emerging to take advantage of contemporary technology. Healthcare marketing has matured significantly, and the quality of healthcare marketing professionals has improved dramatically. The data available today, the analytical techniques, and marketing efforts that rely on contemporary technology (e.g., customer relationship management, predictive modeling) offer capabilities not even imagined by the healthcare marketer of the 1980s. The direct-to-consumer movement is bringing the customer back into the spotlight, which can only be good news for health-care marketers.

During the short history of marketing in healthcare the field has experienced a variety of ups and downs. The appropriateness of the role of marketing in healthcare has always been controversial, and the gains made on behalf of the marketing enterprise during the 1980s and 1990s were hard won. Despite this halting progress, the last years of the twentieth century witnessed the growing acceptance of marketing as a legitimate function of the healthcare organization.

Support for marketing appeared to have plateaued around 2000 after several years of enthusiastic support. This was not necessarily a negative development but demonstrated that the profession was beginning to show maturity. Healthcare marketing had returned to a degree of reasonableness by the end of the twentieth century, leaving behind some of the excesses of the 1980s and 1990s.

Because of the increased pressure on all healthcare organizations (and especially not-for-profits) to maximize the bottom line, most have come to appreciate the importance of marketing. Given the need to attract patients and increase volume in a very competitive environment, progressive organizations place more value on marketing. Nevertheless, some still see marketing as a cost center, not a contributor to the bottom line.

Although healthcare marketing has been slowed by the economic downturn at the beginning of this decade, healthcare does not appear to be affected as badly as some other industries where much more of the corporate budget is devoted to marketing. Healthcare may have experienced a slight pause, but not much more. Healthcare marketing continues to face numerous distractions, and concerns over the impact of bioterrorism were added in 2001. The economic downturn that followed led healthcare administrators to question what they were doing and whether they were making the best use of their resources.

In the post-9/11 environment some healthcare administrators became so focused on survival, both personal and institutional, that marketing became less top of mind (although it probably should have become even more important). Healthcare marketing has fared best within those organizations that had both adopted a market orientation and evinced a determination to stay the course. Those with a true strategic focus have remained strong supporters of marketing, whereas organizations that have not incorporated a marketing mind-set are more likely to waiver in the face of distractions.

Since 2001 some moderation in marketing investment on the part of healthcare organizations has occurred. While a slow down has involved cutbacks in budgets and staffs to a certain extent, the cutbacks appear to be reactions to higher operating costs, more expensive personnel, and the overall increased cost of doing business that have led to a reduction of expenses across the board and not necessarily directed at marketing. Some movement toward the elimination of internal marketing departments and their staffs in favor of outside consultants has occurred, allowing the healthcare organization to replace a long-term investment in staff with a short-term commitment to outside contractors. This does not necessarily mean the total outsourcing of services but rather bringing in outside companies for comarketing, cobranding, and sponsorships.

Shifting to web-based marketing has been one approach taken by many healthcare organizations. Those who have bought into an interactive approach, and have adequate capabilities to support it, have found this to be a successful strategy for the current environment.

Where Healthcare Marketing Is Going

There is every indication that the trend toward greater acceptance of marketing will continue and its role within healthcare will expand. Recognition is growing that marketing is not an optional activity but something that every organization must do. The fact that marketing is being coupled with the business development function means that it will increasingly be an inherent part of corporate operations. The question will no longer be, "To market or not to market?" but it will ask the extent to which marketing will contribute to the success of the organization.

A growing emphasis on grass-roots marketing has been in evidence. Marketers are developing the ability to attract more and "better" customers and are increasingly focusing on improving customer satisfaction. New employees may receive a marketing orientation, and incentive programs at some organizations turn employees into marketers. This means working more closely with the fund-development department, developing marketable facilities, comarketing with the community-relations area, and developing a long-term affinity with the community. These actions have often led to increased business volume, and marketers can increasingly demonstrate that the business came because of the marketing.

Some providers are using this period to take advantage of more technology-based techniques, incorporate more computer capabilities, and adopt sophisticated customer relationship management programs. For example, some healthcare organizations have stopped airing television ads and are moving more to print ads. Direct mail appears to be gaining popularity under the current circumstances.

Trends Affecting the Future of Healthcare Marketing

In recent years the healthcare industry has moved in a direction that fosters, or mandates, marketing. Virtually every development in healthcare suggests dramatic growth for the role of marketing in the future. Consumer choice is reemerging in healthcare as the baby boomers begin to dominate. The emergence of defined contributions is expected to add more fuel to this fire, and we are only beginning to see the effect of the retail aspect of healthcare. If marketers can demonstrate the effectiveness of marketing initiatives, marketing could well become *the* critical function in most healthcare organizations of the future.

Shifting Demand for Health Services

The amount and type of demand for future health services are arguably the most important pieces of information the healthcare marketer can possess. Yet, in healthcare this is an extremely elusive body of knowledge. The demand for health services is influenced by numerous factors both inside and outside healthcare. Some of the emerging demand may be created by the industry as it introduces new products and services; some will be a result of changes in reimbursement patterns or the introduction of regulations. Still more of the change in demand for services will reflect broad social trends that have direct or indirect implications for healthcare.

In one sense it could be argued that the demand for health services in the United States will essentially be flat for the foreseeable future. Population growth is slow, and a limited number of new potential customers are being added to the pool annually. On the other hand, the market for elective procedures is burgeoning; once the economy recovers and middle-aged baby boomers begin to assert themselves, the demand for various elective procedures and vanity products will likely surge.

The demand for inpatient care is already reviving, and many facilities are scrambling to find space for their admissions. Despite the factors restraining the use of inpatient care, demand appears to be increasing; this demand can only grow as the aging baby boomers require increasing amounts of inpatient care. Current demographic trends suggest an increase in gerontological services, women's services, and specialty care for older adults. These trends portend a likely decrease in obstetric and pediatric care but an increase in the demand for gynecological services.

Perhaps more than any other factor, the nature of the future demand for health services will set the direction of healthcare marketing. Healthcare marketers therefore need to develop adequate methodologies for predicting the future needs and wants of healthcare consumers.

Growing Consumerism

Some observers have predicted that the first decade of this century will be the decade of the consumer in healthcare, and ample evidence certainly exists to support this assertion. Periodically, the field has seen the emergence of consumerism as a force for influencing policy and programs, but these movements have always been short lived. The current revival of consumerism, however, appears to have substantial staying power. It is driven by a number of factors, from a backlash against managed care to the introduction of defined contributions by benefit managers to the ascendancy of the baby boom cohort as the dominant population group in U.S. society.

Many see healthcare as increasingly market driven and consumer oriented. A consumer choice environment is emerging, they argue, in which healthcare organizations will be required to increasingly cater to the needs and wants of a population that is heterogeneous in terms of demographics, lifestyles, and health behavior. If defined contributions become a standard part of employee benefit plans, consumer choice will be an increasingly important aspect of the system.

As competition remains strong, healthcare organizations will be forced to vie for the attention, business, and loyalty of the healthcare consumer with an intensity unknown in the past. These trends will require marketers to understand both the customer and the prospective customer better than at any previous time. Target marketing will become increasingly important, and mass customization will become common in marketing. Direct-to-consumer marketing and customer relationship management will be essential techniques for many healthcare organizations in the future.

Increasing Competition

Healthcare organizations can expect continued, and even increased, competition for the healthcare consumer. The capacity of the system continues to exceed demand in most places, and slow growth in demand coupled with the continued entry of new players into the healthcare arena can be expected to raise competition to a level not experienced in the past. The emergence of a new industry around alternative therapies has added another dimension of competition in the healthcare arena as unconventional providers promote goods and services that compete with mainstream providers.

The monopolies that many healthcare organizations maintained in the past have given way to situations characterized by cutthroat competition, and no component of the industry remains unaffected. Hospitals face competition from other hospitals, physicians and other clinicians, and entrepreneurs who enter healthcare from other industries. Physicians face competition from other physicians, hospitals and urgent care facilities, and increasingly alternative therapists. Health plans face heated competition for customers, and the survival of managed care plans depends on their ability to successfully compete for enrollees. Even the pharmaceutical industry has become more competitive as the stakes have gotten higher.

New products and services continue to be introduced, and the healthcare consumer needs to be educated on these issues (and convinced to purchase a particular brand). An industry experiencing such a profusion of new products and services cannot help but be highly competitive. In many instances existing products and services have become increasingly standardized, challenging marketers to be creative in finding ways to differentiate between competing organizations.

The Dominance of Technology

Regardless of the other trends that develop in healthcare, the industry will clearly continue to be technologically oriented. Even as some decry the impersonality of a technology-based system of care, the technological component becomes increasingly dominant. Not only will technology play an increasing role in the provision of care, but it will also be a major factor in the development of new products and services. The widespread acceptance of electronic patient records and the ultimate conversion of clinicians to computer enthusiasts will ensure that the industry is permeated with technology at all levels.

Healthcare marketing will similarly be affected by the ubiquity of technology. Traditional approaches to marketing are being supplanted by often more complex methodologies that capitalize on contemporary technology. Database marketing, customer relationship management, and predictive modeling are all approaches to the target population that have emerged based on information technology.

These developments mean that healthcare marketers must be knowledgeable concerning the technology underlying the provision of care. They will be asked to explain cutting-edge technology to consumers and sell them on the use of these techniques. They will be asked to differentiate these techniques from traditional ones and convey these differences to prospective patients.

Healthcare marketers also must incorporate a range of technology-based marketing techniques into their armamentaria for cultivating the patient population. Techniques being adopted from other industries (e.g., database marketing, customer relationship management) must be understood and championed by the marketer. Even traditional marketing methods such as direct-to-consumer approaches will take advantage of information technology as they become more sophisticated.

Increasing Costs

After a brief period of moderated costs in the healthcare industry, virtually everyone predicts rising costs for the foreseeable future; indeed, some of those increases are already being seen. A number of factors contribute to the higher costs of providing health services and the consequent higher prices charged to consumers. Although consumers have been essentially insulated from the costs of healthcare in the past, the changing insurance environment and the emergence of a large elective-surgery industry are making cost issues central to the concerns of consumers, employers, and anyone else paying for health services.

A lack of price-based competition and the extraordinary role of third-party payers have limited the involvement of healthcare marketers in the pricing component of the four Ps in the past (see Box 4.3 in Chapter 4), but that situation will likely change. Health plans, providers of elective procedures, and other entities are expected to compete increasingly on the basis of price, and healthcare marketers must be in a position to support this marketing angle. Furthermore, marketers will likely be asked to explain to consumers why prices are increasing or why their provider's prices are higher than the competitor's. Thus, a topic that has received limited attention from marketers in the past will become increasingly salient.

Emphasis on Outcomes

Many observers have suggested that the first decade of this century will be the one that focuses on outcomes in healthcare. Driven by concerns over the effectiveness of the healthcare delivery system and persistent disclosures of the level of medical errors during care, healthcare providers are increasingly faced with the outcomes issue. They must defend adverse outcomes reported but at the same time have the opportunity to capitalize on favorable outcomes they can document. Patient safety issues will continue to be paramount, and a considerable groundswell of support for more controls over patient care appears to exist.

Marketers will be increasingly called on to moderate the outcomes issue. They may be asked to develop promotional campaigns based on high surgical success rates or low mortality rates. They may be asked to rationalize low success rates or high mortality rates. In any case marketers will likely be the go-betweens for the provider and the public, regulators, and policy setters.

Growing Labor Force Concerns

Despite the weak labor market of today, healthcare providers continue to face shortages of key personnel. While cyclical labor shortages have occurred in the past, the current shortfall is more extreme than previous ones, and little chance for short-term amelioration of the problem exists. The most highly publicized shortages are for nurses; indeed, this situation appears to dwarf other considerations. However, shortages of many other clinicians and technical staff exist, and some even predict a future physician shortage.

Given an absolute shortfall in trained personnel, most providers must attempt to attract staff from other providers in the short run; much of the energy of marketers has therefore shifted from attracting consumers to attracting skilled personnel. Gone are the days when nurses or other personnel automatically showed up if a job was posted. Marketers must develop aggressive recruitment plans that help differentiate their providers from others competing for the same pool of workers, especially now that it has been conceded that salary is only one factor—and maybe not the most important factor—that drives the decisions of would-be employees.

Healthcare marketers are also faced with the challenge of facilitating the retention of skilled staff. This challenge requires skills in internal marketing and the ability to support administrative efforts to develop an environment that encourages loyalty and retention among nurses and other personnel.

The Erosion of Trust

Perhaps the past decade's most significant development in terms of its effect on the healthcare-consuming public has been the erosion of trust in the healthcare system. Twenty years ago physicians were accorded the status of demigods, and hospitals were held up as examples of efficient and altruistic institutions. Health plans were considered valuable safety nets, and pharmaceutical companies were hailed for their contributions to new therapies. The developments in recent years have served to sully the reputations of most players in healthcare in one way or another. A spate of criminal and civil charges brought against healthcare executives has served to further create an environment of distrust and suspicion.

This is not an easy environment for a healthcare marketer to operate in, and the situation is not likely to improve for the foreseeable future. It behooves the marketer to keep his or her finger on the pulse of public sentiment with regard to healthcare and develop marketing plans accordingly. A major role of the healthcare marketer in the future will likely be trust building as efforts are made to repair the damage that healthcare has inflicted on itself over the past two decades. Marketers will be promoting not only a product or service but also the image and integrity of the entire industry.

Healthcare Marketing: Seizing the Opportunity

Healthcare marketers have a better opportunity to seize the moment in healthcare than ever before. They need to continue to demonstrate the contribution marketing can make to the bottom line and its value in developing and promoting new services. They need to get involved early in the process to influence the development of services and programs and make organizations more customer oriented. They need to demonstrate the potential contribution marketing can make to new ventures and identify trends on which the organization may want to capitalize (e.g., patient safety, empowering consumers). They must ensure that all initiatives have a marketing component and even make some contribution to the clinical side.

The most important action marketers can take is to demonstrate their role in developing, enhancing, and packaging services that meet the needs of the market. The ability to match products to customer needs is a unique contribution marketers can make. The marketer needs to have the ability to persuade decision makers of the critical role of marketing and provide evidence of the success of marketing initiatives; this requires that the marketer develop the ability to see things from the perspective of the decision maker.

Ultimately, healthcare marketing is nothing more or less than defining a community need and facilitating the fulfillment of that need. By focusing on identifying the needs of the community and then striving to meet them, marketers can contribute to the improved health of U.S. citizens while improving the bottom line of their organizations; this means that in many organizations healthcare marketers will have to contribute to redefining the role of marketing.

Today, healthcare marketers have a unique opportunity to shape the future of the field. They are becoming increasingly well positioned to contribute to the success of their organizations, the health and satisfaction of individual healthcare consumers, and the overall health status of the community. (See Box 17.1 for a discussion of some future hot areas for marketing.)

Summary

Because of the youth of the field, most of healthcare marketing's future is indeed in front of it. As the field matures and becomes increasingly tailored to the needs of healthcare, substantial changes can be anticipated. Although healthcare marketing has encountered some fits and starts during its first quarter century, it now appears to be in relative good shape.

There is every indication that the trend toward more acceptance of marketing will continue and its role within healthcare will expand. Recognition is growing that marketing is not an optional activity but something every organization must do. The fact that marketing is being coupled with the business-development function means that it will increasingly be an inherent part of corporate operations. Today, the data available, the

Box 17.1: Hot Marketing Areas for the Decade	Based on the information currently available, it could be argued that the following areas will be targeted by healthcare marketers in this decade. Given the unpredictable nature of healthcare, the hot areas will likely change rapidly, so these should be considered examples of the types of areas to which marketers may want to be open for the foreseeable future.

Eldercare

The continued aging of the U.S. population guarantees that eldercare will be a growing concern for healthcare marketers. Although the health of U.S. seniors has improved over that of previous generations, their numbers alone ensure that geriatric care will be a major industry well into the coming years. Elderly people require both a high level and wide variety of services, and healthcare providers are already beginning to experience increases in the demand for senior services. This trend will only be exacerbated by the baby boom cohort as it enters old age. Marketers should be cognizant of the differences that exist among the elderly and take these differences into consideration in marketing planning. Future developments with regard to Medicare reimbursement will likely have a major effect on service utilization by the senior population.

Older Adult Services

While those 45 to 64 years of age do not require the same intensity of services as the elderly, they are at an age during which chronic conditions arise and symptoms of physical deterioration appear. Not only is physical impairment a factor, but individuals in this age group suffer from conditions related to stress and psychological dysfunction. This is the age of midlife crises, menopause, empty nests, and a variety of other factors that create anxiety for contemporary Americans. These services will become particularly critical as the huge baby boom cohort begins entering its 60s during this decade. Demand for a wide range of specialty services will burgeon, and the elective surgery component of the system can be expected to expand dramatically. The baby boomers will place increasing pressure on existing services while creating demand for a variety of new and different services.

analytical techniques, and the marketing efforts that rely on contemporary technology offer capabilities not even imagined by the healthcare marketer of the 1980s. The nature of the future demand for health services will set the direction of healthcare marketing. Healthcare marketers, therefore, need to develop adequate methodologies for predicting the future needs and wants of healthcare consumers.

Fitness and Sports Medicine

While the growth of the fitness craze in the last couple of decades appears to have leveled off, the wellness, fitness, and sports-medicine industry is not going to go away. Despite reports of an increasingly sedentary population, the demand for fitness programs and equipment, sports medicine, and "nutriceuticals" remains high. Fueled by the huge baby boom cohort, products and services that purport to be healthy or natural will continue to attract a large following. Increased fitness activities mean more sports-related activities among many people who are not used to strenuous exercise; this should increase the demand for the services of orthopedic surgeons, physiatrists, rehabilitation counselors, and a variety of other health professionals in the sports-medicine field.

Ethnic and Minority Healthcare

As early as the 1970s concerns were raised over the ability of the U.S. healthcare system to deal with what at the time seemed like a reasonably diverse population. The ensuing quarter century saw an explosion in the number and variety of racial and ethnic groups within the U.S. population. Burgeoning ethnic groups such as Hispanic Americans, growing racial groups such as Asian Americans, and newly arrived immigrants, along with the significant African-American population, represent untapped areas for health services providers. An increasingly diverse population will call for culturally sensitive programs and creative marketing to address the disparate issues these populations manifest. Our system has come a long way from the one-size-fits-all healthcare system of the 1970s, but it still has a long way to go in adapting to the needs of an increasingly diverse patient pool. Healthcare marketers are beginning to see the opportunities rather than the challenges engendered by this growing racial and ethnic diversity, and many organizations are beginning to adapt their services to cater to these new target audiences. Many ethnic groups carry the potential for significant growth in the demand for health services, and healthcare organizations must position themselves to take advantage of these emerging opportunities.

Vanity Services

The growth in cosmetic surgery, laser eye surgery, and other elective procedures has been dramatic over the past decade; now the baby boomers promise to fuel even greater demand for health services that make them look and feel better. Cosmetic surgery, once the province of older women, is now sought by younger women and increasingly by men. Consumers must pay out of pocket for most of these services, and the discretionary income of baby boomers should contribute to rapid expansion of the elective component of health services. Many of these procedures are practical responses to the physical deterioration that affects everyone, as witnessed by the demand for laser eye surgery and arthroscopic procedures; many are clearly elective, such as facelifts, tummy tucks, and hair transplantation. While the demand for many of these procedures was driven by older women in the past, statistics now indicate that an increasingly younger population is demanding vanity services and that men now equal women in number as clients for these services.

Skin Care

Recent developments in skin care procedures occurred just in time to address the exploding demand by a rapidly aging population. The growth of the senior segment of the population will increase the demand for therapeutic skin care (e.g., for skin cancer), whereas the burgeoning baby boom population will demand "cosmeceuticals" that reduce age spots and keep their skin young looking. From rejuvenating creams to laser skin therapy, the demands for all types of skin care should increase dramatically. Skin care should become a real growth area in this decade, as virtually everyone can benefit from this type of therapy. The demand for skin care will reinforce the demand for vanity services and fitness programs noted above.

Alternative Therapies

While the demand for a wide range of alternative (or complementary) therapies has been increasing steadily for the past quarter century, not until the 1990s was the size of this

Virtually every development in healthcare suggests dramatic growth for the role of marketing in the future. The factors that are likely to affect the future direction of healthcare marketing in the U.S. include growing consumerism, heightened competition, continued technological advances, increasing costs, emphasis on outcomes, labor shortages, and erosion of trust in the system.

Today, healthcare marketers have a unique opportunity to shape the future of the field. They are becoming increasingly well positioned to contribute to the success of their organizations, the health and satisfaction of individual healthcare consumers, and the overall health status of the community. A number of "hot areas" can be identified that will demand the marketer's skill in the future.

industry discovered. By that time U.S. consumers were spending more on alternative therapies than on conventional therapies, and the burgeoning industry supporting such therapies had become well entrenched. Once limited to certain ethnic groups and subsegments of the population, the use of chiropractic, acupuncture, naturopathy, and massage therapy now cuts across virtually all segments of the U.S. population. As the underlying orientation of the U.S. healthcare system has changed and the U.S. public has become more open to unconventional approaches, the demand for various alternative therapies has exploded. The correspondence between the emerging preferences of the baby boomers and other segments of the population and the attributes of holistic care and various alternative therapies ensures that this will be a major growth industry for the foreseeable future.

Mental Healthcare

Although the consciousness of the general public and the medical community was raised with regard to the need for mental health services during the 1960s and 1970s, the surge in interest in this clinical area was short lived. Reductions in reimbursement for mental health services and persistent reluctance to openly address this type of problem had pushed mental healthcare to the back burner of the healthcare system by the end of the century. Today, interest in addressing mental health challenges has been renewed, and reports by the U.S. Surgeon General and the World Health Organization indicate that the future management of mental illness will be a major challenge both domestically and worldwide. As the baby boomers enter a period when they can expect increased prevalence of mental and emotional disorders, they will likely exert considerable influence on the healthcare system; this could result in a level of interest in mental health services never before seen, coupled with some significant changes in the manner in which these services are funded.

Discussion Questions

- What indications do we have that the roller coaster ride that has characterized healthcare for the past quarter of a century is leveling off?
- What are some of the major trends currently characterizing healthcare, and what are their implications for marketing?
- How is marketing uniquely positioned to address some of the more challenging aspects of contemporary healthcare?
- What indications do we have that marketing is becoming more of a core function for healthcare organizations?
- What responsibilities do marketers have in promoting the field of marketing within their organizations?

- What educational role should marketers perform for healthcare consumers?
- What are some of the hot areas for healthcare in the future, and how can marketers respond to these opportunities?

Additional Resources

Siegal, M., and L. Doner. 1998. *Marketing Public Health: Strategies for Promoting Social Change*. Gaithersburg, MD: Aspen.

Society for Healthcare Strategy and Market Development. 2004. *Futurescan: Healthcare Trends and Implications 2004–2008*. Chicago: Health Administration Press and American Hospital Association.

Thomas, R. K. 2002. "How Far Have We Come?" *Marketing Health Services* 22 (4): 36–41.

GLOSSARY

Account management	The mechanism by which an agency interfaces with a client related to a particular marketing campaign
Administrative records	A form of registration system that contains a record of transactions of individuals in the registry
Administrative unit	A bounded geographic area formally defined for administrative purposes, such as a state, county, municipality, school district, or other unit defined for purposes of governance
Advertising	Any paid form of nonpersonal presentation and promotion of ideas, goods, or services by an identifiable sponsor transmitted via mass media to achieve marketing objectives
Agency	An internal or external entity that supports some or all aspects of an organization's marketing effort
Alternative therapy	An umbrella term that refers to a variety of therapeutic modalities used by individuals as alternatives to conventional allopathic medicine; also referred to as complementary therapy
AMA	The American Marketing Association is the primary U.S. organization devoted to the promotion of the field of marketing, including healthcare marketing
Attitude	A position an individual has adopted in response to a theory, belief, object, event, or another person that establishes a relatively consistent, acquired predisposition to behave in a certain way
Audience	People, households, or organizations that read, view, hear, or are otherwise exposed to a promotional message; the target for a marketer's message
Banner ad	An advertisement printed on small "banners" that appear in a newspaper or on a web page

Brand	A name, symbol, or other identifier that marks a seller's goods and/or services and differentiates them from similar goods and/or services offered by competitors
Branding	The process of creating a brand for a company, product or service.
Business-to-business marketing	The process of building profitable, value-oriented relationships between two businesses and the many individuals within them
Call center	A centralized communication center established by a healthcare organization to capture incoming customer inquiries and generate outgoing marketing messages
Call to action	A statement, usually at the end of a marketing piece, encouraging the audience to take action on the good or service being promoted
Causal research	A form of research that attempts to specify the nature of the functional relationship between two or more variables in the situation under study
CDC	The Centers for Disease Control and Prevention is the federal agency charged with monitoring morbidity and mortality in the United States
Census	A complete count of the persons residing in a specific place at a specific time
Census Bureau	The agency within the U.S. Department of Commerce that conducts the decennial census and other data-collection activities
Channel	A formal means of distribution for a good or service (e.g., the provision of family planning information through health department clinics)
Client	A type of customer that consumes services rather than goods; in advertising, the internal or external entity is the customer for the promotional project
Coding system	One of several classification systems used in healthcare for the identification of procedures, therapies, and other healthcare events
Comarketing	An approach in which two or more organizations combine their marketing efforts in the joint pursuit of individual objectives

Commercial data vendor	A private organization established for purposes of collecting, compiling, analyzing, and/or disseminating health-related data
Communication	In healthcare, the materials (usually print) that provide information on the organization and its services to internal and/or external audiences
Communications	Processes used to convey information in print or electronic form to internal and/or external audiences
Community outreach	A form of marketing that seeks to present the programs of the organization to the community and establish relationships with community organizations
Competition	The presence of one or more organizations within the same field vying for the same customers
Composition	The breakdown of a population into relevant traits such as demographic characteristics, lifestyle patterns, and financial payer class
Computerized	Surveys conducted via the Internet or other electronic medium of interviews
Concierge services	Customized health services offered to select customers who pay a premium for the personal attention
Consumer	In healthcare, any individual or organization within the population that is a potential purchaser of goods and services
Consumer behavior	The patterns of consumption of goods and services that characterize healthcare consumers; also refers to the factors that contribute to this behavior and the processes that lead up to a purchase decision
Consumer product	Healthcare product distributed through traditional retail outlets, including the Internet
Consumerism	A movement in healthcare in which consumers take a more aggressive role in defining their healthcare needs and the manner in which these needs should be met
Cosmeceutical	A health or beauty product that has the attributes of a cosmetic and a drug (e.g., anti-aging creams)
Creative department	The component of the marketing department responsible for copy, graphics, and creative content
Cross-selling	A marketing approach for encouraging customers to buy additional products and services

Culture	A society's way of life that reflects its particular worldview, beliefs, values, and norms
Customer	The purchaser or end user of a good or service
Customer relationship management	A business strategy designed to optimize profitability, revenue, and customer satisfaction by focusing on relationships rather than transactions
Customer satisfaction	The consumer's level of satisfaction with a good or service
Database marketing	The establishment and exploitation of data on past and current customers and on future prospect that is structured to allow for implementation of effective marketing strategies
Deferred contribution	A form of employee benefit that involves the allocation of "credits" to the employee's account to be used in a manner designated by the employee
Demand	The extent to which a target population needs and/or wants a particular product
Demographics	The range of biosocial and sociocultural attributes of a population that can be used for determining market potential
Decision making	In marketing, the process of determining a need for a product, evaluating the available options, and making a choice
Descriptive research	A form of research that involves the development of a profile of the community or population being examined, thereby describing but not explaining the phenomenon
Direct marketing	A form of marketing that targets groups or individuals with specific characteristics by transmiting promotional messages directly to them
Direct-to-consumer marketing	An approach that targets the individual end user rather than referral agents or intermediaries
Discretionary purchase	A purchase that involves choice on the part of the buyer (e.g., laser eye surgery, hair transplant), rather than a necessity (e.g., bypass surgery)
Display advertising	A promotional approach that uses posters, billboards, and other signs to present a product to the public

Durable good	A good or tangible product that is used over an extended period of time (e.g., hospital bed)
Early adopter	An individual or group willing to try new products and services before they are accepted by the general public
Effective market	The portion of the potential business within a specified market area that is considered capturable
Elasticity	A characteristic that reflects the tendency for the demand for health services to rise and fall in response to various factors both inside and outside of the industry
Elective procedure	A clinical procedure that is consumed at the discretion of the customer and is not considered medically necessary
Electronic media	Any form in media that conveys a message electronically, primarily including radio, television, and the Internet
End user	The person or organization that ultimately consumes a good or service, regardless of who makes the purchase decision or pays for the product
Enrollee	An individual who is enrolled in a health plan
Environmental assessment	A systematic process of data collection and analysis for purposes of profiling and evaluating the external environment faced by an organization
Epidemiologic transition	A process whereby a population, as a result of increasing average age, undergoes a transition from a predominance of acute health problems to a predominance of chronic health problems
Estimate	The calculation of a figure for a current or past time period using a statistical method, as in an estimate of the population between censuses
Ethical evaluation	An approach to evaluation that emphasizes the marketer's responsibility and accountability to the target audience
Ethics	A code of behavior that proscribes appropriate moral stances, particularly related to the professions
Evaluation	The systematic assessment of the efficiency and effectiveness of a particular initiative

Exploratory research	A form of research aimed at discerning the general nature of a problem or opportunity under study and identifying the associated factors of importance
Focus group	A data-collection technique that involves eliciting opinions and perspectives from a group of individuals who interact under the direction of a focus group leader
Forecast	A form of projection (e.g., for a population) that attempts to account for a wide range of likely future developments
Functional unit	A bounded geographic area formally defined for the carrying out of some practical function such as mail delivery
Gatekeeper	In healthcare, an individual or organization that makes decisions on behalf of an end user or otherwise controls the purchase of goods and services
Geographic information system (GIS)	Computerized application that uses geographically linked data for purposes of spatial analysis and map generation
Geographic unit	A physical area, used for spatial analysis, that is demarcated by defined boundaries
Goal	A generalized statement indicating the desired position of an organization at some point in the future; an ideal state that an organization strives to achieve
Good	A tangible product that is typically purchased in an impersonal setting on a one-at-a-time basis
Government relations	A process through which healthcare organizations maintain liaison with the government agencies that regulate them, determine reimbursement levels, provide funding, and otherwise affect their status
Health	From a traditional (medical model) perspective, a state reflecting the absence of biological pathology; from a contemporary (healthcare model) perspective, the state of overall physical, social, and psychological well-being
Health professional	Generally refers to anyone involved in healthcare in a professional (e.g., physician), administrative (e.g., hospital vice president), or technical (e.g., information technology director) capacity

Healthcare	Any activity, whether formal or informal, performed with the intention of restoring, maintaining, or enhancing the health of an individual or population
Healthcare model	A paradigm for viewing health and illness that involves a broad definition of these concepts and that takes a holistic view, which incorporates the biological, social, and psychological dimensions
Healthcare system	Refers to the combination of facilities, personnel, and services that together constitute the mechanism for the provision of healthcare
Hierarchy of needs	The hierarchical prioritization of personal needs, ranging from basic survival needs at the bottom of the hierarchy to self-actualization needs at the top
HIPAA	The Health Insurance Portability and Accountability Act that limits access to "protected health information" of individuals
Image	The perception of a company, product or service that emphasizes subjective attributes rather than objective attributes (e.g., a caring hospital rather than a well-staffed hospital)
Impact evaluation	An approach to evaluation that assesses the actual changes brought about through the marketing effort
Implementation plan	A plan accompanying the marketing plan that lays out the process for accomplishing the objectives specified in the plan
Incidence	The number of new cases of a disease, disability, or other health-related phenomenon within a population during a specified year
In-depth interview	A data-collection technique that involves one respondent and one interviewer who asks detailed information from the respondent
Industrial product	Product used to produce or support the production of another product
Institution	A pattern of behavior that evolves to meet a societal need; the social and cultural components that constitute the social structure
Institutional advertising	Advertising efforts directed at the promotion of an organization rather than the organization's products

Integrated marketing	An approach to marketing that involves a level of consistency within the promotional strategy and achieves synergy between its component parts
Internal audit	A data-collection process that generates information from the organization's internal records
Internal marketing	Efforts by a service provider to effectively train and motivate its customer-contact employees and all the supporting service people to work as a team to generate customer satisfaction
Internet marketing	A marketing approach that uses the Internet as a means of promoting an idea, an organization, a service or a good
Internet survey	A data-collection technique that involves the administration of a survey instrument via the Internet
Life cycle	The process of maturation from birth to death that characterizes a product or industry
Low-intensity marketing	Promotional activities that involve low-cost, relatively unobtrusive marketing techniques (e.g., banner ads)
Mail interview	A data-collection technique that involves the distribution of a survey instrument via the mail to a predetermined set of respondents who subsequently return the completed questionnaires via the mail
Managed care	A planned and coordinated approach to the financing of healthcare that involves positive and negative incentives for both enrollees and providers for "managing" the services received by a population enrolled in a particular health plan
Market	A real or virtual setting in which potential buyers and potential sellers of a good or service come together for the purpose of exchange
Market area	The actual or desired area (usually defined in terms of geography) from which an organization draws or intends to draw its customers; often used interchangeably with "service area" but more commonly used by for-profit organizations
Market segmentation	A process used to group individuals or households with common characteristics for purposes of target marketing

Market share	The percentage of the total market for a product/service category that has been captured by a particular product/service or by a company that offers multiple products/services in that category
Marketing	The process of planning and executing the conception, pricing, promotion, and distribution of ideas, goods, and services to create exchanges that satisfy individual and organizational objectives (American Marketing Association definition)
Marketing brief	A brief document developed for use by a marketing agency or consultant that presents the specifics of the campaign to the extent that they are known
Marketing budget	The itemization of the resources allocated for a global marketing effort or a specific marketing campaign
Marketing consulting firm	An external firm that provides any of a variety of services to support an organization's marketing function
Marketing management	The analysis, planning, implementation, and control of programs designed to create, build, and maintain beneficial exchanges with target buyers for the purpose of achieving organizational objectives
Marketing mix	Refers to the proportionate roles that product, price, place, and promotion play in the marketing of a particular good or service
Marketing planning	The development of a systematic process for promoting an organization, a good, or a service
Marketing research	The function that links the consumer, customer, and public to the marketer through information used to identify and define marketing opportunities and problems; generate, refine, and evaluate marketing actions; monitor marketing performance; and improve the understanding of the marketing process
Mass marketing	A marketing approach that targets the total population as if it were one undifferentiated mass of consumers, usually uses broad-based approaches such as network television or newspapers
Media buying	The marketing function that involves research, selection, and negotiation of media exposure to support the marketing effort

Media plan	A plan developed for a marketing initiative that outlines the objectives of the promotional campaign, the target audience, and the specific media vehicles that will be used to reach that audience
Media supplier	Any of the commercial television and radio companies, newspapers and magazine owners, poster companies, and other organizations that make media available to the campaign
Medical model	The traditional paradigm characteristic of Western medicine based on germ theory and emphasizes a biomedical approach to health and illness
Medicalization	Process through which a growing number of problems are defined as health problems, an increasing portion of the population is brought under medical management, and the healthcare institution accrues increasing amounts of influence over society
Medicaid	The joint federal-state health insurance program that provides coverage for low-income individuals
Medicare	The federal health insurance program that provides coverage for older Americans
Message	The formal presentation of the information that the marketer is trying to convey; the content of a promotional piece
Micro-marketing	An approach to marketing that breaks the market down to the household or even the individual level in an attempt to target those most likely to consume a product
Mission	The overarching goal of an organization; its reason for being
Monopoly	A situation in which one organization controls the total market for a particular good or service
Mystery shopper	An individual hired to pose as a potential customer for a healthcare good or service to covertly collect information on an organization or operation
NCHS	The National Center for Health Statistics is the nation's leading source of health-related data
Need	A condition of an individual that indicates the need for a health service; an objective determination of medical necessity

Networking	The process of establishing and nurturing relationships with individuals and organizations with which mutually beneficial transactions may be carried out
Niche	A segment of a market that can be carved out based on the uniqueness of the target population, the geographic area, or the product
Nondurable good	A good or tangible product that is used once or a small number of times and then disposed of (e.g., disposable medical supplies)
Nonelective procedure	A clinical procedure that is considered medically necessary
Not for profit	An organization that has been granted tax-exempt status by the Internal Revenue Service to perform certain functions
Objective	A formally designated achievement to be accomplished in support of a goal that is specific, concise, and time-bound
Observation	A data-collection technique in which the actions and/or attributes of those being studied are observed either by another individual or through a mechanical recording device such as a video camera
Oligopoly	A situation in which a small number of organizations dominate a market or an industry
Outcome	Generally refers to the consequences of a clinical episode (e.g., cure, death)
Outcome evaluation	An approach to evaluation that assesses the effectiveness of the marketing effort in reaching its objectives
Packaging	The presentation of a good or service in terms of physical attributes or the positioning of the product
Patient	An individual who has been officially diagnosed with a health condition and subsequently presented himself for formal medical care
Payer (or payor) mix	The combination of payment sources characterizing a population of patients or consumers; the relative proportions of private insurance, government insurance, and self-pay characterizing a population

Personal interview	A data-collection technique that involves the administration of a survey instrument through face-to-face interaction between the interviewer and the respondent
Personal sales	The oral presentation of promotional material to one or more prospective purchasers for the purpose of making sales
Place	The point of distribution of a healthcare good or service
Positioning	The placement of an idea, organization, or product in the minds of the market relative to its competition
Predictive modeling	A statistical method for identifying and quantifying likely future need for health services based on known utilization patterns for a defined population
Predictive research	A form of research that uses known characteristics of a phenomenon under study to predict future characteristics or actions
Prevalence	The total number of cases of a disease, disability, or other health-related condition at a particular point in time
Price	The amount of money that is charged for a product (e.g., doctor's fee, insurance premium)
Primary care	The provision of basic, routine health services, including preventive care
Primary data	Data generated through surveys, focus groups, observational methods, and other techniques for the stated purpose of obtaining information on a specific topic
Primary research	The direct collection of data for a specific use
Print media	Any mechanism for delivering an advertising message that uses the printed word, such as through newspapers, magazines, journals, and newsletters
Process evaluation	An approach to evaluation that assesses the efficiency with which the marketing campaign was carried out
Product	Generally thought of as a "good" or a "service" but also includes ideas or organizations, the product is the object of the marketer's promotional activities

Product advertising	Advertising efforts designed to promote specific goods and services rather than the organization overall
Production	An orientation within an industry that focuses on the production process rather than the distribution process, thereby deemphasizing the use of marketing
Production good	Good (e.g., raw materials) used to produce another good
Professional advertising	Advertising that targets members of a profession such as law, medicine, engineering, or architecture
Projection	The calculation of a future estimate (e.g., for a population) based on the use of one of any statistical techniques for calculating a figure for a point in the future
Promotional mix	The combination of marketing techniques chosen in pursuit of a particular promotional goal
Promotion	Any means of informing the marketplace that the organization has developed a response to meet its needs and includes the mechanisms available for facilitating the hoped-for exchange
Prospect	A consumer who is thought to have an interest in a particular good or service; a potential buyer
Provider	Generic term for a health professional or organization that provides direct patient care or related support services
Psychographics	The lifestyle characteristics of a population, which include such factors as attitudes, consumer purchase patterns, and leisure activities, that can be used for determining market potential
Public relations	A form of communication management that seeks to make use of publicity and other nonpaid forms of promotion and information to influence feelings, opinions, or beliefs about the organization and its offerings
Public service announcement	A free advertisement displayed via print or electronic media in support of a community program as part of the media's responsibility to the public
Quaternary care	Superspecialized care provided in large medical centers for the treatment of complex cases (e.g., organ transplantation, trauma care)

Referral	A unique characteristic of healthcare by which customers are referred to a provider by another provider or organization with, in many cases, a formal referral required before the individual can be treated
Reimbursement	Method of repayment in healthcare in which a third-party payer compensates a provider or patient for the cost of services rendered
Relationship management	An approach to marketing that focuses on the long-term relationship between the buyer and seller and not on a one-time sale
Relationship marketing	An approach to marketing that emphasizes the establishment and nurturing of long-term relationships rather than a one-time sale
Retail healthcare	Aspects of healthcare that are designed to attract discretionary consumption as opposed to medically required consumption (e.g., health spas, "cosmeceuticals")
Return on investment	The benefits—however measured—returned to an organization as a result of its investment in marketing
Sales	An approach to business that emphasizes the transaction aspects of the buyer-seller relationship rather than the more information-oriented approach associated with marketing
Sales promotion	An activity or material that acts as a direct inducement by offering added value to the product or incentives for resellers, salespersons, or consumers
Sample survey	A data-collection method that involves the administration of a survey form or questionnaire to a segment of a target population that has been systematically selected
Secondary care	A level of health services that involves moderate complexity of care and a moderate level of resources and skills
Secondary data	Data that have been previously collected through primary data-collection methods and are now being used for some other purpose such as market research
Secondary research	The analysis of data originally collected for some other purpose than its desired use
Segment	A component of a population or market defined based on some characteristic relevant to marketers

Service	An intangible product that involves an activity or process (or sets thereof) carried out by a service provider that meets the needs of the consumer
Service area	The actual or desired area (usually defined in terms of geography) from which an organization draws or intends to draw its customers; often used interchangeably with "market area" but more commonly used by not-for-profit organizations
Service line	An approach to organizing the services of a healthcare organization along vertical lines to facilitate service management and marketing efforts
Shopping good	A product for which consumers engage in a significant amount of search to compare competing brands on selected attributes such as price, style, or features
SHSMD	Society for Healthcare Strategy and Market Development; a section of the American Hospital Association
Social marketing	An approach to bringing about change in behavior in the general population through the use of marketing techniques such as public relations and advertising
Specialty product	A consumer product, usually a big-ticket item, that consumers seek out, often specifying a particular brand name
Statistical unit	A bounded geographic area formally defined for data-collection purposes such as the geographic units developed by the Census Bureau
Strategic plan	A comprehensive plan for the organization that lays out its strategic direction
Strategy	The generalized approach that is to be taken in meeting the challenges of the market
Support services	The range of nonclinical services that are required for the operation of healthcare organizations, from medical supplies to billing and collections to information management
Survey research	A category of data-collection techniques that involves the use of a questionnaire or survey instrument administered in any one of a number of methods
SWOT analysis	An approach to assessing an organization that examines its strengths and weaknesses as well as the opportunities and threats that confront it

Synthetic data	Data generated in the form of estimates, projections, and forecasts that represent calculated figures as opposed to actual data
Target marketing	Marketing initiatives that focus on a market segment to which an organization desires to offer goods/ services
Telemarketing	The use of telephones for selling by means of either outbound or inbound calls
Telephone interview	A data-collection technique that involves the administration of a survey instrument by an interviewer to a respondent via the telephone
Tertiary care	Specialized health services for the treatment of serious health conditions that require specialized clinicians, equipment, and facilities
Third-party payer	A party other than the provider (seller) and patient (buyer) who pays for the cost of goods and/or services, usually an insurance company or government-sponsored health plan; also referred to as third-party payor
Trade show	The convening of interested parties related to a particular product or industry in which vendors can present their products
Up-selling	A process that involves convincing a buyer to choose a more extensive (and inevitably higher priced) product over the less-complex choice
Utilization	The level of use of health services; various measures of the extent of health services use
Value	Anything that a society considers important, usually an intangible such as youth, economic success, education, or freedom
Vanity services	Health services, usually elective, in response to consumers' desires to improve their physical appearance or functioning (e.g., cosmetic surgery, spa programs)
Want	An expressed desire for a health service based on felt need on the part of the consumer rather than a medically identified need; a health-service want may or may not correlate with a health-service need

INDEX

ABOUT THE AUTHOR

Richard K. Thomas, Ph.D., has been involved in market research and marketing in the healthcare field for more than 30 years. He has experience in both the public and private sectors in healthcare and since 1991 has been primarily involved in consultation with hospitals, clinics, health plans, and other healthcare organizations.

Dr. Thomas holds master's degrees in sociology and geography from the University of Memphis and a doctorate degree in medical sociology from Vanderbilt University. He holds an associate professor (adjunct) appointment in the Department of Preventive Medicine at the University of Tennessee and serves on the adjunct faculties of healthcare administration for the University of St. Francis and Central Michigan University.

Dr. Thomas is active in publishing and speaks on healthcare marketing and related topics. Among his 14 books in the field are *Health Services Planning, 2nd edition; Health Care Market Research;* and *The Demography of Health and Healthcare, 2nd edition.* He has authored dozens of articles on healthcare issues and has done numerous presentations, seminars, and workshops on healthcare marketing. He recently completed a three-year assignment as editor of *Marketing Health Services,* the healthcare publication of the American Marketing Association.

Dr. Thomas is active in various associations for health professionals and is currently on the board of directors of the American Health Planning Association. He has also been active in the American Marketing Association, the Society for Healthcare Strategy and Market Development, the American Public Health Association, and the Population Association of America.